Continuous Quality Improvement in Health Care
Theory, Implementation, and Applications
Second Edition

Curtis P. McLaughlin, DBA
Professor Emeritus of Business Administration
Kenan-Flagler Business School
Professor Emeritus of Health Policy and Administration
School of Public Health
Senior Research Fellow
Cecil G. Sheps Center for Health Services Research
University of North Carolina at Chapel Hill
Chapel Hill, North Carolina
Adjunct Professor
College of Business Administration
University of Tennessee
Knoxville, Tennessee

Arnold D. Kaluzny, PhD
Professor of Health Policy and Administration
Director of the Public Health Leadership Program
School of Public Health
Senior Research Fellow
Cecil G. Sheps Center for Health Services Research
University of North Carolina at Chapel Hill
Chapel Hill, North Carolina

AN ASPEN PUBLICATION®
Aspen Publishers, Inc.
Gaithersburg, Maryland
1999

The author has made every effort to ensure the accuracy of the information herein. However, appropriate information sources should be consulted, especially for new or unfamiliar procedures. It is the responsibility of every practitioner to evaluate the appropriateness of a particular opinion in the context of actual clinical situations and with due considerations to new developments. The author, editors, and the publisher cannot be held responsible for any typographical or other errors found in this book.

Library of Congress Cataloging-in-Publication Data

McLaughlin, Curtis P.
Continuous quality improvement in health care : theory, implementation, and applications /
Curtis P. McLaughlin, Arnold D. Kaluzny—2nd ed.
p. cm.
Includes bibliographical references and index.
ISBN 0-8342-1655-8
1. Medical care—Quality control. 2. Total quality management.
I. Kaluzny, Arnold D. II. Title.
RA399.A3C66 1999
362.1'068'5—dc21
99-20197
CIP

About Aspen Publishers • For more than 35 years, Aspen has been a leading professional publisher in a variety of disciplines. Aspen's vast information resources are available in both print and electronic formats. We are committed to providing the highest quality information available in the most appropriate format for our customers. Visit Aspen's Internet site for more information resources, directories, articles, and a searchable version of Aspen's full catalog, including the most recent publications: **http://www.aspenpublishers.com**
Aspen Publishers, Inc. • The hallmark of quality in publishing
Member of the worldwide Wolters Kluwer group.

Editorial Services: Kathy Litzenberg
Library of Congress Catalog Card Number: 99-20197
ISBN: 0-8342-1655-8

Printed in the United States of America

1 2 3 4 5

To Gordon DeFriese and Kerry Kilpatrick,
who over the years provided the opportunities
and conditions for our exploration of continuous
quality improvement in health care.

TABLE OF CONTENTS

CONTRIBUTORS

EDITORS

Curtis P. McLaughlin, DBA
Professor Emeritus of Business Administration
Kenan-Flagler Business School
Professor Emeritus of Health Policy and Administration
School of Public Health
Senior Research Fellow
Cecil G. Sheps Center for Health Services Research
University of North Carolina at Chapel Hill
Chapel Hill, North Carolina
Adjunct Professor
College of Business Administration
University of Tennessee
Knoxville, Tennessee

Arnold D. Kaluzny, PhD
Professor of Health Policy and Administration
Director of the Public Health Leadership Program
School of Public Health
Senior Research Fellow
Cecil G. Sheps Center for Health Services Research
University of North Carolina at Chapel Hill
Chapel Hill, North Carolina

CONTRIBUTORS

G. Ross Baker, PhD
Associate Professor
Department of Health Administration
University of Toronto
Ontario, Canada

Paul B. Batalden, MD
Professor
Departments of Pediatrics and Community and Family Medicine
Director, Health Care
Improvement Leadership
Development, Center for the
Evaluative Clinical Sciences
Dartmouth Medical School
Hanover, New Hampshire

Milo L. Brekke, PhD, LP, MTh
President
Brekke Associates
Minneapolis, Minnesota

Peter J. Dean, PhD
Senior Fellow
The Wharton School
University of Pennsylvania
Philadelphia, Pennsylvania
Associate Professor
College of Business Administration
University of Tennessee
Knoxville, Tennessee

Susan I. DesHarnais, PhD
Professor and Chair
Department of Health Administration
Medical University of South Carolina
Charleston, South Carolina

Sandra K. Evans, MBA, BSN
Assistant Director of Operations
Vice Chair, Nursing Department
UNC Health Care System
University of North Carolina at Chapel Hill
Chapel Hill, North Carolina

Lucy R. Fischer, PhD
Senior Research Investigator
Health Partners Research Foundation
Minneapolis, Minnesota

Sherril Gelmon, DrPH
Associate Professor of Public Health
College of Urban and Public Affairs
Portland State University
Portland, Oregon

Paul K. Halverson, DrPH
Director
National Public Health Performance Standards Program
Centers for Disease Control and Prevention
Atlanta, Georgia

Russell P. Harris, MD, MPH
Associate Professor of Medicine
School of Medicine
University of North Carolina at Chapel Hill
Chapel Hill, North Carolina

Theresa Hatzell, PhD, MPH
Senior Research Associate
Family Health International, Inc.
Research Triangle Park, North Carolina

Linda Headrick, MD
Professor of Medicine
Department of Medicine
Case Western Reserve University
Cleveland, Ohio

Susan Paul Johnson, PhD
Adjunct Assistant Professor of Operations Management
Goizueta Business School
Emory University
Decatur, Georgia

Linda C. Jordan, MSN, BSN
Director
Clinical Services Division
Rex Healthcare, Inc.
Raleigh, North Carolina

William Q. Judge, PhD, MBA, BSIE
Associate Professor of Management
Department of Management
University of Tennessee
Knoxville, Tennessee

David C. Kibbe, MD, MPH
CEO and President
Future Healthcare, Inc.
Chapel Hill, North Carolina
Adjunct Assistant Professor
Department of Health Policy and
   Administration
School of Public Health
University of North Carolina at
   Chapel Hill
Chapel Hill, North Carolina

Linda Kinsinger, MD, MPH
Assistant Professor of Medicine
School of Medicine
University of North Carolina at
   Chapel Hill
Chapel Hill, North Carolina

Marian L. Knapp, MA
Community Health Improvement
   Consultant
Marian L. Knapp and Associates
Newton, Massachusetts

Thomas E. Kottke, MD, MSPH
Professor of Medicine

Mayo Clinic
Rochester, Minnesota

Rebecca LaVallee, PhD-C, MPH
Department of Health Policy and
   Administration
School of Public Health
University of North Carolina
Chapel Hill, North Carolina

David Levy, MD, MSc, FACPM
Chairman and CEO
Franklin Health, Inc.
Upper Saddle River, New Jersey

Glen P. Mays, PhD, MPH
Research Assistant
Department of Health Policy and
   Administration
Project Director
Center for Public Health Practice
School of Public Health
University of North Carolina at
   Chapel Hill
Chapel Hill, North Carolina

Michael McDade, BS
McLendon Laboratories
UNC Health Care System
University of North Carolina at
   Chapel Hill
Chapel Hill, North Carolina

Duncan Neuhauser, PhD
Professor
Department of Epidemiology and
   Biostatistics

School of Medicine
Case Western Reserve University
Cleveland, Ohio

Linda Norman, MSN, RN
Associate Dean for Academics
School of Nursing
Vanderbilt University
Nashville, Tennessee

Ronald T. Pannesi, PhD, MBA
Adjunct Associate Professor of Operations Management
Kenan-Flagler Business School
University of North Carolina at Chapel Hill
Chapel Hill, North Carolina

Doris Quinn, PhD
Director of Quality Education and Measurement
Vanderbilt Medical Group
Vanderbilt University
Nashville, Tennessee

Lucy A. Savitz, PhD, MBA
Research Assistant Professor
Department of Health Policy and Administration
School of Public Health
University of North Carolina at Chapel Hill
Chapel Hill, North Carolina

Kit N. Simpson, DrPH, MPH
Professor of Pharmoeconomics
College of Pharmacy

Medical University of South Carolina
Charleston, South Carolina

Leif I. Solberg, MD
Associate Medical Director for Care Improvement Research
Health Partners Research Foundation
Minneapolis, Minnesota

William A. Sollecito, DrPH
Research Professor of Health Policy and Administration
Associate Director, Public Health Leadership Program
School of Public Health
University of North Carolina at Chapel Hill
Chapel Hill, North Carolina

William Thar, MD, MPH
Vice President for Research and Product Development
Franklin Health, Inc.
Upper Saddle River, New Jersey

Vaughn Upshaw, EdD, MPH
Clinical Assistant Professor
Department of Health Policy and Administration
School of Public Health
University of North Carolina at Chapel Hill
Chapel Hill, North Carolina

PREFACE

Quality management has come of age in health care. This book presents an interdisciplinary perspective on quality management in health care, taking into account a number of disciplines, including operations management, organizational behavior, and health services research. Graduate students in health services management are the primary audience. This book will also be of interest to those in undergraduate and extended degree programs and in executive education, as well as continuing educational activities involving medicine, nursing, and allied health.

Our approach to quality management is integrative. We have paid special attention to the underlying tools and approaches fundamental to total quality management (TQM)/continuous quality improvement (CQI). The challenges of implementation and institutionalization are addressed in a variety of health care organizations, including primary care clinics, hospital laboratories, public health departments, and academic health centers. TQM/CQI is a "body-contact sport," and any real effort to understand the concept and its application requires studying its implementation in a real setting. The book concludes with seven case studies that track the development of CQI in a variety of settings and show how these organizations have adapted TQM/CQI concepts to their particular needs and strategies. Each case describes in detail the implementation in that context and is accompanied by a case analysis or study guide that highlights important points and links the case back to specific chapters in the text.

The figure illustrated here and in Part I, "Introduction," represents the basic structure of the book. In Chapter 1, we outline the underlying philosophy of TQM/CQI with its structural elements, its health-care-associated elements, and the context within which these elements must

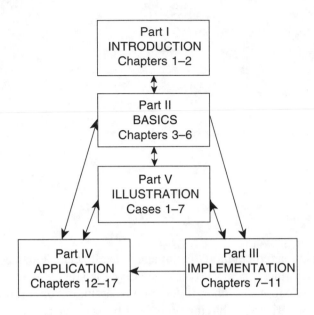

presently function. Chapter 2 summarizes in a balanced way the theoretical and empirical evidence that CQI can work and can improve health care quality.

The remaining chapters are divided into four parts: Part II, "Basics" (Chapters 3–6); Part III, "Implementation" (Chapters 7–11); Part IV, "Application" (Chapters 12–17); and Part V, "Illustration" (Cases 1–7). As presented in the illustration, the book's structure reflects a continuous process in which the basics lead to implementation, and implementation leads to application. Application of TQM/CQI provides an opportunity for further refinement and understanding of the basics through studying illustrative cases and conducting other research.

Part II, "Basics," deals with the underlying tools and approaches fundamental to TQM/CQI. Chapter 3 presents this within an outcomes model. It focuses on the existing quality movement within health care and on the specific measurement issues that health care improvement programs must address. Chapter 4 presents the fundamentals of measurement and statistical analysis applied in CQI efforts. Various techniques are presented here and in the cases in Part V with specific examples taken from the health care setting. Chapter 5 discusses issues of meeting customer satisfaction requirements together with methods and instrumentation required for assessing satisfaction. Again, specific illustrations are presented. Chapter 6 focuses on the role of teams within the context of CQI.

Part III, "Implementation," presents the challenges associated with the implementation and institutionalization of CQI within the health care setting. The five chapters in this part address the challenges that a manager is likely to face in implementing CQI in the professional environment, including managing a number of transitions during the implementation process, ensuring a high level of physician involvement, and providing an appropriate information infrastructure. Chapter 7 outlines the challenge of CQI in a managed care environment and the requirement that, for CQI to meet its expectations, managers and physicians be involved in a "learning organization." Chapter 8 presents some of the challenges of the implementation process. Chapter 9 considers the management information system requirements of CQI and suggests how to set up such a resource. Chapters 10 and 11 suggest that for CQI truly to have an impact, it must be incorporated into professional development efforts, including graduate education.

Part IV, "Application," deals with the specific application of CQI to a variety of health service settings, including primary care (Chapter 12), managed care (Chapter 13), contract research organizations (Chapter 14), public health departments (Chapter 15), and academic medical centers (Chapter 16). Part IV concludes with an assessment of CQI as a tool for disease management and patient-centered care.

Part V, "Illustration," presents a series of seven cases of CQI activity in real settings. All are intended for the purposes of classroom discussion of the philosophy and techniques of CQI as applied in a real context. These case studies both illustrate the applications of the methods and discuss ways of applying the concepts examined in earlier chapters. "CQI Principles for a Personnel Problem" (Case 1) shows how an individual supervisor can use these approaches to attack a serious workload and morale problem coming out of a merger of multiple laboratory functions by applying fact-based management to the situation. "The Family Practice Center" (Case 2) shows how a multidisciplinary team can be used to assess and then improve continuity of care in an academic practice. "Holston Valley Hospital and Medical Center" (Case 3) shows the application of a locally developed industrial TQM model to a community hospital's administrative functions. "West Florida Regional Medical Center" (Case 4) outlines parts of the CQI activity followed by a Hospital Corporation of America hospital in response to serious price competition in its community. "Rex Healthcare and Service Line Teams" (Case 5) illustrates the organizational structure that this institution has been developing to implement productivity improvement that includes both CQI and establishing service line teams. "Dr. Johnson, Market Medical Director" (Case 6) describes the role of a medical director in managing both quality and cost within an overall quality management structure in a very large HMO. "The Patient Transportation Project at University Hospitals" (Case 7) shows how a TQM effort can be managed in parallel with other management steps to improve services and improve employee responsiveness through increased empowerment.

Curtis P. McLaughlin
Arnold D. Kaluzny

ACKNOWLEDGMENTS

Throughout the development of this second edition, we have had the privilege and good fortune of working with many individuals of considerable talent, dedication, and good humor who permitted the chapters to be delivered on target and on time. This group of faculty and student colleagues has brought home to us how fortunate we are to be at a university where interdisciplinary efforts are encouraged and where informal networking is a reality. Specifically, Gordon DeFriese of the Cecil G. Sheps Center for Health Services Research and Kerry Kilpatrick of the Department of Health Policy and Administration, School of Public Health, to whom we have dedicated the book, have helped create the climate that supported this collaboration. It has allowed us to bring together a group of clinicians, health services and management researchers, and health services administrators, all of whom have brought a unique set of skills and points of view to the book.

In addition to working with contributing authors, who some would say "thrive on abuse," we have had extraordinary support from many other individuals—people here in Chapel Hill and elsewhere. The case writing effort was supported in part by a grant from the American College of Healthcare Executives, by the Whelan Fund of the Kenan-Flagler Business School, and by the Physician Executive MBA Program, University of Tennessee, Knoxville. Dr. Paul Batalden of Dartmouth University and Henry Ford Health System has been a frequent visitor to our campus and a powerful intellectual model for this effort. Specific thanks must go to Marlene Sturgill, Kim Vaughn, Christena Maus, Lynette Wyche, Erin O'Rourke, and Janice Pope for their overall assistance in the preparation of the bibliography and various drafts of chapters. Thanks also are due to

Marjorie Satinsky of Rex Healthcare for helping to gather illustrative materials, to Claudia Haglund and Steve Durbin from the Sisters of Providence system for their early consultation as we formulated various ideas, and to numerous participants, colleagues at UNC and Duke, and students in our seminars and courses over these years. Special thanks are given to our initial authors who provided the basis for the current edition—specifically, Jon Jaeger, Kate Macintyre, Carolyn Cable Kleman, Richard Scoville, Rudy Jackson, and Vic Strecher. We also wish to acknowledge the assistance of Cathy Frye, Sandy Cannon, and Kalen Conerly from Aspen Publishers for their overall guidance, suggestions, and periodic time extensions in the production of this book.

PART I

Introduction

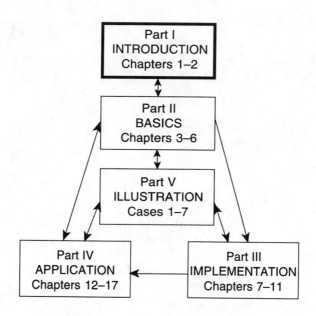

CHAPTER 1

Defining Quality Improvement: Past, Present, and Future

Curtis P. McLaughlin and Arnold D. Kaluzny

Continuous quality improvement in health care comes in a variety of "shapes, colors, and sizes" and is referred to by many names. Don't be confused—whether it is called total quality management (TQM), continuous quality improvement (CQI), or some other term, TQM/CQI is a structured organizational process for involving personnel in planning and executing a continuous flow of improvements to provide quality health care that meets or exceeds expectations. In this book, the two terms CQI and TQM will be used interchangeably: TQM, referring primarily to industry-based programs, and CQI referring more often to clinical settings. The latter term will be used most frequently to encompass all of these efforts and philosophies. While TQM/CQI is known by various names, it usually exhibits these common characteristics: (1) a link to key elements of the organization's strategic plan, (2) a quality council made up of the institution's top leadership, (3) training programs for personnel, (4) mechanisms for selecting improvement opportunities, (5) formation of process improvement teams, (6) staff support for process analysis and redesign, and (7) personnel policies that motivate and support staff participation in process improvement. In the course of that process analysis, rigorous techniques of the scientific method, including statistical process control, are typically applied. The purpose of this chapter is to present the distinguishing characteristics and elements of performance improvement of all types, and their underlying philosophy. TQM/CQI is both an approach and the label for one of the three broad types of performance improvement initiatives that can be undertaken within a given institution:

3

1. localized improvement efforts
2. organizational learning
3. process reengineering

Localized improvement occurs when an ad hoc team is developed to look at a specific process problem or opportunity. *Organizational learning* occurs when this process is documented and results in the development of policies and procedures that are implemented. Examples would include the development of protocols, procedures, clinical pathways, etc. *Process reengineering* occurs when a major investment is made which blends internal and external resources to make changes, usually including the development of an information system effort that radically affects key organizational processes. The lines of demarcation between these three are not clear because performance improvement can occur across a continuum of project size, impact, external consultant involvement, and departure from existing norms.

RATIONALE AND DISTINGUISHING CHARACTERISTICS

As health care organizations develop their own performance improvement approaches, their management must go through a decision process in which activities are initiated, adapted, and then institutionalized. Organizations embark on CQI for a variety of reasons, including accreditation requirements, cost control, competition for customers, and pressure from employers and payers. Linder (1991), for example, suggests that there are three basic CQI strategies: (1) conformance to requirements, (2) competitive advantage, and (3) true process improvement. Some institutions genuinely desire to maximize the quality of care provided as defined in both technical and customer preference terms. Others wish simply to increase their share of the local health care market. Still others wish to do whatever is necessary to maintain their accreditation status with bodies such as the Joint Commission on Accreditation of Healthcare Organizations (Joint Commission) and the National Committee on Quality Assurance (NCQA) and then return to business as usual. As you might imagine, this book is written for the first group, those who truly wish to excel in the competitive health care market by giving their customers the quality care that they deserve.

Although CQI comes in a variety of forms and is initiated for a variety of reasons, it does have a set of distinguishing characteristics and functions. These characteristics and functions are often defined as the essence of good management. They include: (1) understanding and adapting to the organization's external environment; (2) empowering clinicians and managers to analyze and improve processes; (3) adopting a norm that customer preferences are the primary determinants of quality and that the term *customer* includes both the patients and the providers in the process; (4) developing a multidisciplinary approach that goes beyond conventional departmental and professional lines; (5) adopting a planned, articulated philosophy of ongoing change and adaptation; (6) setting up mechanisms to ensure implementation of best practices through planned organizational learning; and (7) providing the motivation for a rational, data-based, cooperative approach to process analysis and change.

What is perhaps radical vis-à-vis past health care improvement efforts is a willingness to examine existing health care processes and rework these processes using state-of-the-art scientific and administrative knowledge and relevant data-gathering and analysis methodologies. Many health care processes have developed and expanded in a complex, political, and authoritarian environment, acquiring the patina of science. The application of data-based management and scientific principles to the clinical and administrative processes that produce patient care is what CQI is all about.

CQI is simultaneously two things: a management philosophy and a management method. It is distinguished from other philosophies and methods by the recognition that customer requirements are the key to customer quality and that ultimately customer requirements will change over time because of changes in education, economics, technology, and culture. Such changes, in turn, require continuous improvements in the administrative and clinical methods that affect the quality of patient care. This dynamic between changing expectations and continuous efforts to meet these expectations is captured in the Japanese word, *kaizen*, translated as "continuous improvement" (Imai 1986). Change is a fundamental of the health care environment, and the organization's systems must have both the will and the way to master such change effectively.

The use of the term *customer* presents a special challenge to many health professionals. It is a term that runs contrary to the professional model of health services and the idea that "the doctor knows best." Some health professionals would prefer terms that connote the more dependent roles of *client* or *patient*. In CQI terms, *customer* is a generic term that refers to the end user of a group's output or product. The customer can be external or internal to the system—a patient, a payer, a colleague, or someone from another department. User satisfaction then becomes one ultimate test of process and product quality. Consequently, new efforts and new resources must be devoted to ascertaining what the customer does want through consumer surveys, focus groups, interviews, and a wide variety of ways of gathering information on customer preferences, expectations, and perceived experiences. If one encounters resistance and challenges to the use of words such as customer, perhaps the best strategy is to demur, since the real issue is the concept and not the labels.

CQI is further distinguished by its emphasis on avoiding personal blame. The focus is on managerial and professional processes associated with a specific outcome. The initial assumption is that the process needs to be changed and that the persons already involved in that process are needed to help identify how to approach a given problem or opportunity.

Therefore, CQI moves beyond the ideas of participative management and decentralized organizations. It is participative in that it encourages the involvement of all personnel associated with a particular work process to provide relevant information and become part of the solution. CQI is also decentralized in that it places responsibility for ownership of each process in the hands of its implementers, those most directly involved with it. Yet this level of participation and decentralization does not absolve management of its fundamental responsibility; in fact, it places additional burdens on management. Where the problem is with the system (the usual case), management is responsible for change. CQI calls for significant amounts of management thought, oversight, and responsibility.

CQI inherently increases the dignity of the employees involved because it not only recognizes the important role of each member of the process improvement team, but also involves them as partners and even leaders in the redesign of the process. In some cases, professionals can also serve as consultants to other teams and to management itself. Not surprisingly, organizations using CQI often experience improvements in morale. With the level of quality that is being measured, workers can more rightly take pride in the quality of the work they are producing.

Another distinguishing feature of CQI is the rigorous belief in fact-based decision making captured by the saying: "In God we trust. All others send data." Facts do include perceptions, and decisions are not delayed to await the results of scientifically correct, double-blind studies. Everyone involved in CQI activities, however, is expected to study the multiple causes of events and to explore a wide array of systemwide solutions. It is surprising and rewarding to see a team move away from the table-pounding, "I'm right and you're stupid" position (with which so many meetings in health care start), by gathering data, both hard and soft, to see what is actually happening and why. Multiple causation is assumed and the search is started to identify the full set of factors contributing to less than optimal system performance.

Later in this book we will also refer to some of the built-in stresses that accompany CQI implementation. These include the tension between the professionals' need for autonomy and control and the objectives of organizational learning and conformance to best practices. Organizations can also oversimplify their environment as sometimes happens with clinical pathways. Seriously ill patients often do not fit the simple diagnoses assumed in developing pathways. There may also be a related tendency to try to "overcontrol" processes. Health care is not like manufacturing, and it is necessary to understand that patients (anatomy, physiology, psyche, and family setting), providers, and diagnostic categories are inherently highly variable and that variance reduction can only go so far. One has to develop systems that properly handle the inherent variability (called *common cause variability*) after unnecessary variability (called *special cause variability*) has been removed.

ELEMENTS OF CQI

Together with these distinguishing characteristics, CQI is usually composed of a number of elements:

1. Philosophical elements, which for the most part mirror the distinguishing characteristics cited above
2. Structural elements, which are usually associated with both industrial and professional quality improvement programs
3. Health-care-specific elements, which add the specialized knowledge of health care to the generic CQI approach

The philosophical elements are those aspects of CQI that, at a minimum, have to be present in order to constitute a CQI effort. The structural elements also are usually associated with CQI, but are not defining and might occasionally be omitted for one reason or another. The health-care-specific elements are those not often included in lists of elements of CQI initiatives, but that are particularly relevant to the health care setting.

Philosophical Elements

The philosophical elements that are representative of continuous quality improvement include:

1. Strategic focus—emphasis on having a mission, values, and objectives that performance improvement processes are designed, prioritized, and implemented to support
2. Customer focus—emphasis on both customer (patient, provider, payer) satisfaction and health outcomes as performance measure
3. Systems view—emphasis on analysis of the whole system, providing a service, or influencing an outcome
4. Data-driven analysis—emphasis on gathering and using objective data on system operation and system performance
5. Implementer involvement—emphasis on involving the owners of all components of the system in seeking a common understanding of its delivery process
6. Multiple causation—emphasis on identifying the multiple root causes of a set of system phenomena
7. Solution identification—emphasis on seeking a set of solutions that enhance overall system performance through simultaneous improvements in a number of normally independent functions
8. Process optimization—emphasis on optimizing a delivery process to meet customer needs regardless of existing precedents and on implementing the system changes regardless of existing territories and fiefdoms. To quote Dr. W. Edwards Deming: "Management's job is to optimize the system"
9. Continuing improvement—emphasis on continuing the systems analysis even when a satisfactory solution to the presenting problem is obtained
10. Organizational learning—emphasis on enhancing the capacity of the organization to generate process improvement and foster personal growth

Structural Elements

Beyond the philosophical elements cited above, a number of useful elements could help structure, organize, and support the continuous improvement process. Almost all CQI initiatives make intensive use of these structural elements, which reflect the operational aspects of CQI and include:

1. Process improvement teams—emphasis on forming and empowering teams of employees to deal with existing problems and opportunities
2. Seven tools—use of one or more of the seven quality tools frequently cited in industrial and health quality literature: flow charts, cause-and-effect diagrams, checksheets, histograms, Pareto charts, control charts, and correlational analyses
3. Parallel organization—development of a separate management structure to set priorities for and monitor CQI strategy and implementation, usually referred to as a *quality council*
4. Top management commitment—top management leadership to make the process effective and foster its integration into the institutional fabric of the organization
5. Statistical analysis—use of statistics, including statistical process control, to identify and reduce unnecessary variation in processes and practices
6. Customer satisfaction measures—introduction of market research instruments to monitor customer satisfaction at various levels
7. Benchmarking—identification of best practices in related and unrelated settings to emulate as processes or use as performance targets
8. Redesign of processes from scratch—ensuring that the end product conforms to customer requirements by using techniques of quality function deployment and/or process reengineering

Health-Care-Specific Elements

The use of CQI in health care is often described as a major management innovation, but it also resonates with past and ongoing efforts within the health services research community. The health care quality movement has had its own history with its own leadership and values that must be understood and respected. Thus, in health care there are several additional approaches and techniques that health managers and professionals have successfully added to the philosophical and structural elements associated with CQI, including:

1. Epidemiological studies, coupled with insurance payment and medical records data
2. Involvement of the medical staff governance process, including quality assurance, tissue committees, pharmacy and therapeutics committees, and peer review
3. Use of risk-adjusted outcome measures
4. Use of cost-effectiveness analysis
5. Use of quality assurance data and techniques and risk management data

THE PAST AND FUTURE OF HEALTH CARE QUALITY MANAGEMENT

Quality has been and continues to be a central issue in health care organizations and among health care providers. The works of Avedis Donabedian, Robert Brook, and Len Rosenfeld, to name a few, are legendary and have made major contributions to the definition, measurement, and understanding of health care quality.

The "corporatization" of health care in the United States (Starr 1982), however, and health care change have redefined and will continue to redefine how we manage quality. Given the increasing proportion of the gross national product being allocated to health services and the redefinition of health care as an "economic good," health care organizations are influenced to a growing extent by organizations in the industrial sector. As part of this process, health care organizations have become increasingly isomorphic with the organizations that finance most of the services that they provide. This conformity is reflected by the increasing tendency to refer to hospitals as "corporations"; the development of "product lines" rather than service areas; the replacement of planning by marketing; the use of titles such as President, Chief Executive Officer, or Chief Operating Officer rather than Administrator; and, in the area of quality, by a nomenclature and perspective known as total quality management (TQM). Although the components of this approach are not antithetical to the way that quality has been defined and managed within health services, neither are the two completely isomorphic. This chapter will trace the development of TQM and then discuss its application as continuous quality improvement (CQI) in health service organizations.

In the 1960s and 1970s health care was still considered a cottage industry. That implied that health care was being delivered by individual professionals who practiced a craft or art , who learned by apprenticeship, worked independently in a decentralized system, tailored their craft to each individual situation using processes which were not recorded nor explicitly engineered, and were personally accountable for the performance and financial outcomes.

During the 1980s and 1990s, there has been a decided change, which is often described as the "industrialization of health care" (Kongstvedt 1997). The usual suspects for those unhappy with these changes are the HMOs and managed care, but many types of consolidation and integration have been affecting almost all aspects of health care delivery. These changes have affected the ways that risks are allocated, how care is organized, and how professionals are motivated and incentivized. Figure 1–1 outlines this industrialization process utilizing the dynamic stability model of Boynton, Victor, and Pine (1993). One route, marked A, follows the traditional route of industrialization as illustrated by the bundling of cataract operations into a few high-volume, specialized centers. Most health care activities, however, have followed the B route, bypassing mass production due to the high variability in patient needs and using techniques of CQI and process reengineering.

The Victor and Boynton (1998) model for the organization suggests an appropriate path for organizational development and improvement. As presented in Figure 1–2, health care processes and product lines have begun to move from the craft stage to positions in all of the other four stages of that model. Each of these stages requires its own approach to quality.

1. Craft requires that the individual improve with experience and use the tacit knowledge produced to develop a better individual reputation and group reputation. A community of cooperating and teaching craftspersons can leverage craft activities to a limited extent.
2. Mass production requires the discipline that produces conformance quality in high volume at low cost.

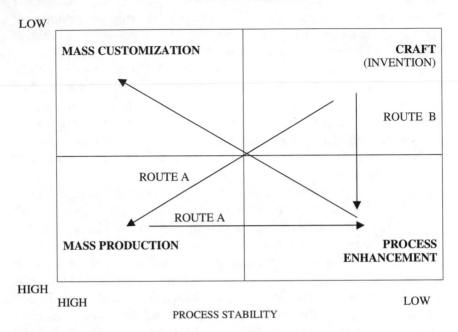

Figure 1–1 Adapting the Boynton-Victor-Pine Dynamic Stability Model to Health Care

3. Process enhancement requires that processes be analyzed and modi-fied to develop a best practice approach using worker feedback and process-owning teams within the organization.

4. Mass customization requires that the organization takes that best practice, modularizes and supports it independently, and then uses those modules to build efficient, low-cost processes that are respon-sive to individual customer wants and needs.

5. Co-configuration involves continuous adaptation to customer intelli-gence, changing the product to match changing customer needs and wants.

Because health care is a complex, multiproduct environment, various types of care can be found at each of the five stages, depending on the state of the technology and the strategy of the delivery unit. The correct place to

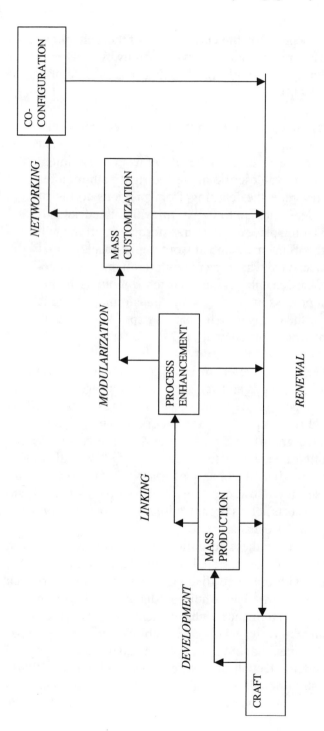

Figure 1–2 The Right Path Transformations Are Sequenced Along the Way

be along that pathway depends on the current state of the technology. The revolution in health care organizations is driven not only by economics, but also by the type of knowledge work that is being done. As described in Victor and Boynton (1998):

> Managers take the wrong path when they fail to account for the fact that: (1) learning is always taking place, and (2) what learning is taking place depends on the kind of work one is doing. The learning system we describe along the right path requires that managers leverage the learning from previous forms of work. . . . If managers attempt to transform without understanding the learning taking place . . . then transformation efforts will be at best slightly off the mark and at worst futile. In addition, if managers misunderstand what type of work (craft, mass production, process enhancement, or mass customization) is taking place in a given process or activity when transformation starts, then they may use the wrong transformation steps (development, linking, modularization, or renewal). (129)

These authors, however, were referring to a single commercial firm with a relatively limited line of goods and services. In health care we can find examples of multiple stages in a single organization such as a hospital. This is because so many different products are produced there. The various DRG (diagnosis-related group) systems offer almost 500 categories and we know that those often are not precise enough. Having these rather loose product designations has been the basis of managed care and disease management, because they allowed us for the first time to collect and compare outcomes and costs across organizations and processes for many purposes, including process enhancement.

As already stated, however, these definitions are not very precise. Even where clinical pathways are institutionalized one hears complaints that these refer to patients with only one diagnosis, whereas most very sick patients, especially the elderly, have multiple diagnoses. Therefore, the prevailing quality and performance enhancement systems have to be prepared to handle much greater levels of variability—variability in patient problem constellations, anatomy, physiology, and preferences as well as variability in provider potentials and preferences (McLaughlin 1996).

Figure 1–3 suggests how this has and will occur in health care. As scientific information about a health care process accumulates, it shifts

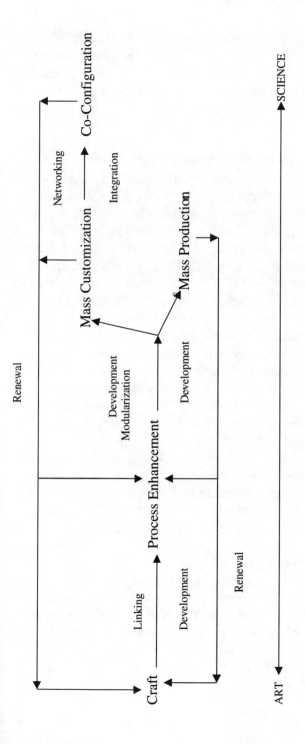

Figure 1–3 Revised Boynton and Victor Model for Health Care

from the craft to the process enhancement stage. After the process is codified and developed further, it may shift into the mass production mode if the approach is sufficiently cut and dried, the volume is high, and the patients accept this impersonal mode of delivery. If there is still too much art or lack of science to justify codification, the enhanced process can be returned to the craft mode or move on to the mass customization and co-configuration pathways.

Even in the craft mode there are multiple delivery alternatives. If one commissioned an artist to make a custom work of art, one could specify two ways of controlling it. The first is to say, "You are the artist, do your thing and I will pay whatever it costs." This is fee-for-service indemnity. The other is to say, "You can decide what to do, but here is all that I can afford to pay." That is capitation. In both cases, the grand design and the execution is still in the hands of the artist. That does not preclude the artist, however, from learning either by doing or from vendors of materials and equipment or from observing and collaborating with colleagues. One does not commit to a one best way to do things, however, because one is not able either to articulate or agree on what is the best way.

The mass customization pathway is the way that is best suited to the production of satisfied health care customers at low or reasonable relative costs. The organization develops a series of modular approaches to prevention and care, highly articulated and well supported by information technology, so that they can be deployed efficiently in a variety of places and configurations to respond to customer needs. Clinical pathways represent one example of modularization. They represent best practice as known to the organization and are applied by a "configuror" (the health care professional) to meet the needs of the individual patient. This requires an integrated information system to give the configuror, usually a generalist, access to specialized information, to full information about the patient's background, medical history, and status, and to synchronize the implementation of the service modules being delivered.

In a sense, mass customization represents a process that simulates craft, but is highly science-based, coordinated, integrated with other process flows, and efficient. How does this differ from the well-run modern hospital or clinic? As described by Victor and Boynton (1998):

The tightly linked process steps developed under process enhancement are now exploded, not into isolated parts, but into a dynamic web of interconnected modular units. Rather than the sequential assembly lines . . . work is now organized as a complex, reconfigurable product and service system.

Modularization breaks up the work into units that are inter-changeable on demand from the customer. And everything has to happen fast. . . . Modularization transforms work by creating a dynamic, robust network of units. Within some of these units . . . there may still be active craft, mass production, or process enhancement work taking place, but all the possible interfaces among modules must be carefully designed so that they can rapidly, efficiently, and seamlessly regroup to meet customer needs. (12–13)

Where does science come in? Victor and Boynton refer to architectural knowledge, a much deeper process understanding than that needed for earlier stages of their model. Also at a practical level it takes hard science to legitimize the conformance by providers required to make such as system work.

The remaining and most futuristic stage of this model is what they call *co-configuration*—a system in which the customer is linked into the network and customer intelligence is accessed as readily as the providers'. Perhaps it is significant that the example that they use is Oticon, a Danish hearing aid manufacturer perfecting a hearing aid that digitally adapts to the wearer's acoustical environment and personal preferences. In the future, one should be able to include the patient in the decision-making network to a high degree.

The History of Continuous Quality Improvement (The Performance Enhancement Stage)

The explosion of medical and technical knowledge in the last 50 years has moved much of medicine away from art and toward science. This movement has occurred at a very uneven pace, however. Even within a single disease entity, the scientific bases for diagnosis, treatment, and aftercare may be at quite different levels. Therefore, some activities in the organization are still very much an art form and still suited to the craft approach. Others have become so routine and are done in such high volumes that the Centers of Excellence and focused factories that are the health care equivalent of mass production seem appropriate. The recent past, the present, and still much of the future of health care, however, focus on performance enhancement. This has resulted in the adaptation of the total quality management approach from industry, especially the work of W. Edwards Deming, Joseph Juran, and others. Here the tacit craft knowledge in use is examined, codified, compared to best practices elsewhere, reworked and tested (often using a variant of the PDCA cycle outlined below), implemented, and then institutionalized. Such efforts produce individual and group learning and, if properly implemented, promote organizational learning.

Because this TQM/CQI process takes a great deal of time to implement and relies on information available only to the participants, including that of benchmarking, and the skills inherent in the organization, some organizations have adopted the business process reengineering approach. This approach calls for much bigger investments, especially in outside information technology talent, to provide a better process faster, but at a much greater financial and organizational cost. These processes use teams of inside and outside individuals to produce totally new processes on relatively tight timetables. Both the TQM/CQI processes and the reengineering processes can produce tightly articulated processes and procedures, such as clinical protocols, clinical pathways, and clinical guidelines.

The processes under consideration can be administrative and/or clinical. The approaches to clinical process enhancement have many names, including the currently popular clinical quality improvement, evidence-based medicine, outcomes management, and disease management. Each of these terms represents a reliance on clinical epidemiology and joint organizational and professional learning.

Approaches to organizational forms for delivery and strategies of implementation vary widely. HMOs and other managed care organizations are very much involved in process enhancement, especially where decision making is based on continuous review of best practice and of billing, costing, and patient record files. They often are guilty, however, of applying a one-size-fits-all control system to all levels of art and science. Figure 1–4 illustrates that control mechanisms need to vary at the very least with the degree of art versus science involved.

Delivery Mode Continuum	Individual Choice of Methods (Craft)	Organizational Learning (Mass Customization)
Disease Knowledge Status Continuum	Continuous Quality → Improvement	
ART	• Professional autonomy needed • Fits well with either fee-for-service (PPO) or capitation • High cost/high quality • Apprenticeship effective	• Conflict over autonomy and efficiency • Conflict over costs • Highly variable quality • Peer review effective
SCIENCE	• High costs • Highly variable quality • Conflict over autonomy versus efficiency • Continuing medical education effective	• Best practice protocols • Managed care fits well • Low cost/high quality • Procedural inservice training effective

Figure 1–4 Relationship between Delivery Mode and Degree of Disease Knowledge

EMERGENCE OF TQM

The fundamentals of TQM are based on the Scientific Management movement developed at the turn of the century. This movement emphasized "management based on facts," with management assumed to be the master of the facts. It believed that management was responsible for specifying one correct method of work for all workers and for seeing that personnel executed that method to ensure quality. Gradually that perspective has been influenced by the human relations perspective and by the recognition of the importance and ability of the people in the organization. Building on those perspectives, Figure 1–5 presents the major U.S. contributors to the emergence of TQM.

Shewhart

Most histories of TQM credit statistics pioneer Walter Shewhart, at Bell Laboratories, with the first published efforts in this area. His best known contributions are the control chart and the Plan, Do, Check, Act (PDCA) cycle illustrated in Figure 1–6. Although the PDCA cycle is often attributed to Deming, Deming himself attributes it to Shewhart (Deming 1986).

Shewhart was aware of and promoted the idea that price alone was no indication of value. He wrote that price, without an understanding of quality, was meaningless. Shewhart taught that decisions based on price alone were almost certain, in the long run, to be more expensive than

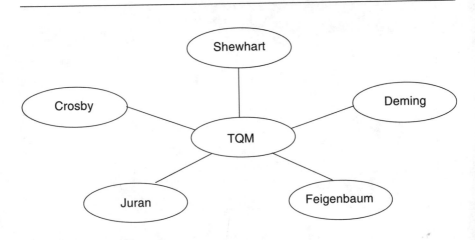

Figure 1–5 Major U.S. Contributors to TQM

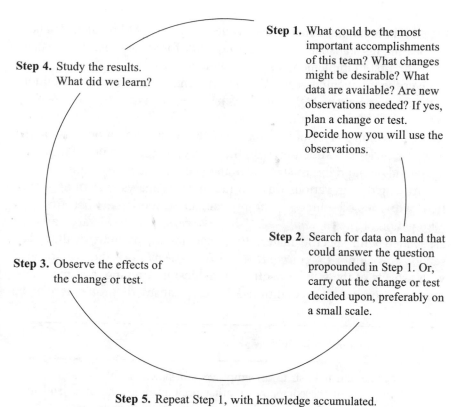

Step 1. What could be the most important accomplishments of this team? What changes might be desirable? What data are available? Are new observations needed? If yes, plan a change or test. Decide how you will use the observations.

Step 4. Study the results. What did we learn?

Step 2. Search for data on hand that could answer the question propounded in Step 1. Or, carry out the change or test decided upon, preferably on a small scale.

Step 3. Observe the effects of the change or test.

Step 5. Repeat Step 1, with knowledge accumulated.
Step 6. Repeat Step 3, and onward.

Figure 1–6 Shewhart's PDCA Cycle

necessary and to lead to undesirable results. He also was aware that there were inherent difficulties in defining quality, although he felt that reasonable people could develop operational definitions, that is, standards.

Furthermore, it was Shewhart's idea that statistical control (also called *statistical process control*) of stable or "in control" processes is the foundation of all empirical CQI activities. If a process exhibited variation, then the cause of that variation had to be discovered and removed. Determining variation and analyzing its causes in order to remove them is one primary function of TQM.

Deming

W. Edwards Deming is the best known of the proponents of TQM. In 1950 he was invited by representatives of Japanese industry to suggest how they might best rebuild their war-ravaged economy. Although he had been advocating his statistical approach to quality for some time, the Japanese were the first to implement his ideas widely.

Over the intervening years, Deming has made enormous contributions to the development of TQM, and he is perhaps best known for the 14-point program of recommendations that he devised for management to improve quality (Exhibit 1–1). But his focus has always been on processes (rather than organizational structures), on the ever-continuous cycle of improvement, and on the rigorous statistical analysis of objective data.

Arraying data in various ways to facilitate its analysis, Deming identified two types of sources for improvement in processes. The first was elimination of *special causes of process variation*: unnecessary variation associated with specific material(s), machine(s), or individual(s). The second was elimination of *common causes of variation*: those associated with aspects of the system itself such as design, training, and materials, machines, or working conditions. Special causes of problems can be

Exhibit 1–1 Deming's 14-Point Program

1. Create and publish to all employees a statement of the aims and purposes of the company or other organization. The management must demonstrate constantly their commitment to this statement.
2. Learn the new philosophy, top management and everybody.
3. Understand the purpose of inspection, for improvement of processes and reduction of cost.
4. End the practice of awarding business on the basis of price tag alone.
5. Improve constantly and forever the system of production and service.
6. Institute training.
7. Teach and institute leadership.
8. Drive out fear. Create trust. Create a climate for innovation.
9. Optimize toward the aims and purposes of the company the efforts of teams, groups, and staff areas.
10. Eliminate exhortations for the work force.
11a. Eliminate numerical quotas for production. Instead, learn and institute methods for improvement.
11b. Eliminate management by objective.
12. Remove barriers that rob people of pride of workmanship.
13. Encourage education and self-improvement for everyone.
14. Take action to accomplish the transformation.

addressed by those working directly with the process, whereas common causes of problems are the responsibility of management to correct.

Deming believed that management has the final responsibility for quality. Employees work in the system; management deals with the system itself. He also felt that most quality problems are management controlled rather than worker controlled. This was the basis for his requirement that TQM be based on a top-down, organizationwide commitment.

Feigenbaum

Building on Deming's statistical approach, Armand F. Feigenbaum and Joseph M. Juran provided theoretical constructs for TQM. Feigenbaum coined the phrase *total quality control*, which he defined as an effective system for integrating the functions of quality development (conception, planning, design, set-up), quality maintenance (production, distribution, service), and quality improvement (training, data analysis, user feedback). These functions cut across all activities in the organization (including marketing, production, and finance) and involve all system phases (inputs, transformation, outputs, and outcomes). Both suppliers and customers are drawn into the total quality concept. The goal of quality, according to Feigenbaum (1983), is to meet satisfactorily whatever customers believe to be their requirements for the service or product. (Note that factors outside the organization—cultural, attitudinal, and technological changes—can make customers dissatisfied with a once satisfactory outcome, thereby continuously motivating new quality improvement cycles.)

Juran

Joseph M. Juran, like Deming, was involved with the Japanese in the 1950s. He argued that the quality improvement process is a never-ending spiral of progress, or "fitness for use," as defined by customers. He argued that management must focus on two levels within the organization. The first level is the mission (always fitness for use), which is determined by design requirements and by the degree of conformance to the specifications of that design's availability, reliability, and maintainability. The second level is the mission of the individual departments and units within the organization to do their work according to the specifications that have been designed to achieve fitness for use. That is, they should go about their work in a way that maximizes the organization's overall attainment of fitness for use. (This may mean that some units must suboptimize their performance in order for the organization as a whole to optimize its performance. This is often a difficult concept for professional personnel to accept.) Juran emphasized the interdependency of all units in achieving the ultimate outcome.

Juran's writings parallel Deming's concepts of classifying process variations, separating them into *sporadic* and *chronic*. *Sporadic problems* occur when production falls below acceptable standards; chronic problems are inherent in the work setting and require intervention by management. Improvements in chronic problems he calls "breakthroughs" (Juran 1988).

Furthermore, Juran insists that quality goals be specific. Vague statements such as "We are dedicated to improving quality" or "Quality is Job One" are unacceptable. Instead, he insists on a specific goal such as "We will reduce the number of medical records uncompleted after two weeks to one percent of total discharges by January 1 of next year."

Juran's followers in health care also emphasize Juran's "Quality Trilogy" of basic quality processes: (1) quality planning, (2) quality control, and (3) quality improvement. These must be supported by an "infrastructure" of measurement systems, buyer-user-supplier relationships, education and training, and information management. These quality processes must rest on a "foundation" of customer focus, management involvement, and strategic planning that links all quality efforts back to the firm's key business goals (Juran 1988).

Crosby

Philip B. Crosby, working in the 1980s, developed a different theoretical perspective on quality improvement based on changing the corporate culture and attitudes. He departed from his predecessors' focus on statistical process control techniques and emphasized the concept of "zero defects." He emphasized organization and management theories rather than the application of statistical tools.

Crosby asked two questions: What is quality? and What standards and systems are needed to achieve quality? He answered with four *absolutes of quality*. The first absolute requirement is "conformance to requirements," often referred to as "Do it right the first time." The second is "Defect prevention is the only acceptable approach." The third is that "zero defects" is the only performance standard, and the fourth is that the cost of quality is the only measure of quality. (This led to the often-quoted title of his 1979 book, *Quality Is Free*, meaning that the costs of producing quality (zero defects) are less than the losses associated with nonquality defects.) His approach, like Deming's, is to implement a 14-step process, but a process that stresses changes in the organization's culture and attitudes. Crosby's 14 steps (1979) are listed in Exhibit 1–2.

Crosby believed that the quality program should go forward on two fronts. On the one hand, management needs to master a set of skills, including his 14 steps, and to develop the necessary implementation and support systems. At the same time, individuals will need training in a variety of tools, including process and systems modeling, statistical techniques, experimental design, problem solving, and error prevention. Crosby's writings emphasize developing an estimate of the "cost of nonconformance," also called the "cost of quality." This involves identifying and assigning values to all of the unnecessary costs associated with waste and wasted effort when work is not done correctly the first time. This includes the costs of identifying errors, correcting them, and making up for the customer dissatisfaction that results. Estimates of the cost of quality range from 20 to 40 percent of the total costs of the industry, a range also widely accepted by hospital administrators and other health care experts.

Exhibit 1–2 Crosby's Fourteen Steps

1. Management commitment
2. Quality improvement team
3. Quality measurement
4. Cost of quality evaluation
5. Quality awareness
6. Corrective action
7. Establish an ad hoc committee for the zero defects program
8. Supervisor training
9. Zero defects day
10. Goal setting
11. Error cause removal
12. Recognition of success
13. Quality councils
14. Do it over again

Source: Adapted with permission from P. Crosby, *Quality Is Free: The Art of Making Quality Certain*, pp. 135–139, © 1978, The McGraw Hill Companies.

Crosby's concept of the cost of quality is a good one to use when the top management has not yet accepted the philosophical arguments of CQI. They often can be impressed by arguments that show the specific cost items that poor quality generates, especially when the presenter also shows how these faults can be addressed using standard quality improvement techniques.

The Japanese

All the individuals mentioned up to this point have been Americans (although their ideas were largely ignored in the United States until about 1980). The Japanese, however, have made numerous original contributions to CQI thinking, tools, and techniques, especially since the 1960s. The most famous of Japanese experts are Genichi Taguchi and Kaoru Ishikawa. Taguchi emphasized using statistical techniques developed for the design of experiments for quick identification of problematic variations in a service or product, and focused on what he called *robust* (forgiving) design. He also emphasized evaluating quality from both an end-user and a process approach. Ishikawa and other Japanese quality engineers refined the application of the foundations of CQI and added:

1. total participation by all members of an organization (quality must be companywide)
2. identifying the next step of a process as its *customer* just as the preceding step is its *supplier*
3. the necessity of communicating with both customer and supplier (promoting feedback and creating channels of communication throughout the system)
4. a participative team emphasis, starting with *quality circles*
5. an emphasis on education and training
6. quality audits, e.g., the Deming Prize
7. rigorous use of statistics
8. "just in time" processes

New approaches, refinements of older concepts, and different combinations of ideas are occurring almost daily. As more organizations adopt CQI, we are seeing increasing innovation and experimentation with CQI thinking and its applications. This is especially true of the health care arena, where virtually every organization has had to work hard to adapt CQI to its own clinical process.

APPLICATION TO HEALTH CARE ORGANIZATIONS

Around the mid-1980s, CQI was applied in several health care settings. Most notable was the early work done by three physicians: Paul Batalden at the Hospital Corporation of America (HCA), Donald Berwick at Harvard Community Health Center, and Brent James at Intermountain Health System, all following the principles outlined by Deming.

One of Deming's major premises (1993) is that management needs to undergo a transformation. To respond successfully to the current challenges facing our organizations and their environments, the way to accomplish that transformation (which must be deliberately learned and incorporated into management), is to pursue what he calls *profound knowledge.* The key elements of his system of profound knowledge are (1) appreciation for a system, (2) knowledge about variation, (3) theory of knowledge, and (4) psychology.

A Deming approach, formerly used by HCA, is illustrated in Figure 1–7. HCA referred to it as FOCUS-PDCA. It provided the firm's health care workers with a common language and an orderly sequence for implementing the cycle of continuous improvement.

The Deming process is especially useful in health care because professionals already have knowledge of the subject matter and have a set of values and disciplines that fit the Deming philosophy. What training in Deming methods adds is knowledge of how to build a new theory using insights about systems, variation, and psychology; plus it focuses on the answers given to the following basic questions (Batalden and Stoltz 1993):

1. What are we trying to accomplish?
2. How will we know when that change is an improvement?
3. What changes can we predict will make an improvement?
4. How shall we pilot test the predicted improvements?
5. What do we expect to learn from the test run?
6. As the data come in, what have we learned?
7. If we get positive results, how do we hold onto the gains?
8. If we get negative results, what needs to be done next?

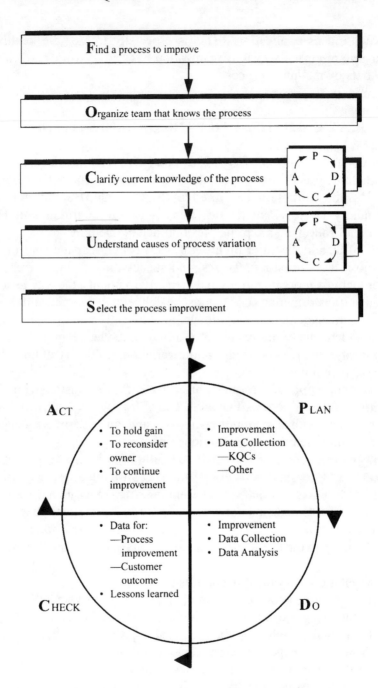

Figure 1–7 The FOCUS-PDCA® Cycle

9. When we review the experience, what can we learn about doing a better job in the future?

A number of hospitals began to experiment with applications of CQI, some of which began to receive public notice in the late 1980s. Several of those mentioned early in the literature and at professional meetings were Meriter Hospital, Madison, Wisconsin; University of Michigan Hospitals, Ann Arbor, Michigan; Alliant Health System, Louisville, Kentucky; Henry Ford Health System, Detroit, Michigan; and West Paces Ferry Hospital, Atlanta, Georgia.

COMPARING INDUSTRIAL AND HEALTH CARE QUALITY

Quality has been a fundamental issue within health services, and therefore some might question the value added by CQI. A comparison of quality from an industrial perspective versus quality from a health care perspective reveals that the two are surprisingly similar and that both have strengths and weaknesses (Donabedian 1993).

The industrial model is limited in that it: (1) ignores the complexities of the patient-practitioner relationship; (2) downplays the knowledge, skills, and motivation of the practitioner; (3) treats quality as free, ignoring quality/cost trade-offs; (4) gives more attention to supportive activities and less to clinical ones; and (5) provides less emphasis on influencing professional performance via "education, retraining, supervision, encouragement and censure" (Donabedian 1993, 1–4). On the other hand, Donabedian suggests that the professional health care model can learn the following from the industrial model:

1. new appreciation of the fundamental soundness of health care quality traditions
2. the need for even greater attention to consumer requirements, values, and expectations
3. the need for greater attention to the design of systems and processes as a means of quality assurance
4. the need to extend the self-monitoring, self-governing tradition of physicians to others in the organization
5. the need for a greater role by management in assuring the quality of clinical care

6. the need to develop appropriate applications of statistical control methods to health care monitoring
7. the need for greater education and training in quality monitoring and assurance for all concerned (1993, 1–4)

In reality, there is a continuum of TQM/CQI activities, with manufacturing at one end of the continuum and professional services at the other (Hart 1993). The TQM approach should be modified in accordance with its position along this continuum. Manufacturing processes have linear flows, repetitive cycle steps, standardized inputs, high analyzability, and low worker discretion. Professional services, on the other hand, involve nonstandardized and variable inputs, nonrepetitive operations, unpredictable demand peaks, and high worker discretion. Many organizations, including health care organizations, have processes at different points along that continuum that should be analyzed accordingly. The hospital, for example, has laboratory and support operations that are like a factory and diagnostic and treatment activities that are professional services. The objective of factory-like operations is to drive out variability to conform to requirements and to produce near-zero defects. At the other end, the objectives of diagnosis and treatment are to do whatever it takes to produce customer health and satisfaction and maintain the loyalty of customers and employees.

PROBLEMS, CHALLENGES, AND ISSUES IN HEALTH CARE

As is the case with any new approach to the management of organizations, difficulties and conflicts with prior concepts need to be anticipated.

Defining Quality

Although there are many definitions of quality, there are essentially three levels of quality commonly talked about today. These levels are cumulative, with the difficulty in achieving quality increasing with each one:

1. Conformance quality—conforming to specifications; having a product or service that meets predetermined standards

2. Requirements quality—meeting total customer requirements; having perceived attributes of a service or product that meet or exceed customer requirements
3. Quality of kind—quality so extraordinary that it delights the customer; having perceived attributes of a product or service that significantly exceed customer expectations, thereby delighting the customer with its value (Dumas et al. 1987).

CQI is not the same as quality assurance (QA), which focuses on conformance quality, although at times the concepts overlap. The confusion that surrounds the use of the two terms CQI and QA stems in large part from the difference in quality as conceptualized in the work of early leaders in the health care quality movement and the somewhat simplistic popularization of TQM by health care groups and organizations. If one reads carefully the initial quality efforts in health care, such as Donabedian, there is surprisingly little difference between that conceptualization of quality and what TQM leaders in industry have written.

Quality has been an issue in health care for many decades. Quality is inherent in the professional standards, guidelines, and codes of the myriad professions involved in health care, the many associations that represent these professionals, and the health care organizations themselves. A concern for quality is also evident in the many statutes enacted over the years at the local, state, and national levels to "protect" the quality of health care provided to the public. This results in several significant problems. First, conflict can develop between the standards of one group and the standards of another group. Second, there can be conflict between the professionals and the health care organization in which they are working. Third, all these standards can be viewed as "floors" or lowest acceptable limits for quality: as thresholds where quality becomes acceptable but where there is no recognition that some quality levels are better than others. Finally, these standards tend to be static and therefore counter to the "continuous improvement" philosophy of CQI.

Who Defines It?

Akin to the potential differences among the quality standards set by professional groups is the tendency of health care professionals, particularly physicians, to think of themselves as operating individually, authoritatively, and situationally. In practice, professionals are contributing members of a group, each of whose members is empowered to correct the actions of others for the good of the customer. Similar difficulties will be encountered between management and those involved in any participative process.

Will It Help with Malpractice Suits?

There are legal as well as organizational issues involved in CQI. It is not clear whether CQI efforts will be viewed positively or negatively in tort cases, such as malpractice suits. Most states have laws that shield from discovery proceedings in malpractice cases quality assurance studies done on behalf of the institution's board of trustees. Some laws are being amended to cover, under the same principles of law, CQI program data as well. The legal status of practice guidelines and their use is less clear. According to Holzer (1990, 78): "Although it is possible that such policies and guidelines could be admitted into evidence to show that a provider breached a legal duty or standard of care owed a patient, it is uncertain whether these risk control standards could ultimately pass the evidentiary rules of relevancy or materiality in a given law suit." Borbas et al. (1990) cite the use of the argument in Minnesota that solid data are more effective for defending physicians' practices than are expert witnesses.

Although many observers express concern about the use of continuous quality improvement data in discovery proceedings associated with malpractice suits, Holzer (1990, 78) suggests that it is more likely that "the consensus-based process of creating clinical standards and guidelines specifically for controlling professional liability losses is itself a powerful and emerging standard for health care risk management programs." This would be especially important should the initial data suggest that the quality of care is generally enhanced by the use of health care protocols per se.

How Much Will It Cost?

Another challenge is how to determine the economic impact of quality improvement on health care organizations. Meaningful cost-benefit and cost-effectiveness studies are often difficult to do. Yet, as previously indicated, there are costs associated with implementing quality improvement. Boards, third parties, employer groups, and government entities will want to know what the payoff is for CQI. The costs of quality have typically fallen into four categories. Two are somewhat easy to determine: the cost of prevention (training, team activities, communication, etc.) and the cost of appraisal (testing and inspection). The other two are difficult to determine: the cost of internal failure (waste, rework, downtime, disruption, etc.) and the cost of external failure (patients go elsewhere, litigation, ill will, etc.). There is also the problem of determining when too much is being done.

How Do We Achieve It?

A number of implementation issues emerge when CQI is examined within an organizational context. Some issues are beginning to be investigated by researchers. For example, what can be done to improve the acceptance of TQM/CQI by first-line supervisors, the group that seems to have the hardest time adjusting to the changes that CQI calls for? What is the role of busy clinicians in the information process? What are the implications of CQI for clinical outcomes? Many of these "how to" issues will be addressed in subsequent sections of this book.

CHAPTER 2

Does TQM/CQI Work in Health Care?

Curtis P. McLaughlin and Kit N. Simpson

Despite widespread enthusiasm for total quality management/continuous quality improvement (TQM/CQI), whether and how it works in health care remain legitimate concerns. Health care organizations are paradoxical, large, and complex. Yet at their core they involve a fundamental relationship between providers and patient. Moreover, if this were not a sufficient challenge, the structure and process of providing care face unprecedented uncertainty and change, making the measurement of any single effort very difficult, if not impossible.

This chapter reviews the evidence to date on the effectiveness of TQM/CQI in health care at a system level. Although evidence is beginning to accumulate from both controlled trials (Solberg 1993; Goldberg et al. 1998) and survey data (Shortell et al. 1993) on the implementation process and perceived impact, much of the evidence remains anecdotal (Arndt and Bigelow 1995; Bigelow and Arndt 1995). Concerns about whether and how TQM/CQI works in health care remain. Below we consider the evidence currently available.

LESSONS FROM THE NATIONAL DEMONSTRATION PROJECT

The National Demonstration Project in Quality Improvement in Health Care, reported on by Berwick et al. in *Curing Health Care* (1990), was the initial effort to launch quality improvement within health services. Although it did not give evidence on the costs and benefits of CQI, this eight-month demonstration project clearly showed that the quality improvement techniques that have succeeded in industry could be applied to the health care setting. The project provided 10 key lessons to guide subsequent efforts, namely:

1. Quality improvement tools can work in health care.
2. Cross-functional teams are valuable in improving health care processes.
3. Data useful for quality improvement abound in health care.
4. Quality improvement methods are fun to use.
5. Costs of poor quality are high, and savings are within reach.
6. Involving physicians is difficult.
7. Training needs arise early.
8. Nonclinical processes draw early attention.
9. Health care organizations may need a broader definition of quality.
10. In health care, as in industry, the fate of quality improvement is first of all in the hands of leaders. (Berwick et al. 1990, 145–157)

In the book's afterword, Garvin (1990) suggests that a number of unanswered questions continue to pose problems. These problems include the indirect relationship between input and outputs (and especially outcomes) in health care, the lack of clear quality standards, and the professionally separate organizational structures of the health care institutions. He also cites the following differences between the quality assurance model and the industrial quality model:

1. Variation may be viewed differently.
2. Prevention is better than successful inspection.
3. The system, not the individual, is the unit of analysis.
4. The focus is on the customer.
5. The definition of quality extends beyond the technical dimensions.

EMPIRICAL EVIDENCE

The health care literature indicates that there are a number of specific benefits associated with quality improvement and related measures such as customer satisfaction. These benefits include profitability, employee satisfaction, reduced costs, improved patient survival, and better continuity of care. Below, some of the evidence is presented about each of these criteria.

Profitability

There appears to be a clear relationship between profitability and customer satisfaction in hospitals. Harkey and Vraciu (1992), for example, report on the relationship among the 82 HealthTrust hospitals. They suggest a quality-profitability model that is shown in Figure 2–1. This model shows profitability affected by increased market share and better prices on the market gains side and reduced costs due to productivity improvements and reduced lengths of stay. They reviewed the literature, which had reached varied conclusions on cost/quality relationships. Then they compared the gross margins of the HealthTrust hospitals with the results that were achieved on the company's standardized customer quality surveys in prior years. These surveys were sent to active medical staff, discharged patients, employees, and community members. Each hospital surveyed all of its active medical staff annually by mail with a 60 to 65 percent response rate; 350 discharged patients every six months by mail with a 60 to 65 percent response rate; most employees annually with an 86 percent response rate; and up to 300 randomly selected residents in the

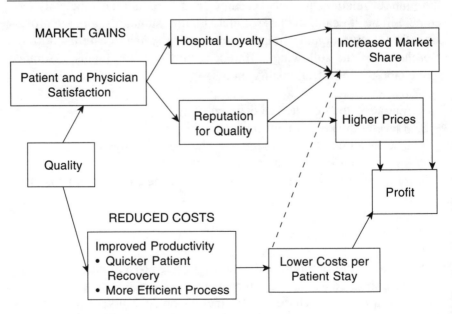

Figure 2–1 Relationship between Costs and Quality

hospital's market area annually by telephone survey. Financial performance was defined as the net operating income of the hospital, excluding interest, depreciation, employee stock ownership plan (ESOP) expenses, and corporate management fees. These researchers took the results of all these surveys and looked at the relationship between questionnaire values and financial performance.

Factor analysis was used to determine whether a quality factor could be developed from the many quality questions. Two quality factors developed from 10 questions. The first seven questions, based on employee, patient, and physician responses, made a very strong factor accounting for 39.4 percent of the variance. The second quality factor was made up of three community responses about the hospital's image and explained 11.1 percent of the variance. The questions used for these two factors are shown in Table 2–1. Other factors developed to control for other attributes of the hospitals were wealth of the community and bed size. Given a reliable factor for quality based on the first seven questions above, the researchers then used regression analysis to estimate the relationship between a quality factor score and net operating margin. The reported regression model uses this quality factor and two other variables—"percent Medicare" and "percent managed care"—to explain 29 percent of the variance in net operating income. The quality factor was positively associated with net operating income and significant at the 0.02 level in this model. The other two dependent variables were negatively associated and significant at the 0.01 level. The authors concluded that the perceptions of quality by employees, patients, and physicians were in strong agreement and that the perception of quality, when controlled for payer mix and managed care, added to profitability.

Nelson et al. (1992) also have reported that patients, employees, and physicians have correlated quality perceptions. They determined that quality ratings by 15,095 patients at 51 Hospital Corporation of America (HCA) hospitals explained 10 to 29 percent of the variation in net operating revenue and return on assets. Both the HCA and the HealthTrust organizations use similar questionnaires, which are described in Chapter 5, to measure customer satisfaction.

The finding of a link between perceived quality and profitability is important in justifying CQI. Other research can find other intermediate relationships, but it is this "meta-relationship" that will be of great interest to boards of trustees and to senior management.

Table 2–1 Questions and Responses

Respondent	Question	Response Used	Mean Value (%)
Employee	"Are you proud of the overall quality of care provided by your hospital?"	Yes (of 5)	34.9
Employee	"Is good service to physicians a high priority for this hospital?"	Yes (of 5)	59.4
Employee	"Do you feel the community views the quality of medicine provided by your medical staff as being generally high?"	Yes (of 5)	24.9
Physician	"My patients typically give positive reports about their experiences at this hospital."	Strongly or somewhat agree (of 5)	78.8
Physician	"The nursing care delivered to my patients is typically good (competent and caring)."	Strongly or somewhat agree (of 5)	79.0
Patient	"How well did our nursing staff do their job (skill, competence, helpfulness, and friendliness)?"	Excellent or very good (of 5)	74.6
Patient	"How would you rate the hospital's overall care?"	Excellent or very good (of 5)	74.2
Community	"HealthTrust has the best physicians." (Yes or No or Don't Know)	Yes	14.1
Community	"HealthTrust has the best care." (Yes or No or Don't Know)	Yes	18.6
Community	"HealthTrust has the most modern technology (Yes or No or Don't Know)	Yes	12.5

Employee Satisfaction

Rush-Presbyterian-St. Luke's Medical Center in Chicago surveyed 5,174 employees (out of a possible 7,400) in 1990, two years into an extensive TQM program. About half of these employees had participated in that effort. After adjusting for demographic differences in the participating and nonparticipating groups, the hospital found a statistically significant improvement in intrinsic job satisfaction, in the general opinion of the hospital as a place to be a patient and to work, and in a number of positive attitudes toward TQM. Because of the large sample, statistical significance was relative easy to achieve. Particularly large changes in scale values (1–5) were achieved in the areas of higher organizational standards, worker and management involvement, and especially TQM awareness (the objective of the program) (Counte et al. 1992).

Reduced Costs

The University of Michigan Medical Center in Ann Arbor, Michigan, monitored its savings and its costs from 19 teams between July 1987 and June 1991. Seventeen of the 19 teams showed a positive net cost saving. The implementation costs were estimated at $2.5 million, of which $1.3 million represented programmatic costs. The combined two-year savings and additional revenues attributed to these teams were $17.7 million. Teams focusing on the turnaround of the center's operating rooms led to added revenues of about $13 million. These were direct costs and did not include the time of the team members while in training or carrying out the team efforts. The time spent in training was valued at $1.5 million. Including the training costs, the return was 4.5 times the investment. One might still ask about the cost of employee time in team activities, but the reported return would be highly favorable, even if that cost were included (Gaucher and Coffey 1993).

Other efforts have also recorded cost savings. Baptist Medical Center in Columbia, South Carolina, found that the suppliers of contrast media solution for radiology were packaging the solution in volumes greater than each patient needed to drink. The team asked the vendor to repackage the material in smaller volumes. The waste avoided came to about $200,000 per year. Yet the bigger part of the saving may be in hundreds of day-to-day small changes. The West Florida Regional Medical Center case discussed later in this book shows a reduction in inpatient antibiotic costs of more than $200,000 per year. Additionally, Bluth et al. (1982) report that one team reduced outpatient "stat" lab delays by 76 percent, reduced patient waiting time 62 percent, and made a one-time saving of $225,000 and annual recurring savings of $40,000.

Improvements may not come quickly in the beginning, and may occur in spurts as the approach is internalized and then reoriented. Consultant Thomas H. Breedlove, senior vice president of Crosby Associates, argues against a time estimate for full implementation of TQM, since he sees it as always evolving. He does argue, however, that with full consultant experience, the hospital should be getting a three-to-one payback within six months (Burrus 1993a). Northwest Hospital in Seattle, Washington, found this out when its director decided that CQI was a philosophy and not just a procedure. The director began to develop 40 to 45 teams around product lines, representing what he calls "the molecular structure," and to emphasize statistical process control. In the first few months of the change, the hospital saved about $3 million and the average length of stay dropped one day. A number of middle management positions have been eliminated, as has the contract management company, at a savings of $750,000 annually (Burrus 1993b).

Improved Patient Survival and Continuity of Care

Reduced costs are not the only outcome of CQI efforts. At the University of Utah, for example, the development of a protocol supported by computer systems to control life support equipment has increased the survival rate of adult respiratory distress syndrome (ARDS) patients from 12 percent to 42 percent. A double-blind study was conducted to compare two types of equipment to see which would improve the patient survival rate. To the researchers' surprise, the improvement occurred with both sets of equipment, indicating that the improvement was the result of the rationalized system, not of the equipment choices (Morris 1992).

Other benefits associated with quality improvement include increased capacity utilization and improved continuity of care. For example, the Joint Commission on Accreditation of Healthcare Organizations' (Joint Commission) book, *Striving toward Improvement* (1992), describes the CQI efforts of six hospitals. These hospitals report improved operating room utilization, a 78 percent reduction in food waste on the pediatric service, increased utilization of transportation orderlies, and reduced admission and discharge waiting times. The cases in this book show increased utilization of capacity, lower supply costs, increased physician continuity, reduced laboratory costs, reduced hospitalization for low-back pain, more satisfied obstetric patients, and reduced inpatient antibiotic costs. West Paces Ferry Hospital also reports how empowered employee teams implemented an $83,000 reduction in antibiotic waste. Finally, Kibbe et al. (1993) shows how CQI techniques were able to improve continuity of care in an academic medical practice.

Costs of Quality

Crosby (1979) talks about the *cost of quality*, meaning the cost of poor quality. Knowledgeable administrators do not hesitate to say that the cost of nonconformance and waste in health care is in the same range—20 to 40 percent of total costs—that has been seen in American industry. As much as 25 percent of the cost of care goes into billing, collections, and handling of claims, and the Florida Health Care Cost Containment Commission warns the public that some 90 percent of hospital bills contain errors. As we will discuss later, there are also the costs of clinical errors and of waste as individual employees and groups of employees act to protect themselves from unpleasant situations due to variation in the system. One can legitimately include in that set of unnecessary costs both malpractice costs and defensive medicine costs. With the costs of health care estimated at about 14 percent of GNP, the size of these unnecessary costs is staggering (*Fortune*, December 21, 1998, p. 154).

So why then do people often question the investment costs of a CQI program? First, the data cited above indicate potential savings, thus raising the issue of the probabilities of achieving them. Consultants report that the likelihood that hospital CEOs will maintain a CQI effort is probably about 50–50. Moreover, there appears to be a moment of truth about 18 months into the process when the CEO suddenly realizes that the process does not involve simply changing the corporate culture, but involves a fundamental change in the way managers, including the CEO, make decisions. Some CEOs never reach that level of understanding; some do and still cannot make the transition.

Another factor limiting the payoff is the fact that only a limited number of quality improvement teams or task forces can be underway at any given time. Even though everyone may be trained in the basics of CQI, only a smaller subset are actually practicing CQI at one time. The effective increased capacity for change emphasized above is limited, then, by the number of teams that can be maintained at one time: probably five to a dozen teams, depending on the size of the institution. The limit on the number of teams is related to the capacity of the facilitators to fully train and support the teams as well as to the number of processes that can be in flux at one time without confusing people. Thus, although the investment in developing the program and doing the awareness training for large numbers of staff occurs early, the returns come later, mostly in the third year and beyond.

Although the savings on the cost side are relatively easy to quantify, the effects of increased competitiveness are harder to document. An increased occupancy rate quickly improves the bottom line, but one usually cannot tell why a patient came to a hospital, and one hears almost nothing about the one who didn't come because a neighbor told him or her that the hospital was unfriendly or poorly run. That is why the relationship between customer satisfaction and financial performance is important. The competitive effect cannot be justified based on specific events, as can the waste avoidance and cost savings effects. Furthermore, any analysis of competition effects can be confounded by the offsetting marketing efforts of competitors. Hospital A may enhance its image in the community by way of continuous improvement, but it may be countered by a heavy advertising campaign by Hospital B or special equipment purchases to attract physicians at Hospital C. Right now, we are virtually in the dark about the relative effectiveness of those three strategies or combinations thereof, so it is virtually impossible to compare the impact of a dollar spent on CQI against the impact of a dollar spent on other market-oriented activities.

Because CQI is new, there is little information about how effective such an effort will be after 5 or 10 years. Prior approaches, such as quality circles, often started with good results but declined over time as motivation waned. Certainly, it is possible in the early years to "pick the low-hanging fruit"—to clear up the obvious quality problems and to show some immediate improvements That is not likely, however, to be the overall rate of return over several years of activity. One may experience diminishing returns, or one may find a learning effect at work in which teams and management with experience gradually develop sufficient confidence to tackle major issues with high potentials for payoffs, such as admissions and discharge. We predict that the program will produce savings immediately, then have a decline in savings or contribution to earnings, and later on, as clinicians become more involved and management more assertive in looking for high-potential areas, will experience some increasing returns. The comparison of CQI investment and payoffs over time displayed in Figure 2–2 shows how these costs and benefits might interact.

Quality efforts can affect the process directly and lead to improvements and reduced costs. They should also lead to improved physician and patient satisfaction with the institution, leading to more admissions, more patients, more patient days, and an increased share of the market. Improved quality might also lessen the pressure for reduced prices to compete against other institutions. All of these together could be contributing to the observed profitability by both lowering unit costs and increasing volume and revenues.

The costs of a CQI program are not trivial. The organization may pay $20,000 to $200,000 for program development, training materials, trainers, and workshops for senior managers, board members, and key clinicians. Then there is the cost of the facilitators and the time lost by employees attending training sessions and engaging in team tasks. In addition to these costs, there are opportunity costs for the resources that went into the program that might have been used for something else. These efforts are not cheap and are not to be undertaken lightly. Much of the opposition to the Joint Commission requirement for a continuous improvement process has been couched in terms of the costs involved and how they might exceed the returns.

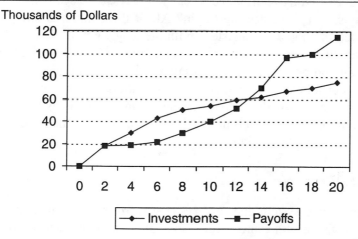

Figure 2–2 Comparison of Investment and Payoffs of CQI over Time

CQI and Changing Clinical Processes

As CQI has moved from administrative to clinical process change, the question has been raised about its effectiveness in working with medical staff. Goldberg et al. (1998) report on a clinical trial of academic detailing (AD) and CQI in improving chronic disease guideline compliance and clinical outcomes. Academic detailing involves visits by educators much in the manner that drug companies send detailers to call on physicians. CQI was not a stand-alone alternative in this study, but an add-on to academic detailing. Their rationale was "We chose this design because we believed most organizations would find it feasible to implement AD. It was important, therefore, to examine the value added by what was hypothesized to be a more complex and labor-intensive CQI program." (133) Their results were inconclusive and they end up citing the confounding factors of local differences in organizational cultures, specific personnel, and disease conditions involved. Chapters 7 through 11 will deal further with changing physician practice patterns and the barriers to such change.

Here again, there are many success stories in the literature, but few which show systemwide effects, a mixture of all types of outcomes. The reasons for this are many. The two most important ones are: (1) nomenclature and (2) confounding variables.

Nomenclature

Where does CQI leave off and clinical pathways, disease management, action teams, and reengineering begin? All of these can and have been implemented in a manner consistent with the way we have defined CQI, while others have gone at them with a command-and-control orientation. Many change programs that may or may not fit the CQI mold have been adopted by consultants and health care organizations. The reporting in the literature, however, usually focuses on one term and sticks with it. With this proliferation of efforts, it is increasingly hard to assess the systemwide effects of any one intervention.

Confounding Variables

The health care system does not stand still for the implementation of CQI. One major health center with a long-standing commitment to CQI also decided to downsize and knock out one whole layer of middle management. Unfortunately, this layoff included many of those responsible for implementing CQI teams. Was it the layoff or the CQI approach that was at fault for the temporary faltering of the CQI effort? Who can tell? One can go to extremes and claim all of the benefits of clinical pathways for CQI or claim none, whereas the truth lies somewhere in between. Westert and Lagoe (1995) reported on the relatively straightforward variable of length of stay for total hip replacement in Syracuse and Onondaga County, New York and Enschede and the Twente region of the Netherlands. In both cases, quality interventions reduced the length of stay, but there was also evidence that a secular downward trend prior to the intervention and the pressure of the reimbursement system in both countries also affected the length of stay.

Coddington et al. (1996) looked at a number of large integrated systems and concluded that there were specific team efforts that led to savings in the millions and that also worked to link clinical pathway implementation to multidisciplinary teams and CQI-based processes. But they also observed a number of issues to be dealt with, namely:

- Legal reservations have to be overcome.
- Supporting information systems must be in place.
- Lack of financial incentives to improve clinical performance can slow down the processes.
- Clinical guidelines are hard to implement unless physicians are organized.
- CQI teams may become too encumbered with processes to achieve results.
- Some must be ready and able to blast through turf battles.
- Processes will lose momentum unless the chief quality officer (CQO) pushes continuously and is a strong proponent of CQI. (84)

Similarly, Weingart (1998) reports that efforts at Beth Israel Deaconess in Boston to involve house officers in CQI were fruitful, but required strong faculty leadership to achieve results because of resident rotations, long hours, urgent demands, and lack of training in CQI methods. The measurement of system outcomes, therefore, has been difficult and not as enlightening as we would have hoped. The economics of quality, however, are rapidly changing, anyway. The issue associated with quality will soon be organizational survival rather than return on investment.

ADVANTAGES OF CQI APPLICATION IN HEALTH CARE

Health care personnel are likely to focus on the differences between their service sector and other parts of the economy and society. Therefore, it is incumbent upon advocates of CQI to explain why and how it works in health care. Intelligent and articulate professionals need answers to the question, "What is behind the assumption of 'value added' from a health care organization participating in CQI?"

A number of factors contribute to the sustained interest and enthusiasm for CQI for health care, despite the limited empirical evidence regarding impact and cost. The first argument for CQI is its direct impact on quality, usually a net gain to the customer and to the organization. The second is that systems can often be designed or redesigned to result in lower costs at the same time and with the same techniques used for quality improvement. The third argument relates to the set of benefits associated with a plan that empowers employees in health care through participation in decision making.

Although some benefits of participatory programs are well understood, the managerial benefits in health care generally come from five sources, several of which are particularly relevant to CQI:

1. increasing the intrinsic motivation of the work force
2. capturing the intellectual capital already developed by the work force
3. reducing the managerial overhead necessary to induce managerial change
4. vastly increasing the capacity of the professionally dominated organization to do process analysis
5. creating lateral linkages across highly specialized organizational units to increase effectiveness and reduce the process irresponsibility inherent in most health care settings.

These five benefits are discussed below, with particular emphasis on the provision of health services.

Intrinsic Motivation

The vast majority of health care workers believes in progress and would like to see improvements and take credit for making them happen. Allowing personnel to work on their own processes, permitting them to "do the right thing," and then rewarding them for that behavior is almost sure to increase their intrinsic motivation, if done properly. It is a classic case of job enrichment for health care workers.

Capturing the Intellectual Capital of the Work Force

Industrial managers are increasingly recognizing that front-line workers know their work processes better than the management does. Therefore management encourages workers to apply that knowledge and insight to the firm's processes. This is especially true in health care, where the professionals employed by or practicing in the institution control its technological core. Management that does not capitalize on this available pool of professional and specialized knowledge within the organization is naive at best.

Reducing Managerial Overhead

Some companies have been able to remove layers of management as work groups have taken responsibility for their own processes. The redesign work that the work force performs can also lead to reduced investment in industrial engineers, quality control specialists, and other overhead staff services. Health care organizations actually are already limited in the number of staff positions, since it is the professionals rather than the corporate staff who have clinical process knowledge.

Increasing Capacity for Process Analysis

The health care institution's management often lacks in-depth knowledge of the technological core (medicine, nursing, laboratory chemistry, etc.) of most of its activities. Therefore, management representatives, such as industrial engineers, if they are on the staff, are usually restricted to areas where they have full knowledge and legitimacy, namely administrative activities. By imparting many of those skills to professional staff in their respective departments, units, and centers, CQI can vastly increase the effective capacity of the organization to examine its processes and introduce change. This expansion comes both in personnel hours available and in the areas of operation. For example, a management engineer can participate in and facilitate the process, but would not normally presume to study these processes in the normal hospital setting. Figure 2–3 shows this capacity effect in parallel with the quality program effect. This figure shows how quality efforts and process improvement efforts are mutually reinforcing and how the added capacity induced by involving professionals in process improvement also contributes to the support of the quality effort and ultimately can improve both cost and quality in parallel.

Lateral Linkages

Health care organizations are characterized by their many medical specialties, each organized into its own professional fiefdom. Galbraith, for example, suggests that specialization is but one response to an information overload in the organization. By specializing, each unit learns more

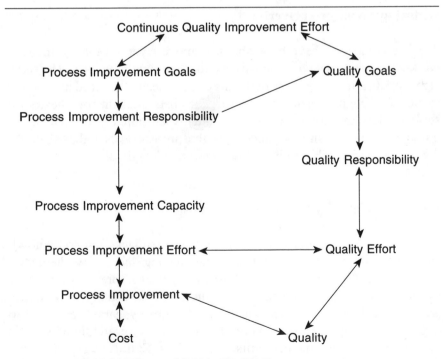

Figure 2–3 Multiple Effects of CQI in Health Care

and more about less and less. One way to offset the effects of this specialization is to provide lateral linkages—coordinators, integrating mechanisms—to get the information moving across the organization as well as up and down the chain of command (Galbraith 1973; Lawrence and Lorsch 1967). So far, that has proved very difficult in health care institutions. CQI, however, through its use of interdisciplinary task forces and its focus on a broader definition of process and system as it affects customers rather than professional groups, presents one way to establish linkages. The technology of CQI focuses as much on coordination of the change process as on its motivation.

QUALITY AND ORGANIZATIONAL SURVIVAL

Once health care organizations have successfully addressed the gross inefficiencies and cost containment, the competitive challenge will shift from one of price to one of value, the combination of cost and quality. In that context we can expect both the visibility and cost of quality problems to rise. More and more report cards will be issued for and by stakeholder organizations. These will be more readily available because of the Internet, and they will be used more frequently by consumers and their proxies to make decisions and choices about sources of health care. Oshel et al. (1997) report that there were already more than 6,000 users of the National Practitioner Data Bank for Adverse Information on Physicians and Other Health Professionals, maintained by the federal government. The users of this disclosure information, when surveyed, reported very high rates of use of the adverse action reports, formal reports of licensure disciplinary actions, or actions against clinical privileges or professional society relationships. A majority of the users reported that this information affected their health care decisions. More employer and regulatory organizations are requiring and publicizing patient satisfaction measures, and various oversight and accrediting bodies, including National Committee for Quality Assurance (NCQA) and the Joint Commission, are insisting on the use of benchmarking systems, including quality-of-care measures such as readmission rates, mammography, and Pap smear coverage.

Increasingly the surviving health care organizations will be asked to justify their existence on the basis of providing good care at reasonable cost. They will be asked to submit information according to standardized data sets. Current examples include the Oryx system required by the Joint

Commission and the Health Plan Employer Data Information Set (HEDIS®)* measures developed by the NCQA. These systems are a combination of organization-specific criteria, such as waiting times, and required outcome measurements, such as HEDIS. The health care organization is required to meet its own criteria and to report its performance on the required outcome measures. It is likely that over time the self-selected criteria will be replaced by more standardized reporting requirements.

Oryx

The Joint Commission requires that the health care organizations it accredits select a series of measures for evaluating their performance. Because some institutions felt that the Joint Commission had been heavy-handed in requiring the use of CQI in order to maintain their accreditation, in January 1997 the Commission's Board of Commissioners approved a plan and timetable for integrating outcome measures into the accreditation process for hospitals and long-term care organizations. Oryx allows the institution to select a set of standardized performance measures from a list of sets approved by the Joint Commission. According to the Joint Commission:**

> The Oryx initiative is intended to be a flexible and affordable approach to progressively increasing the relevance of accreditation and an important building block for supporting quality improvement efforts in accredited organizations. The use of performance measures as an integral feature of the new accreditation process should significantly enhance its value to health care organizations and to those who rely on accreditation information. Today, a growing number of accreditation organizations are finding it necessary to have objective, quantifiable information about their own performance which they can use externally to demonstrate accountability. . . .
>
> Specifically, by March 2, 1998, each accredited hospital and long-term care organization must select (or already be participating in) one or more performance measurement systems that have been accepted by the Board of Commissioners as having met the initial requirements for inclusion in the accreditation process,

*HEDIS® is a registered trademark of the National Committee for Quality Assurance (NCQA).

**Source: © Performance Measurement. Oakbrook Terrace, IL: Joint Commission on Accreditation of Healthcare Organizations, 1998, http://www.jcaho.org/perfmeas/oryx/dearcol.htm, 11/15/98. Reprinted with permission.

and that have signed a contract with the Joint Commission. There are currently 211 such systems, of which 163 contain clinical measures relevant to hospitals and 72 include measures relevant to long-term care organizations. These measures will be the subject of the additional requirements described below.

Secondly, and also by March 2, 1998, each accredited hospital and long-term care organization must select from its performance measurement system(s)—for future reporting purposes— at least two clinical measures that relate to at least 20 percent of its patient or resident population. Each accredited organization will be asked to provide to the Joint Commission the identity of its performance measurement system(s) and the clinical measures that it has selected by March 2, 1998.

Finally, each accredited hospital and long-term care organization will be required to begin submitting data, through their selected measurement systems, to the Joint Commission relative to its selected measures no later than the first quarter of 1999. Because the Joint Commission will need comparative data for monitoring purposes, it is expected that actual data submissions will be performed by the participating performance measurement systems. . . .

We fully understand that organizations are at varying stages in mastering the collection and use of measurement data. Our intent is to provide the support necessary to permit all accredited organizations to make successful transitions to the new requirements. Various resources have been developed to support this effort, and the Joint Commission will hold a series of regional briefings to help organizations in understanding and meeting the Oryx initiative expectations. (Joint Commission 1998)

It is also apparent that the Joint Commission's intent is to ratchet up these quality reporting requirements over time. For example, the Oryx system will be undergoing a phased expansion over the next several years as illustrated in Table 2–2.

HEDIS

The NCQA has been involved in the development of a standardized set of performance measures called HEDIS for use by the group purchasers of

Table 2–2 The Oryx Initiative Planning Schedule

Select by Date	Minimum number of clinical measures	Required # of measures or % of patients	Initial quarter of data collection	Data to be submitted to Joint Commission by
March 2, 1998	2	5 measures or 20%	Third of 1998	3/31/99
December 31, 1998	4	8 measures or 25%	First of 1999	7/31/99
December 31, 1999	6	10 measures or 30%	First of 2000	To be determined
December 31, 2000	8	12 measures or 35%	First of 2001	To be determined

health care coverage. NCQA is a nonprofit organization developed by managed care industry to develop such an information set in close cooperation with the Health Care Financing Administration (HCFA) for Medicare and Medicaid beneficiaries and with the Managed Health Care Association (MHCA), an organization of more than 80 FORTUNE 500 companies. The HEDIS system is under continuous refinement. HEDIS 3.0, when issued in 1996, included 71 reporting variables and a "Testing Set" of 42 other variables subject to further evaluation and refinement. The 1999 reporting set for HEDIS includes the types of measures shown in Exhibit 2–1.

NCQA also issues a data set called *Quality Compass* that consumers can use to compare health plans. It has an agreement with HCIA, Inc., a hospital-discharge database company, to market this information product. "*Quality Compass* not only saves us an inordinate amount of time collecting data, it provides vital information our employees can use to make better plan selection decisions. Having comparable data allows us to make apples-to-apples comparison between health plans, identify strengths and weaknesses and establish realistic performance expectations".*

Baldrige National Quality Award for Health Care Organizations

An interesting new development is the emergence of a health care version of the Malcolm Baldrige National Quality Award for health care organizations (Hertz et al. 1994). A pilot evaluation was conducted in 1995 with 46 health care organizations as well as with a group of 19 educational

---

*Source: Reprinted with permission from the National Committee for Quality Assurance; "1999 Reporting Set for HEDIS." http://www.ncqa.org/news/h99meas.htm, 11/15/98.

Exhibit 2–1 1999 Reporting Measures for HEDIS

EFFECTIVENESS OF CARE DOMAIN
  Childhood Immunization Status (A)
  Adolescent Immunization Status (A)
  Advising Smokers to Quit
  Flu Shots for Older Adults (A)
  Breast Cancer Screening (A)
  Cervical Cancer Screening (A)
  Prenatal Care for the First Trimester (A)
  Low Birth Weight Babies (V)
  Checkups after Delivery (A)
  Beta Blocker Treatment after Heart Attack (A)
  Cholesterol Management after Acute Cardiovascular Events
  Eye Exams for People with Diabetes (A)
  Comprehensive Diabetes Care (V)
  Follow-up after Hospitalization for Mental Illness (A)
  Antidepressant Medication Management
  The Health of Seniors
ACCESS/AVAILABILITY OF CARE
  Adults' Access to Primary/Ambulatory Health Services
  Children's Access to Primary Care Providers
  Initiation of Prenatal Care
  Low Birth Weight Deliveries at Facility for High-Risk Deliveries &
    Neonates
  Annual Dental Visit
  Availability of Language Interpretation Services
SATISFACTION WITH THE EXPERIENCE OF CARE
  HEDIS/CAHPS 2.0H Survey (Adult Medicaid, Commercial) (A)
  HEDIS/CAHPS 2.0H Child (Medicaid, Commercial)
  HEDIS/CAHPS 2.0 (Medicare)
HEALTH PLAN STABILITY
  Disenrollment
  Practitioner Turnover
  Years in Business/Total Membership
  Indicators of Financial Stability
USES OF SERVICES
  Frequency of Ongoing Prenatal Care
  Well-Child Visits in the First 15 Months of Life
  Well-Child Visits in the Third, Fourth, Fifth, and Sixth Year of Life

continues

Exhibit 2–1 continued

> Adolescent Well-Care Visits
> Frequency of Selected Procedures
> Inpatient Utilization—General Hospital/Acute Care
> Ambulatory Care
> Inpatient Utilization—Nonacute Care
> Discharge and Average Length of Stay—Maternity Care
> Caesarean Section Rate
> Vaginal Birth after Caesarean Rate
> Births and Average Length of Stay—Newborns
> Mental Health Utilization—Inpatient Discharges and Average
>   Length of Stay
> Mental Health Utilization—Percentage of Members Receiving
>   Inpatient, Day/Night Care, and Ambulatory Services
> Chemical Dependency Utilization—Inpatient Discharges and
>   Average Length of Stay
> Chemical Dependency Utilization—Percentage of Members
>   Receiving Inpatient, Day/Night Care, and Ambulatory Services
> Outpatient Drug Utilization
>
> COST OF CARE
> Rate Trends
> High-Occurrence/High-Cost DRGs
> Board Certification/Residency Completion
> Practitioner Compensation
> Arrangements with Public Health, Educational, and Social Service
>   Organizations
> Total Enrollment
> Enrollment by Payer (Member Years/Months)
> Unduplicated Count of Medicaid Members
> Cultural Diversity of Medicaid Membership
> Weeks of Pregnancy at Time of Enrollment in Health Plan

(A) Measure or survey instrument required for reporting in Accreditation '99.
(V) Voluntary

Note: Where measures are not relevant for a given population, plans are not required to report that measure.

institutions. At that time the health care organizations did not score as well on the criteria as the educational institutions nor as well as a comparison group of applying industrial firms (Mayer and Collier 1997).

Because the Baldrige awards are a private-public partnership, it required several years after the pilot to raise the private and public monies to implement the award process. The 1998 criteria for the award process, which were available for self-assessments prior to the start-up of the award process and serve as the criteria for the 1999 award competition (See Appendix A.) These criteria are very similar to those of the current private-sector manufacturing and service company awards, with the following exceptions: the "Organizational Performance Results" category replaces the "Business Results" category and the "Focus of and Satisfaction of Patients and Other Stakeholders" category replaces the "Customer and Market Focus" category. They are included here so that the reader can evaluate whether or not they are the most appropriate criteria for judging a quality system in health care organizations. It is clear that further refinement will be necessary to become more health care specific, especially in terms of specifying the outcome measures to be used. The reader is urged to consult with the National Institute of Standards and Technology for updates of the criteria.

If and when a health care organization receives the award, such an occasion could spark considerable interest in the health care award as a competitive weapon and could lead to a marked increase in the number of organizations that apply for the award in hopes of gaining a dominant market position. After all, only one or two health care organizations could win the award in a single year, making it a government-sponsored claim to being the best in the country. The Baldrige Award criteria are also used for health and education awards in 35 states, and the addition of the national award would certainly push that number higher.

CONCLUSION

This chapter has summarized some of the theoretical arguments for and empirical evidence about CQI in the health care environment. There is no certainty that a continuous improvement program at a given institution will enhance quality for the patient and the providers and reduce costs for all concerned. If CQI is managed properly, however, it can and will provide such benefits. The challenge is to design, implement, and lead a CQI effort that is successful for a given institution. It also is clear that such a program is essential to survival in the current regulatory and competitive climate. Later chapters will also identify the need to have such programs and measures in place to respond to the demands of the increasingly hostile health care market.

PART II

Basics

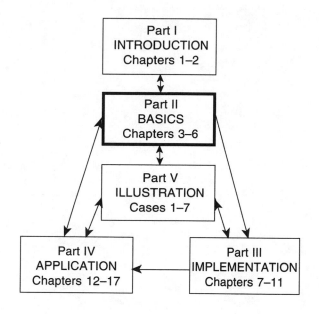

CHAPTER 3

The Outcome Model of Quality

Susan I. DesHarnais and Curtis P. McLaughlin

A critical question facing most health care continuous quality improvement (CQI) efforts is "Who should evaluate clinical performance, and how?" Controversy often arises over issues of quantity of work performed and its quality. Issues of quantity are relatively easy to address objectively. Issues of quality, however, are much more difficult, both politically and in terms of measurement. The objectives of this chapter are to provide a brief historical assessment of quality measurement in health care, much of which predates the widespread use of CQI; to outline a conceptual framework for analysis in health care quality management and procedures for monitoring health outcomes; and, finally, to examine the institutional responses available for addressing quality issues in health care within the context of patient care, teaching, and research.

CLINICAL QUALITY

Although there is much current interest in using measures of patient outcomes (clinical responses to treatment) to evaluate the quality of clinical care, this focus is not new. In the 1860s, Florence Nightingale developed and used a systematic approach to collecting and analyzing information on differences in mortality rates across hospitals. She evaluated the effects of introducing improvements in cleanliness and nutrition on the death rates of the sick and wounded soldiers treated during the Crimean War. Fifty years later, Dr. E.A. Codman reported on his study of the end results of care in the United States. "This famous study emphasized the same issues that are being discussed today when examining the quality of care, including . . . the necessity of taking into consideration the severity or stage of the disease; the issue of co-morbidity (two or more illnesses present at one time); the health and illness behavior of the patient, and economic barriers to receiving care" (Graham 1990, 6–7).

Society did not, however, move in a straight path toward using outcome measures to evaluate the quality of care. Outcome measures were not used more because there were both technical and historical/political problems. The technical problems related to data availability and data processing. In the second half of this century, it became much easier to monitor the outcomes of hospital care using computers and large databases and to develop more sophisticated techniques for modeling risk factors affecting the outcomes of care. Improved access to data will be discussed shortly; however, a more basic issue will be discussed first: the history and politics of quality assessment in the United States.

THE POLITICS OF QUALITY ASSESSMENT

In 1913, the American College of Surgeons (ACS) was formed to develop minimal essential standards of care for hospitals as a first step toward the provision of quality care in American hospitals. The work of this group led in 1918 to the implementation of the Hospital Standardization Program, which developed into an accreditation process that set minimum standards for medical staff credentialing, privileging, and monitoring functions and for adequate medical records and equipment. At that time, virtually no hospital could meet even those minimal standards, although by 1951 some 3,000 hospitals were accredited by the Hospital Standardization Program. In 1951, the Hospital Standardization Program became the Joint Commission on Accreditation of Hospitals (JCAH). The JCAH, created as a private, not-for-profit, voluntary agency, assumed responsibility for the accreditation process, initially using the ACS standards. The JCAH standards were later expanded to cover administrative issues. The JCAH program gained political acceptance, and accreditation was required for licensure and for Blue Cross participation in many states, and eventually for participation in the federal Medicare and Medicaid programs.

The JCAH emphasized establishing a proper environment for providing high-quality care, rather than determining whether high-quality care was actually being provided. Over many years, that focus shifted from structure to process. By the 1980s, hospital quality assurance personnel were asked to identify problems, set goals, focus on errors in the process of care, and demonstrate that they had met their own goals. The standards, however, did not indicate how potential problems were to be identified or addressed. As a result, many hospitals and other facilities focused on issues that could be readily resolved, or on problems that did not reflect the major clinical activities of the department or service (McAninch 1988).

Because the Joint Commission on Accreditation of Hospitals and its successor, the Joint Commission on Accreditation of Healthcare Organizations, assumed a central role in the accreditation of hospitals, many hospitals structured and focused their quality assurance activities primarily toward compliance with the Joint Commission quality assurance survey/guidelines. Quality assurance was defined as a function carried out by clinicians within the hospital. The Joint Commission approach to quality assurance largely reflected the values of society. Since the beginning of this century in the United States, society has delegated the establishment of quality standards to the medical profession. As Starr (1982) points out:

> Physicians and other professionals have a distinctive basis of legitimacy that lends strength to their authority. They claim authority, not as individuals, but as members of a community that has objectively validated their competence. The professional offers judgments and advice, not as a personal act based on privately revealed or idiosyncratic criteria, but as a representative of a community of shared standards. The basis of those standards in the modern professions is presumed to be rational inquiry and empirical evidence (12).

Caper (1988) has summarized the effect on the medical profession of this delegation of authority: "Being the perceived custodian of its own standards has distinct advantages for professions such as medicine. First, it has permitted medical professionals to attain, and retain, a very high level of autonomy, both for themselves as a group and for their individual members. Second, it has allowed them largely to determine working conditions and terms of payment. Third, it has helped turn medical decision making into a 'black box,' relatively immune to outside examination" (51).

Much work took place in the mid-1900s in studying quality and in developing criteria, standards, and protocols, as chronicled by Donabedian (1982). In addition, a substantial amount of research occurred documenting variations in medical care practice (Wennberg and Gittelsohn 1973; Paul-Shaheen et al. 1987), unnecessary surgery (Leape 1987), and preventable complications (Adams et al. 1973; Brook et al. 1975; Roos et al. 1985). These studies, along with others, demonstrated a need to monitor and improve medical care practice. There has, however, been strong resistance by many members of the profession when it comes to measuring quality, particularly if the evaluations are performed by nonphysicians, even if the evaluators are using explicit protocols that were developed by physicians. In a recent editorial, Chassin (1991, 3,472) pointed out that "many physicians think about quality of care the way Justice Stewart characterized his ability to recognize pornography: 'I shall not today define the kinds of material I understand to be embraced within that shorthand description [hard-core pornography]; and perhaps I could never succeed in intelligibly doing so. But I know it when I see it.'" Chassin goes on to note that "a growing armamentarium of new quality assessment tools renders this proposition dangerously obsolete" (1991, 3,473).

By the 1970s and 1980s conditions had changed. As rapid advances took place in medical technology, as the cost of medical care rose in an unprecedented manner, and as evidence began to accumulate about severe quality problems, the government and the public took a growing interest in measuring the quality of care. During this same period, data on health care use and costs became increasingly available to consumers and regulators, as well as to physicians and hospitals. This change in data availability was significant, making it possible for both professionals and others to compare the performance of various providers.

A variety of factors created a demand for and promoted the availability of data on quality, outcomes, and costs of care from hospitals and professionals:

- A 1963 legal case (*Darling* v. *Charleston Community Memorial Hospital*) established that a hospital governing body is responsible for knowing about problems in patient care and the actions staff have taken to resolve them. This case established the concept of *corporate liability*, meaning that the hospital can be held independently liable for its negligence in failing to establish a system of safe practices, as defined by the industry. *Darling* generated demands for information on the part of hospital administrators and board members.

• Corporatization of medicine: HMOs, preferred provided organizations (PPOs), and multisite systems became much more prevalent in the 1970s and 1980s. These types of organizations demanded data on costs, use patterns, and practice patterns because such information was crucial in managing care in these systems. It was also essential to evaluate the costs and quality of care given by the providers with whom these organizations contracted.

• A broader concern with quality developed in industry: Many industries in the United States became highly concerned with methods of measuring and controlling the quality of the products and services they produced. There was a growing focus on using scientific methods, harnessing the energy and creativity of all levels of personnel in an organization. Many U.S. industries adopted total quality management (TQM) principles. In many communities, industries using TQM were represented on hospital boards as well. TQM concepts were introduced into hospital management and eventually began to change the way certain hospitals approached quality.

• Hospitals wanted information on physician performance for appointment and reappointment decisions. Hospitals often lacked the ability to compare physician performance in terms of outcomes produced or resources utilized. As cost-containment pressures increased alongside of concerns for quality, many hospitals wanted objective information on physician performance as part of decision making on privileges.

• In this more competitive climate, hospitals wanted information on both quality and costs for planning and marketing. If a hospital knows that it is either effective or ineffective in producing certain kinds of services, it can make planning and marketing decisions accordingly.

• Hospitals are developing information systems that integrate medical records, risk management, quality management, and financial management systems as part of a new competitive climate under the Medicare Prospective Payment System. Many hospitals are developing integrated management information systems that provide data on both inputs and outcomes for various types of patients and for individual providers.

- Hospitals have become interested in measuring patient outcomes as a defense against mortality data released by the Health Care Financing Administration (HCFA). In some communities, hospitals have received publicity as having high mortality rates since HCFA began releasing such information to the public in the mid-1980s. Because the methods HCFA used to derive these rates had flaws, in many cases the negative findings were invalid. Hospitals needed to defend themselves against such data releases.

- Specialty societies wanted to set standards for certain procedures and conditions to ensure that good care was provided. They wanted information on variations in practice to identify areas where there were problems or uncertainties. Such information could then be analyzed in order to promulgate standards for better practice of medicine within the specialty. In addition, some professional societies wanted information on practice patterns for setting standards for board certification.

The increased availability of data on the use, cost, and outcomes of medical services also enabled consumers, insurance companies, and regulatory agencies to analyze independently trends in the use and costs of health care services and to draw their own conclusions. Employers, unions, consumers, and insurance companies began to demand access to such data for several reasons:

- Unions and industry demanded such information as they negotiated contracts. As new benefits were added, it was necessary to analyze whether they were worth what they cost. In some cases, it was necessary to evaluate the performance of providers such as HMOs in order to decide whether to offer certain plans as options to workers.

- Companies that self-insured needed to develop information on use, costs, and outcomes in order to better manage their insurance plans. Local providers that used excessive resources or had consistently poor outcomes could pose a real problem for such plans.

- PPO contracts also required that the contracting agency exercise care when designating preferred providers. If these providers were producing poor outcomes, marketing of the plan would be impossible, and the PPO could face legal problems.

- Consulting firms that advised insurance companies, labor, industry, or hospitals desired good data on costs and outcomes so that they could analyze choices and provide useful information to their clients.
- Insurance companies needed such information in order to market their products successfully in a more competitive environment. An example of the significance of this issue is the importance they attach to certification by the National Committee on Quality Assurance (NCQA).

In order to provide standardized data sets on costs and outcomes, insurance commissioners and state legislators in many parts of the country (California, Florida, Iowa, Maine, Massachusetts, New Hampshire, New York, Vermont, Washington, West Virginia, and others) mandated that hospitals report these data. Several states prescribed the specific data elements that were required. In many cases, new data elements were mandated beyond the common data set used for billing purposes, at considerable cost to hospitals.

Federal regulators (peer review organizations, HCFA) began to find new uses for data on cost and outcomes of medical care. The federal government used the information for developing changes in payment systems, both for hospitals (diagnosis-related groups [DRGs]) and for professionals (relative value scales). It also became clear that the federal and the state programs were paying large amounts of money for treatments and procedures that might not be the most effective means of caring for patients. By the 1980s, the federal government began to allocate research dollars for "effectiveness research" to learn more about the most effective treatments in areas where great variations in medical practice were discovered.

Also, consumers began to take a much more active role in their own health care. The women's movement in the 1960s and 1970s emerged as a force that was critical of many medical practices. Other consumer interest groups also came forth to question the effectiveness of various practices. Individual consumers, if they had to share costs, get second opinions, select providers from panels in HMOs, and make decisions concerning treatment options, became interested in obtaining accurate and useful data on costs in relationship to the outcomes of care.

Interest in evaluating the quality of care thus moved from the professional domain to the public domain. The medical profession was under attack from the outside as government and consumers sought to measure and evaluate quality. In particular, these groups sought to measure the value received for their money, to evaluate the relative effectiveness of various treatments, and to compare the quality of care provided by different hospitals (Iezzoni et al. 1995; Localio et al. 1995). This interest led to or paralleled the development of more sophisticated, complex, and useful models of medical decision making, including computerized decision-making systems, complex treatment protocols for various diseases, and risk-adjusted measures of hospital performance (DesHarnais et al. 1997).

FRAMEWORK FOR QUALITY MANAGEMENT

Definition of Quality

Quality may be defined in many ways and from many perspectives. The U.S. Office of Technology Assessment (OTA) has defined quality of care as "the degree to which the process of care increases the probability of outcomes desired by the patient, and reduces the probability of undesired outcomes, given the state of medical knowledge" (U.S. Congress, Office of Technology Assessment 1988, x).

Donabedian (1980, 1982, 1986) has observed that definitions of quality ordinarily reflect the values and goals of the current medical care system and of the larger society of which it is part. He has distinguished several aspects of care that one might choose to measure:

- Structure: resources available to provide health care
- Process: extent to which professionals perform according to accepted standards
- Outcome: change in the patient's condition following treatment

In addition, he has broadened the definition of quality to include not just technical management, but also management of interpersonal relationships, access, and continuity of care. One can begin to assess and measure quality using Donabedian's concepts and models, presented in the matrix in Figure 3–1, as a framework. Within each square of the matrix, one can define aspects of quality for which measures and standards can be developed. For example, in the "Structure/Accessibility" cell, one might measure the scope and nature of services provided, provisions for emergency

	Structure	Process	Outcome
Accessibility			
Technical Management			
Management of Interpersonal Relationships			
Continuity			

Figure 3–1 Donabedian's Matrix for the Classification of Quality Measures

care, or geographic factors, such as the distance to the nearest center fully equipped to deal with a given problem. Within "Process/Technical Management," one might measure the adequacy of diagnostic workup and treatment for a particular condition, using a checklist or "branched" criteria. The value of this matrix is that it helps us to define quality broadly and to identify the components that we might wish to measure throughout the health care system.

Why might one choose to monitor structure, process, and outcomes? There are advantages and disadvantages to using each of these approaches. It is relatively simple to monitor structure. In many cases, one can simply do an inventory using a checklist. The Joint Commission took this approach in its early days because there was some agreement that certain structural elements were needed as minimal standards to ensure an environment in which good care was possible. It is obvious, however, that adequate inputs alone do not ensure good outcomes. McLaughlin (1998) suggests the use of the matrix as a diagnostic for analyzing the control mechanisms in an HMO contract as illustrated by Table 3–1. It is evident that this Medicaid program has focused its controls quite heavily on technical quality and access, but could consider ways to beef up the other categories.

Process measures take into account professional performance and would seem to be more closely correlated with better outcomes. It should be obvious, however, that outcomes are not determined solely by professional performance. Other factors such as the patient's condition at the time of treatment, patient compliance, patient age, and chance also enter into the

Table 3–1 Mechanisms for Control Classified According to Donabedian's Matrix

	Resources	Process	Outcome
Access	Readability Less than 2,000 members per FTE provider More than one acute bed per 727 enrollees Specialists available Reinsurance Transport Interpreters Referrals (including WIC)	Nondiscrimination requirement Appointment availability Appointment waiting times Member service department Member orientation required	Encounter data
Technical quality	24 hour per day, 7 day per week coverage Physician medical director Identify services to be given Utilization management (over and under)	24 hour per day, 7 day per week authorization No incentives to withhold care New member physicals Utilization review Quality Monitoring Focused care studies Medical record standards and audits Prenatal care rate EPSDT reviews	Focused care data available 60%–80% compliance with EPSDT standards Audited rates of specific procedures Rates of newborns <1,500–2,000 g by aid category HEIDS data available and within targets

Table 3–1 continued

Resources	Process	Outcome
Affect/relationsip quality	25% of enrollment from community	Enrollment/disenrollment Monthly transfers Grievances/complaints
Continuity of care	3-year contract Include current providers to indigent Conversion privilege	

Note: FTE, full-time equivalent; WIC, Women's Infant's and Children's; EPSDT, early and periodic screening, diagnosis, and treatment; HEDIS, Healthplan Employer Data Information Set.

equation. Nevertheless, it is often easier to measure provider performance than it is to measure patient outcomes for many diseases. One can use process measures to determine whether the professional has performed adequately for those conditions where (1) there is substantial agreement on what constitutes acceptable care, and (2) where the technology is reasonably effective.

Health care leaders would also like to monitor the outcomes of care to determine treatment effectiveness, that is, to measure the effect the treatment has had on the patient's condition. It should be noted, however, that it is much more difficult to gather specific outcome data on patients than it is to measure structure or process. Ideally, one would like to obtain data on patient health status before and after treatment for a large national sample of hospitals. Instead, what is in our available databases is information on variations in rates of adverse consequences of treatment across hospitals, under the questionable assumption that hospitals with the lowest rates of adverse events are producing better patient outcomes.

To construct measures of hospital outcomes, two separate but related problems must be solved: (1) how to take into account differences across hospitals in the type of patient treated, and (2) how to take into account differences in the severity of illness in the patients within type treated across hospitals. These issues will be discussed in more detail below.

Procedures for Monitoring Outcomes

Criteria and standards must be developed in order to monitor outcomes. Such standards may be developed in three different ways:

1. Absolute (normative): determined by clinical trials and/or consensus conferences. Standards developed in this manner by academic health centers reflect the ideal practice of medicine, or the best possible outcomes that can be achieved under optimal circumstances, that is, the most skilled surgeon, the best possible equipment, and the best trained team assisting. Although it is useful to know the theoretical efficacy of a treatment, or the best possible result one could achieve, such standards may not be realistic under ordinary circumstances of practice.
2. Empirical: relative to other institutions treating similar patients. Standards developed by comparing oneself to other institutions treating similar patients may be useful to help identify problem areas. If,

for example, a hospital is experiencing 20 percent more unanticipated readmissions than other hospitals when treating a specific type of patient, that could be a signal that some correction is needed. On the other hand, it is possible that the "average" care in the community is poor. Such comparisons are only relative to the level of quality in the institutions used for comparison.

3. Institutional: based on self-comparisons over time. Such standards are often used in conjunction with both quality assurance and CQI. One collects observations of the same phenomenon over time to determine if a process is in control (small random variations) or out of control (major fluctuations). This information uses the institution as its own "control," and can be coupled with the goal of continuously raising standards in the institution. Although this approach is useful, some external comparisons are required to understand how to prioritize problems. One needs such external comparisons—*benchmarks*—to decide which processes to address first.

The Need for Risk Adjustment

Although mortality rates and measures of adverse events are potentially useful to providers and possibly to patients as one way to measure quality of care, such information can be misleading and potentially damaging if misused. This is particularly important when considering how the government or the public might use such "report cards." Such information must be compiled and interpreted correctly. Several studies have demonstrated that raw death rates, without adjustment for differences in case mix and case complexity, lead to misleading comparisons among hospitals, with those hospitals that treat "riskier" patients appearing to provide poorer care (Moses and Mosteller 1968; Wagner et al. 1986; Pollack et al. 1987; Knaus et al. 1986). These findings demonstrate clearly that death rates must be risk-adjusted and interpreted carefully along with other indicators of quality. This is especially important to academic health centers, with their tendency to receive the cases with the highest risk and complexity, either through referral networks or through dumping.

Hospital-Level Adjustments

In a general sense, differences in outcomes across hospitals (patients' responses to treatment) can be viewed as a result of several different factors that may influence health outcomes. Figure 3–2 illustrates that this is a complex situation. To measure the effect of provider performance on outcomes with accuracy, it is necessary to control for all the other factors. This is clearly not possible, given the existing data sets and measurement tools. Because "report cards" on providers are going to be produced, however, it is essential to develop as valid an approach as possible for risk adjustment.

Historically, two different approaches have been used to perform risk adjustment of hospital mortality data: hospital-level variables to adjust crude death rates and indirect standardization of patient-level data. Hospital-level data were used in several early studies. In a 1968 study by Roemer et al. (1968), hospital-level aggregate measures of patient characteristics (e.g., average age, percentage nonwhite, and percentage of cancer deaths), along with hospital characteristics (e.g., control, occupancy rate, and technology level), were modeled in an attempt to understand whether these proxies for case mix and case complexity were related to the observed differences in crude death rates among hospitals. The authors reasoned that

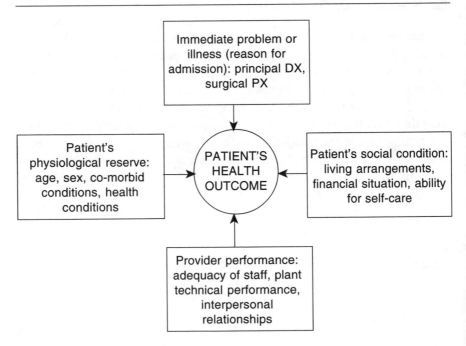

Figure 3–2 Schematic Diagram of Some Factors Related to Health Outcomes.

if these hospital-level proxy measures were related to the crude death rates, they could be used to adjust the rates more accurately to represent each hospital's performance.

This early risk adjustment, as the authors acknowledged, was rather crude. They justified the approach by pointing out that detailed patient-level data on diagnosis and severity of illness were then not available. They adopted hospital-level proxy measures as an indirect approach to estimating case mix and case complexity. The authors stated: "Ideally, one would like to examine the exact diagnosis of each patient admitted and classify it according to a scale of gravity, which might be based on case fatality rates derived from a general literature of clinical investigation. . . . But it is obvious that such a task of calculating average case severity by such an analytic process could present formidable problems of data collection" (Roemer et al. 1968, 98). It certainly would have been difficult in the 1960s, given the limited availability of computers, to model the risks of death for all types of hospital patients using large data sets, even if such information had been available.

Discharge-Level Data

Because hospital-level data are of limited use as proxy measures to account for differences in case mix and case complexity across hospitals, there is no apparent reason to use hospital-level data today. Discharge-level data are now available and are much more sensitive for measuring differences in case mix and case complexity across hospitals. The techniques of using adjusted discharge-level outcome data are documented in early studies, such as the National Halothane Study in the 1960s (Moses and Mosteller 1968), the Stanford Institutional Differences Study in the 1970s (Flood et al. 1982), and work by Luft and Hunt (1986) on the relationship of surgical volume to mortality. In an article summarizing many of the methodological issues in the risk adjustment of outcome data, Blumberg (1986) described indirect standardization, the principle technique used for risk adjustment of discharge-level data:

> Indirect standardization is the method most widely used for risk-adjusted outcome studies. It requires estimates of the expected outcome in a study population, based on the outcome experience

of a standard population. To estimate expected outcome, the numbers of cases in the study population with risk-related attributes are multiplied by the probability of the outcome in a standard population with matching attributes. These expected outcomes in the study population are then compared with the observed number having that outcome in the same study population. . . . The first step involves the development and testing of a risk-prediction model, while the second step is a study of the residuals of the observed less the expected outcomes in the study population (384).

Severity Adjustment: Concepts and Methods

Vladeck (1988, 103) observed that "recent concerns with the quality of health services have focused largely on questions of measurement, comparison, public disclosure, and incentives and disincentives." In order to make valid measurements, and then valid comparisons across institutions, it is essential to account for the differences in types, severity, and complexities of illnesses among the patients treated at each institution. Otherwise those institutions that treat the less severely ill patients may appear to be the "best," while those institutions treating very sick patients may appear to be the "worst." As Iezzoni (1991b) points out:

The goal of "severity standardization" or "risk adjustment" is to control for the confounding influence of patient severity in comparisons of outcomes that might be related to severity . . .[T]he major presumption underlying standardization is that severity is connected to outcome in a way beyond the reach of medical therapeutics. . . . Severity adjustment thus theoretically minimizes the potential for misjudgments about quality due to poor outcomes that are outside the control of the health care provider (179).

In addition to allowing for better comparisons across institutions, severity adjustments are also needed for making comparisons over time for the same health care provider. For example, a hospital may discover it is producing unacceptably high rates of postobstetrical infections. Using methods based on CQI, the hospital may then redesign the process of caring for these patients. In order to assess whether the process redesign actually resulted in a significant reduction in the infection rate, it is important to determine if the patients served before and after the intervention differed at the time of admission in any way that was related to the probability for such infections to occur. For example, if the proportion of obstetrics patients with diabetes or difficult presentation problems requiring instrumentations was greater in the period after the intervention, then these differences should be explicitly taken into account when evaluating the effect of the process redesign.

One of the difficulties in performing severity adjustments is in defining the concept of *severity* that is relevant to a specific need. The definition that one uses must correspond to the purpose that one is pursuing. The purposes of case-mix and severity classification are many, depending upon who the user of the information is—policymakers, administrators, clinicians, health service customers, or patients—and what question the user is trying to answer (DesHarnais et al. 1997).

- Policymakers need definitions of severity that are related to decisions in the following areas:
  1. reimbursement formulas that recognize the differences in resources needed to produce different mixes of outputs across hospitals
  2. planning information that is sensitive to changes in the demand for specialized facilities, personnel, and equipment within a service area
  3. program evaluations, which require information on the impact of services on the health status of the population served
- Administrators need definitions of severity that are related to decisions they must make in the following areas:
  1. quality control, which requires screening criteria that are high in both sensitivity and specificity
  2. institutional planning and budgeting, where information on shifts in case type is needed in order to manage personnel allocations (Hornbrook 1982)
  3. risk management, which requires a classification of cases according to their potential for adverse events leading to liability
- Clinicians need definitions of severity for very different purposes, including:
  1. managing their workload, which requires information for estimating surgical case complexity to predict the time and effort needed

2. ensuring the adequacy of staffing and technology needed to support their activities
3. judging the effectiveness of their treatments in producing desirable health outcomes for their patients
4. assessing the adequacy and equitability of reimbursement systems
5. assessing the difficulty and unpredictability of the clinical management with their patient mix (Kelleher 1993)
6. assessing the prognoses for patients, based on comparisons to groups of patients with similar risk factors in terms of clinical and demographic characteristics

- Groups of customers (insurers, clinicians, potential patients) need definitions of severity to help them:
  1. make contracting decisions, based on information concerning both costs and patient outcomes
  2. make choices among individual providers at the time that care is needed, using comparative data on outcomes

- In addition, there are various dimensions of severity as viewed from the perspective of the patient. Although these severity measures are employed less frequently, they are associated with the patient's satisfaction with the technical aspects of care, which may often be based on information related to:
  1. their subjective assessment of the severity of their illness, and their accompanying expectations regarding pain (degree and duration), stress and anxiety, and the out-of-pocket costs they incur
  2. their subjective assessment of the severity of their illness with respect to the quality of life that they expect following treatment, including residual impairment of senses, loss of independence, and judgment concerning the amount of effort required for rehabilitation

There are surely other definitions and dimensions of *severity*, but the preceding examples do give an idea of the diversity of perspectives and purposes for which one may wish to define and measure *severity*. The challenge, then, is to define one's perspective and purpose first, and then to find a measure that is valid for that particular purpose, that is, a method that has both high predictive validity and explanatory power. These two criteria are valued differently by various people. Clinicians are likely to insist on severity classification methods that have high explanatory power that is consistent with their medical definitions of disease processes. Gonnella (1981, 610) states that a disease definition would, ideally, meet the following four criteria:

1. The disease must be defined in terms of the organ(s) involved.
2. The disease must be specified in terms of some pathophysiological change in the organ(s).
3. An etiological factor or factors hypothesized to be the cause of the disease must be provided.
4. The severity of the pathophysiological changes must be identified.

Several of the severity classification systems presently in use were developed using a clinical perspective, where panels of physicians worked to define severity measurements. These systems include Horn's Computerized Severity Index (CSI) (Horn and Horn 1986), Gonnella's Staging (Gonnella 1981), and Young's PMCs (Young 1984). Other classification systems started with a clinically based disease classification system, but then focused on further breakdowns within each disease grouping, based on empirical methods for identifying risk factors associated with a particular outcome of care such as mortality. Examples include DesHarnais' Risk-Adjusted Mortality Index (DesHarnais et al. 1988), or resource consumption by Fetter et al. (1989) using DRGs. Although strictly empirical approaches to severity adjustment are possible and may be reasonably acceptable to many consumer groups and administrators, they are generally not acceptable to clinicians. Clinicians generally reject a simple association among variables (predictive power) without adequate clinical relevance (explanatory power).

Any one concept of severity cannot and will not meet the needs of all of the parties mentioned earlier, or even all of the needs of any one of the parties. It should be evident that the same cases that will be relatively high on one of the severity scales will be low on another. For example:

- A normal delivery may be low on severity scales focused on mortality or difficulty of case management, but high on scales focused on pain and discomfort as perceived by the patient.
- An appendicitis case may be somewhat high on a severity scale focused on difficulty of clinical management, but relatively low in terms of the resources used or the probability of readmission.

- A psychiatric patient with alcohol problems may be fairly low on severity scales focused on resource use or probability of death, but fairly high on scales that focus on the probability of readmission.

The difficulty is that many of the severity adjustment methods currently available to researchers, administrators, policymakers, and clinicians are not explicit about what they are supposed to do, and/or have not been validated as to whether or not they do what they are supposed to do. This makes it very difficult to determine which method of risk adjustment or severity adjustment should be used for a given purpose. This situation has resulted in much confusion within a very competitive marketplace (Iezzoni 1991a). The level of understanding about the purposes and details of the many severity systems is very low among many consumers, as well as among many administrators and policymakers. Nevertheless, requirements to use various systems for measuring severity are being mandated by many information users—regulators, insurers, and customers—throughout the health care system. In some geographic areas several different systems are being mandated simultaneously with no clear purposes either stated or pursued.

The good news is that we will gradually gain an understanding of which systems work better for which purposes, and how well each works. Many recent studies have examined the performance of various severity classification systems with respect to specific dependent variables, such as in-hospital mortality, readmission rates, resource use, and complication rates. As we gain a better understanding of these different concepts of severity, and how well various systems work toward helping us with each concept, we will be able to use these methods more effectively to help us accomplish the various purposes discussed earlier in this chapter. Because the severity systems used will have an important impact on patient care, it is essential that the various severity classification systems be evaluated and understood. As Iezzoni (1991a, 3,007) says, "Opening the black box is only the first step. We need to guarantee that the information generated is valid, and used in a safe and effective way."

Risk-Adjusted Outcome Studies

Eight early risk-adjusted outcome studies are summarized in Table 3–2. The scope of these studies was limited to very specific types of cases,

Table 3-2 Examples of Outcome Studies Based on Patient-Level Data

Author(s)	Data Source	Scope	Adjustment Variables	Iatrogenic Disease
Pollack et al. (1987)	Prospectively collected from 9 pediatric ICUs in teaching hospitals	Pediatric ICU patients	Age; clinical service; emergency or scheduled; Physiological Stability Index Score	Excluded
Knaus et al. (1986)	Prospectively collected from 13 tertiary ICUs	ICU patients	APACHE II scores	Excluded
Sloan et al. (1986)	CPHA	Seven surgical procedures	Age; sex; LOS; procedure-specific indices of severity; multiple vs. single dx; operation within 6 hours; payer	Included in multiple dxs
Luft and Hunt (1986)	CPHA	Cardiac catheterization	Age (three groups); dysrhythmia (Y,N); heart failure (Y,N); other single secondary dx; multiple secondary dx (Y,N)	Included as any other secondary dx
Flood et al. (1982)	CPHA and chart reviews and patient and provider interviews from 17 hospitals	15 surgical categories	Physical status apart from principal disease; stage; age; sex; emergency status; cardiovascular status; interaction terms	Excluded
Wennberg et al. (1987)	Medicare claims (Maine) and provincial claims (Manitoba)	Prostatectomy (population approach)	Previous history of hospital/SNF treatment; age; type of operation; secondary cancer; secondary cardiovascular; secondary other	Included as secondary dxs
Kelly and Hellinger (1986)	NCHSR (HCUP)	Four surgical groups	Age (five groups); sex; stage; number of dxs; Medicaid or no insurance (Y,N)	Included as number of dxs
Hebel et al. (1982)	100% of hospital records from four hospitals (all hospitals in one city)	All cases in four hospitals	Age; race; sex; payer; 83 MDCs; any secondary diagnoses (Y,N); any surgery (Y,N)	Included in secondary dxs

except for the study by Hebel et al. (1982), which was comprehensive insofar as it included all types of hospitalized patients. The database used by Hebel and colleagues for indirect standardization was limited, however, to four hospitals in one community. Large and representative data sources are essential if indirect standardization is to be valid. Each study in Table 3–2 used a different set of variables for risk adjustment. Age was measured in various ways and was found to be significant in predicting risk of death in all the studies. Other factors, such as emergency status of the patient when admitted, race, sex, and Medicaid status (as a proxy for poverty), were used in some of the studies to predict risk of death.

Patient-Level Data

One of the more difficult problems each of these researchers faced was how to define operationally the severity and the complexity of each case. Several of the studies (Flood et al. 1982; Luft and Hunt 1986; Sloan et al. 1986; Wennberg et al. 1987; Kelly and Hellinger 1986) that focused only on a limited number of specific conditions were able to use panels of clinicians to define severity for those conditions and for relevant co-morbidities. Some of these investigators adopted various existing instruments for severity measurement, such as APACHE II, Disease Staging, and the Physiologic Stability Index Score (see Table 3–2). Others, however, used rather simplistic measures of complexity, such as the existence of any secondary diagnosis or the number of other diagnoses. This was an insensitive way to measure complexity because secondary diagnoses can range from minor conditions that do not increase the risk of death at all to major problems such as cardiac arrest. Also, it seems likely that the riskiness of various secondary diagnoses will vary depending on the primary diagnosis.

Since then, many systems have emerged to classify patients according to severity and risk. Many of these are commercially available and can be programmed for computer analysis. These include the several DRG systems for hospital admissions, the ambulatory care groups (ACG) system, and several systems for the classification of severely ill, intensive care patients–APACHE III, Therapeutic Intervention Scoring System (TISS), and Simplified Acute Physiological Score II (SAPS II). APACHE III and TISS are highly correlated (Stitt et al. 1998), although only the latter handles ages less than 18. Both of these systems are complex, although a simplified, 28-variable version of TISS is available, so some have turned to the less complex SAPS II (Miranda et al. 1996; Clermont et al. 1998). For a broader range of institutional coverage many turn to the DRG systems for adjustments. The original DRG system, however, was designed for Medicare patients and had relatively unsophisticated classifications involving co-morbidities. These include the Refined DRGs (RDRGs) developed at Yale with more than1,200 categories, the New York All Patient DRGs (AP-DRGs) and the 3M APR-DRG system. The latter created more than 1,400 categories by creating four complexity subclasses for most DRG classes. Much of the subclassification can be done on the basis of standardized summary discharge form information. There are many situations, however, where one might want to augment the DRG analysis with outpatient data adjusted using the Johns Hopkins ACG.

Condition-Specific Risk Factors

Certain interactions resulting from co-morbid conditions are undoubtedly more dangerous than others. Ideally, condition-specific risk factors should be used. Moreover, studies that defined a risk factor simply as the presence of any secondary diagnosis often included iatrogenic events as patient risk factors. This was clearly not intended, because the purpose was to measure the patient's risk factors at the time of admission, not to confound risk factors with hospital performance. Although it is not always possible to separate preexisting co-morbidity from complications that occurred during the hospital stay, some attempt should be made to exclude the more obvious complications (e.g., postoperative wound infections or a foreign object left in a surgical wound) when these conditions appear as secondary diagnoses.

Patient-Specific Risk Factors

To measure the effect of provider performance on patient outcomes, we must control for all factors that may affect patient outcomes to the extent possible. Given our existing data sets and measurement tools, it is clearly not possible to control for all of these other factors, especially those risk factors related to the patient's social condition or health behavior. It is possible, however, to use the information contained in existing databases to develop some reasonable proxies for some of the risk factors, other than provider performance, related to patient outcomes. One can use the information readily available in hospital discharge abstract data to assess the risk of various adverse outcomes associated with patients' diagnoses (principal and secondary), ages, and surgical procedures. Once we control for these risk factors, we can obtain much better (although not perfect) comparisons of hospital performance (DesHarnais et al. 1990, 1991, 1997).

A Risk-Adjustment Procedure

It is essential to use risk-adjusted measures for outcome variables to allow valid comparisons across hospitals. The following steps must be followed:

1. In order to ensure consistency in the analysis of risk-adjusted data, do a preliminary assessment of data quality, including coding rules, compliance with coding rules, editing for errors, inconsistencies, and uniform rules for exclusions.
2. Collect data.
3. Using the risk-adjustment models, assign the predicted probability of each relevant adverse event to each case.
4. Develop reports for each hospital, comparing predicted frequencies for each category of adverse event to the observed frequencies.
5. As part of these reports, perform statistical tests on the differences between predicted and observed frequencies to determine whether the differences are statistically significant or merely represent random variations.
6. Using these reports, develop systems profiles, comparing hospitals within a defined subset or the system using these multiple risk-adjusted measures.

We can use these profiles for a "first cut." Hospitals with unusual (significant) patterns of adverse occurrences should examine records and perform peer reviews to determine whether there are problems with the process of care and whether administrative actions may be required at a system level.

What Not To Do

Several kinds of things should not be done with outcome measures:

- Do not try to rank hospitals as "good" or "bad" simply on the basis of the scores on these indexes. Recognize the limitations of these measures, which are derived from discharge abstracts and billing data. Relevant in-depth clinical information may be missing. We cannot always determine time sequences: for example, whether pneumonia or another upper respiratory infection developed while the patient was in the hospital, or whether the infection was already present at the time of admission. We cannot take into account patient compliance, an obvious factor for predicting readmissions.

- Do not assume that data quality is good or uniform across hospitals. Problems with data quality will definitely affect hospital scores on these measures. Poor coding of co-morbidities can make a hospital look worse; good coding of complications can make a hospital look worse.

- Do not assume that a hospital that does well on one measure is necessarily doing well on the other measures. There is no evidence that this is true.

Aggregation of Different Measures of Adverse Events

A valid index of hospital performance must encompass the multiple aspects of hospital care. It may not be possible, either conceptually or technically, to construct a single, all-inclusive index of the quality of hospital care. It is possible, however, to construct several indexes that validly measure important aspects of quality and then to examine the relationships among the various measures to see if they are correlated. For example, APACHE III was found to account for 92 percent of the variation in length of stay for critically ill trauma patients at the institutional level, but only 23 percent at the patient level (Muckart et al. 1997). It requires data on variables usually recorded only in critical care units. If the various indicators are highly correlated, we eventually may be able to construct an overall— *unidimensional*—quality measure. If they are not correlated, we can conclude that the various components measure distinct dimensions of quality and that the separate measures are all necessary in obtaining a valid impression of a hospital's performance.

A 1991 study by DesHarnais et al., for example, analyzed the relationships among three measures that seem to be *intrinsically valid*, in that they clearly are outcomes to be avoided. The three indicators—mortality, unscheduled readmissions, and complications—were adjusted for some of the clinical factors that are predictive of the occurrence of deaths, readmissions, and complications. Risk factors were established empirically within each disease category for each index. The authors demonstrated that hospitals' rankings on the three indexes were not correlated. This result provides some evidence that these different indexes appear to be measuring different dimensions of hospital performance. Thus the three indexes should not be combined into a *unidimensional* measure of quality, at least not at the hospital level of analysis. Neither should any one measure be used to represent all three aspects of quality.

One cannot simply choose one hospital-wide measure, such as a "death rate," to validly represent a hospital's performance. Neither can one simply add up occurrences of different types of adverse events and then claim to have a unidimensional measure of hospital performance. Those hospitals that rank well in terms of mortality rates do not necessarily do well on the other measures and may have excessive readmissions or complications.

Can these different types of adverse events be weighted in a meaningful way so that they can be combined and used as a tool to rank hospitals? Probably not. Even after careful risk adjustment and data quality control, one is still left with the problem of how to weight a death in importance relative to a return surgery or an unscheduled readmission. Clearly, they are not of the same importance, and it would not make sense to treat them as if they were.

INSTITUTIONAL RESPONSES

Given that the management of a health care organization understands the history and politics of quality of health care, has an appropriate conceptual model of quality, and develops suitable risk-adjusted quality measures, what does it then do about quality? The first step is to make sure that everyone shares a quality strategy. The second step is to see that the strategy is implemented consistently across all the major programs of the institution: delivery of care, research, and education.

Linder (1991) suggests that there are three basic strategies, which she calls *models*, that institutions can adopt on quality of care, specifically outcomes measurement. No one is against quality by definition, and no one is about to argue for unreasonable prices. Therefore, all three favor cost control and quality. Linder (1991) describes them as:

- *Status quo organizations targeting reasonable quality at a reasonable price.* They tend to have medical staff as the dominant group, with individual physicians left to provide quality leadership. Outcomes information in these organizations tends to center on routine compliance-oriented data prepared by medical librarians and nurses.
- *Administrative control organizations targeting reasonable quality at an excellent (high) price.* Administration tends to take predominant responsibility for quality and focuses on outliers of quality and resource utilization (cost). Nurses tend to constitute the quality assurance staff, and reports tend to focus on identifying outliers.
- *Professional network organizations targeting for excellent quality at a reasonable price.* These organizations tend to have strong medical leadership and a partnership with the administrative leadership to provide excellent service. The emphasis is on ad hoc studies to inform consensus conferences using the skills of both clinical researchers and information analysts.

About the latter group, Linder (1991) writes:

> Twenty percent of the hospitals had begun to take a very different approach. The administrative and medical staffs joined forces to form an organization that held quality as its first purpose. In contrast to Model 2 (Administrative Control), they believed that financial success would follow from medical effectiveness. Their intent was not to manage the external image of quality, but to continuously assess and improve the organization's actual quality. They believed that the way to achieve this goal was through the free and open discussion of medical effectiveness among professionals. In other words, they used an informed, professional peer network, rather than an authority structure, to manage the organization's performance. The network included administrators, nurses, and physicians, and it addressed both financial and clinical issues (27–28).

It would be foolish to try to classify an entire health care organization into any one of those three categories. That is one of the handicaps of big institutions in attempting to adapt to environmental pressures. They are loosely coupled organizations that seldom respond as a whole, but rather piece by piece (Weick 1976). One department, or even a division of a department, may be in the status quo stage while another is in the professional network stage. For example, at a large academic medical center, one teaching hospital may be in the administrative control stage and another working toward professional networking.

We believe that a forward-thinking health care organization is best served by moving toward the professional networking approach as rapidly as its leadership can take it there. The administrative control approach will not be acceptable to patients or to professionals over time. It does not fit with their concepts of professional autonomy or governance or leadership. Sooner or later, it will lead to a revolution on the part of the staff. The status quo approach, however, appears at worst to set the institution's sights too low for long-run survival and at best to become vulnerable to unpleasant regulatory interventions. That leaves the professional network approach as the only viable alternative for the long run. Getting there, however, will take real medical leadership. There are leaders in medicine who argue that the status quo approach is the prevailing set of professional norms (Cotton 1991).

One fear often expressed by members of the medical profession is that those focusing on health care guidelines are developing protocol-oriented medical automatons or, in other words, promoting "cookbook medicine." Reed and Evans (1987, 3,280) warn that "as bureaucratic protocols based on cost containment seek to homogenize heterogeneous conditions and events, and the organizational penalties for being wrong or not conforming to the uniformity in the system multiply, there will be a devaluation of concepts such as initiative, innovation, or the utilization of experientially based clinical hunches."

Clinicians need to adapt to the changed environment in several ways:

- They need to overcome some of their resistance to accountability to nonphysicians (administrators, government, consumers) and form working alliances with these powerful groups.
- To cooperate, they need to develop the behavioral skills required to function in interdisciplinary teams.

- They need to develop a reasonable degree of sophistication with the methods and tools used to assess/measure quality and a critical appreciation of their strengths and weaknesses.

If these changes occur, it is even possible that physicians can be empowered to actively participate with others in improving the quality of care (Headrick et al. 1991). There can be a change in role and function, but potentially a gain in the ability of physicians to work with others to produce better results. Reed and Evans (1987) point out that the alternatives are either a situation where professionalism inevitably disappears, as our society follows its course of economic and organizational evolution, or a situation where "physicians can be much less the prisoners of history." Physicians can choose to "either act creatively, quickly, and decisively in the interests of their profession and their society, or acquiesce to changes planned by others" (3,282).

Authority Patterns

McLaughlin and Kaluzny (1990) emphasize the autonomy and authority barriers that must be overcome in introducing quality concepts into clinical practice. The debate between Berwick (1990, 1991) and Zusman (1991) shows two contrasting points of view. Berwick (1991, 420) emphasizes the TQM approach, with its multidisciplinary emphasis, arguing that clinical care is "a network of deep interdependencies involving other professionals, nonprofessional staff, information systems, policies and procedures, physical systems, and other influences on their own work and on the patients they serve. Sometimes physicians indeed act alone. But usually not." Zusman (1991) argues that quality assurance (QA) is a well-developed, stable approach that deals adequately with clinical quality, but should not consider cost of care as a quality issue, because cost is a responsibility of the utilization management staff. In his ideal hospital, administration "leaves monitoring of the quality of professional care to the QA system (or more strictly, leaves to the QA system that care that falls under the medical staff privileging system) while it monitors the quality of all other services and products that the hospital either purchases or produces" (418).

The current structuring of medical schools and teaching hospitals supports the "traditional" system outlined by Zusman. Yet the results leave much to be desired from a clinical, cost, and patient perspective. It is time for the management of today's health care organizations to take a strong position in this controversial arena. Consider the outcomes management approach taken by the Greater New York Hospital Association.

Greater New York Hospital Association: One Approach to Outcomes Management

The Greater New York Hospital Association's (GNYHA) Quaesitum Measurement System (QMS) was developed in response to the demand by GNYHA's member institutions for better and more affordable comparative performance information. QMS analyzes key quality, financial, and efficiency indicators and seeks to show the relationships among these indicators. The reports provide a comprehensive picture of institutional performance. QMS reports provide comparative information concerning the performance of (1) the hospital, (2) customized peer groups selected by each hospital, (3) a benchmark group of top-performing hospitals, and (4) all hospitals in the downstate New York region.

A team of national experts in hospital financial, efficiency, and operations management; quality improvement; *medical informatics*; and risk-adjustment methods produced the QMS under the direction of a technical advisory group consisting of clinicians, administrators, quality improvement directors, and finance and managed care experts from GNYHA member facilities. Using state-of-the-art analytical techniques, QMS reports offer hospital chief executive officers, chief financial officers, medical directors, and other senior clinicians and managers greater insight into how their institution performs compared to its peers. In addition, QMS reports can lead to opportunities for improving quality, operations, and managed care contracting and provide information with which to respond to external, published performance reports.

QMS Uses Risk-Adjustment Method

QMS uses a risk-adjustment technique that has been developed and validated for application to discharge abstract databases. The risk-adjustment method accounts for numerous risk factors that influence each specific patient outcome and resource utilization measure. These include age, sex, race, number of major co-morbidities, number of major diagnostic categories with minor co-morbidities, transfer in from a long-term care facility or another acute care facility, and presence of any diagnosis of cancer or of AIDS. In contrast, severity systems tend to be less refined insofar as they typically group patients into severity levels within a disease category by using only one risk factor—the presence or combination of co-morbidities.

The QMS method computes a predicted probability of mortality, a probability of one or more complications, length of stay, and cost per case based on each patient's specific risk factors, using the appropriate regression equations and weights derived from each disease cluster/outcome combination. Nearly 1,000 individual regression equations were estimated in order to achieve the best possible predictive model for each outcome within each disease category. In comparison, severity systems customarily assign patients to one particular severity level and then use the score associated with that severity level as the basis for predicting all outcomes.

Once predicted probabilities/values are assigned to each case, patients are grouped by hospital and then aggregated by clinical service line, procedure, diagnosis, and payer. The predicted probabilities/values are summed to derive expected rates/values for each hospital, which are then compared to the actual rates/values. Appropriate statistical tests are performed to determine whether the differences between actual and expected rates/values are statistically significant. By contrast, severity systems typically cannot estimate predicted probabilities of mortality, etc., with the same level of precision because their reference is the mean performance value for all patients in a particular disease cluster/severity level. Because of its approach, QMS yields statistically significant differences that are more meaningful than those identified by many other systems.

QMS's Distinguishing Features

Several features distinguish QMS from other performance measurement systems. These include the following:

- *Comprehensive performance measurement through the integration of New York State's discharge abstract database known as SPARCS (Statewide Planning and Research Cooperative System) and the insti-*

tutional cost report database. Through a unique "charge mapping" and "payer mapping" process, QMS builds a bridge between the SPARCS and institutional cost report databases to create an integrated database. This first-of-its-kind integrated database permits quality, financial, and efficiency analyses to be performed at the clinical service line, diagnosis, procedure, and payer levels—a capability that is unique for information derived from administrative databases.

- *Peer group comparative performance.* QMS allows performance comparisons with customized peer groups. Users can select a default peer group for all analyses, or they can tailor peer groups for each clinical service line, procedure, diagnosis, or payer group.

- *Risk-adjusted performance analyses.* QMS assesses the performance for each clinical service line, selected procedures and diagnoses, and payer groups according to four risk-adjusted indicators: (1) mortality rates, (2) complication rates (postsurgical and postobstetrical), (3) length of stay, and (4) cost per case. Some performance measurement systems analyze these indicators using one of several patient severity classification schemes. QMS differs from these systems in two important respects:

  1. The *clinical profile* provides a comprehensive picture of hospital performance for various clinical service lines and selected diagnoses and procedures. For the 1995 report, QMS analyzed quality, efficiency, and financial performance for 23 adult and 8 pediatric clinical service lines, 16 procedures, 11 diagnoses, and 8 payer groups. The quality performance measures consist of risk-adjusted mortality and complication rates, while the efficiency performance measures consist of risk-adjusted length of stay and cost per case. The financial analyses focus on profitability within the specified clinical service lines for all payers combined and selected payer categories (i.e., Medicare fee-for-service, HMO, etc.) and within the specified procedures and diagnoses for all payers combined.

  2. The *payer profile* provides comparative performance information for selected payer categories. Information in this section focuses on four risk-adjusted measures (mortality, postsurgical/postobstetrical complications, length of stay, and cost per case) and profitability for each payer category. A sample of a clinical profile follows as Figure 3–3.

Columns provide comparative information across hospital groups. Differences in expected mortality rates noted in this column, for example, may be explained by differences in patient complexity, data quality, or clinical quality.

RISK-ADJUSTED PERFORMANCE MEASUREMENT (1995)

CLINICAL SERVICE LINE: | ONCOLOGY |

OMS PERFORMANCE MEASURE: | RISK-ADJUSTED MORTALITY RATE |

Rows report information for the hospital or group of hospitals indicated. In other words, the hospital and each hospital group shown has its own actual and expected rates and risk-adjusted indexes.

		Total Number of Cases	Actual Rate			Expected Rate		Risk-Adjusted Index (a)
			Rate (%)	Range (%)		Rate (%)	Range (95% C.I.)	
				Min.	Max.			
Hospital #		1,758	6.3	—	—	8.5	7.2–9.8	0.74*
Peer Group (b)		14,385	5.6	3.7	11.2	6.4	5.9–6.7	0.58*
Benchmark Group (c)		28,053	6.7	9.9	15.5	7.7	7.4–8.0	0.74*
NVC Metropolitan Region		65,536	9.0	0.0	25.8	9.0	8.8–9.2	1.08

Key measure: hospital's actual mortality rate is 26% lower than expected (6.3 + 8.5). In this case, the difference is statistically significant based on a 95% confidence interval.

(a) Risk-adjusted index is computed as the actual rate – the expected rate. In general, values < 1 indicate that the hospital(s) is performing better than expected, values > 1 indicate that the hospital(s) is performing worse than expected.

(b) As selected by the hospital, the peer group is composed of the following hospitals: Hospital A, Hospital B, Hospital C, Hospital D, Hospital E, Hospital F, Hospital G.

(c) The "benchmark" is the group of hospital(s) performing at the top of the performance measure.

(d) Indicates that the study hospital is in the benchmark group.

* Indicates that the actual rate is significantly outside the excepted range.

If the hospital's risk-adjusted mortality index had been higher than expected (> 1.0) and statistically significant (p = .05), this signals an opportunity for data and/or clinical quality improvement.

Figure 3–3 Sample QMS Clinical Profile

CONCLUSION

Quality is something that all health care providers favor. It is not, as many would like to believe, something that happens without planning and conscientious effort. The outside world is demanding health care organizations of the highest quality at a reasonable price. Information with which to assess outcome performance in health care is becoming widely available. Providers can fight to maintain professional autonomy by pushing the lay assessors back, or they can take the lead by becoming expert on quality assessment and applying those skills to ongoing operations. They can then educate the public in how to interpret the impact of age, co-morbidity, and other factors on outcomes measures. The profession can incorporate the measures developed in its research into its teaching and into its delivery of care. It can educate its learners in how to participate in the process of quality improvement, to cooperate with other disciplines and professional groups, to lead the way in analysis and process design, and to develop consensus about what is currently known and what warrants further study. It can go much further in empowering all its constituents to follow the scientific method at a pragmatic level in all aspects of medicine and in all settings to the benefit of its consumers. It can move from being on the defensive about consumer-oriented quality and how it is measured toward being its primary advocate.

CHAPTER 4

Measurement and Statistical Analysis in CQI

Susan Paul Johnson and Curtis P. McLaughlin

A slide that is used in a number of continuous quality improvement (CQI) training programs reads: "In God we trust, all others send data." Measurement is a central element of any CQI effort. Health care institutions are full of data, but they are also full of "factoids," opinions, and anecdotes masquerading as facts and as data. Using a scientific approach requires using data to evaluate the current situation, analyze and improve processes, and track progress. The methods used to analyze data include both those originally developed for industrial models of quality management and those developed in the specialties of biostatistics, economics, epidemiology, and health services research.

Recently, the industrial statistical tools have been widely tested on health care models. One conclusion of the National Demonstration Project in Quality Improvement in Health Care (see discussion in Chapter 2) was that these tools are both transferable and meaningful to quality improvement efforts in health care. They are easy to understand and simple to use. The information that they convey shows how consistent the current process is (or is not), points out sources of errors and variation, and indicates where improvements can be made most effectively.

There is no one specified point in the CQI process where one needs to use a given method of measurement and analysis. They should be used on a continuous basis. In the context of the Plan, Do, Check, Act (PDCA) cycle, data and analytical tools are used throughout the Do, Check, Act

Source: Adapted with permission from S.I. Desharnais and C.P. McLaughlin, Clinical Quality, Risk-Adjustment, and Outcome Measures in Academic Medical Centers, in *Managing in an Academic Health Care Environment*, William F. Minogue, Ed., American College of Physician Executives, Tampa, Florida, © 1993.

portions. Different tools will be more helpful at different stages of each improvement project, from the initial analysis to monitoring changes that have already been instituted. This chapter will assist you in understanding what each industrial tool reveals about the process being improved, when to use it, and how to use it.

VARIATION: WHAT IS IT AND WHY ELIMINATE IT?

In the CQI arena, *variation* is the fat in the system that needs to be reduced. It is important first to understand variation and how it affects both administrative and clerical processes. Variation is the extent to which a process differs from the norm. It is related to the statistical concept of variance and standard deviation, familiar to most medical professionals. One can think of variation as a band of outputs around the central measure of a process. If, on average, it takes 10 minutes to complete a test, but it often takes from 8 to 12 minutes, this range indicates the extent of the variation of the process.

Variation exists in every process and always will. This is particularly evident in clinical medical processes. Since every patient is different, the processes used to treat individual patients will have to vary. This is an important characteristic of the health care environment. Any approach to quality in health care must accept and deal with this variability due to the human condition.

The innate nature of variance in processes allows us to identify two general categories of variance: (1) *common cause* and (2) *special source*. *Common cause variation* is that inherent variance in the process that is a result of how the process is performed. It is often referred to as systemic or internal variation. This type of variation is usually random in nature. *Special source* (or externally caused) *variations* are those that can be attributed to a particular source. This type of variation is, therefore, nonrandom.

Another way of understanding variation is to think about the predictability of a process. Can anyone tell a patient entering a health care process what to expect with a high degree of certainty? Can anyone tell the patient how long it will take, whom they are likely to see, and what decisions they might need to make along the way? These are the questions management would like to be able to answer with a "yes." More than just replying yes, CQI tools enable you to back up your answer with facts about the length of time and the potential for errors. The amount of certainty in the answer will depend on the amount of variation that has been observed in a process. The less variation that exists, the more certain management can be about answers and vice versa. Thus, the goal is to decrease variability in the process in order to eliminate uncertainty and the steps that people take to protect themselves against uncertainty. For example, in one hospital where six obstetricians were practicing, some specified one IV solution for a normal delivery and the other physicians specified another type. Since the nurses were uncertain about which physician would perform the delivery and therefore, which IV would be the "right" one, they protected themselves against uncertainty by hanging both units. The result was increased cost of health care induced by variation.

A process that displays little variation, or variation only under predictable circumstances, is considered *under control*. Bringing a process under control is often a goal of CQI efforts. Keeping a process under control requires continuous effort as well as the use of simple monitoring techniques.

PROCESS CAPABILITY

Being under control in health care is only a relative term. There is a great deal of variability in the human condition and in the wide variety of activities undertaken by a health care organization. Therefore, those involved must have a sense of what that inherent variability is. This requires a *process capability study*. In such a study the variable or attribute to be studied is measured and characterized. One of the first questions would be "Is the process inherently stable?" Scatter plots and histograms are often used to look at the natural variability of a process before trying to bring it under control.

If a process is chaotic or unstable, probably due to a number of special causes affecting it from moment to moment, those special causes must be dealt with first and then the underlying process can be understood. Once a process is stable, the investigators can determine its shape (normal or nonnormal), its central tendency (true mean), and its standard deviation. This gives those concerned an idea of what is going on and what can be achieved in a quality improvement effort. This type of process knowledge will be useful at all four stages of the PDCA cycle.

During the *Plan* stage, management compares the natural variability with the requirements of the situation to see how good or bad the situation is. During the *Do* stage, the plan is tested on a small scale to see what effect it might have. During the *Check* phase, data are collected on the impact of the change to see whether it brings the process into better alignment with the desired outcomes. Finally, during the *Act* phase, the process is monitored to make sure the gains are held.

HOW DOES CQI DIFFER FROM QA?

In order to apply these techniques, it is useful to understand the differing views of CQI and quality assurance (QA) with respect to variation. CQI focuses largely on the internal sources of variation, in an effort to reduce the random variation in the system. Although the variation is considered to be random, it can often be reduced by streamlining or changing the process so that there are fewer opportunities for random variation to occur.

QA on the other hand often emphasizes the special source variation. It looks for the anomalies that occur in the process and cause variation so that it can identify the sources and prevent them from affecting the process any more. The emphasis of QA seems to be on dealing with the *outliers* rather than on changing the process mean or variation. Figure 4–1 illustrates these two points of view (Teboul 1991). Segment 2 shows the QA point of view of looking for outliers, and Segment 3 shows the process improvement approach.

In general, CQI activities follow a logical four-step sequence. First, the process is described and sources of variation identified. This initial step is followed by in-depth analysis that will help clarify both the sources and extent of problems. Then the team weighs the alternatives and makes decisions about how to reduce variation. Finally, the team will try one of the alternatives and measure its effect on the process. Once improvements are made, the organization will continue to monitor progress over time to ensure that the process remains in control.

TOOLS FOR QUALITY IMPROVEMENT

In order to improve quality, it is important to measure quality, both before and after improvement efforts. Most writing on TQM/CQI will discuss or illustrate what are commonly referred to as "the seven tools of quality improvement." These tools are a set of statistical methods used in process analysis that are basic to the application of an approach. Most writers usually agree on at least 6, although not necessarily on all 7 of these

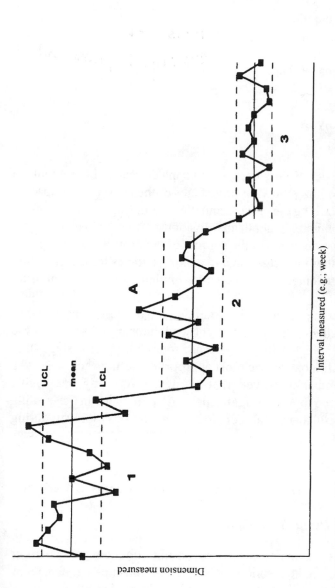

Figure 4-1 Teboul-Type Diagram. This figure illustrates the concept of variation and the results of efforts to reduce variation and improve the process. In Segment 1, we see evidence of a lot of variance in the process as indicated by wide swings. The bands indicate the normal range. Since the process is often outside this normal range, the process at the start would not be considered "under control." When this situation is rectified, as noted where the process tends to stay within the bands, the process has been brought under control. In Segment 2, point A indicates single source variation. Additionally, the overall mean has decreased, signifying improvement (though the variation is still the same). In Segment 3, the mean and variation have both decreased, and the process appears to be under control.

tools; while others will discuss as many as 9 or 10. We chose to report on eight tools that are commonly included in this famous set. They include:

1. flowcharts or diagrams
2. cause-and-effect diagrams
3. checksheets
4. Pareto diagrams or charts
5. histograms
6. run charts
7. regression analyses
8. control charts

tools of quality improvement

In order to guide our discussion, we will consider each of these tools in turn in the context of the following four stages of the continuous improvement cycle: (1) describing the process and identifying sources of variation; (2) performing a concrete, in-depth analysis of the situation to clarify what the team has thus far identified as the sources of the problem; (3) weighing alternatives for further investigation and making choices for changes; and (4) measuring improvements as changes are implemented and monitoring progress achieved.

The remainder of this chapter will examine each of these steps or stages and will introduce the tools as they might well enter into that part of the process analysis. Table 4–1 illustrates these four CQI process stages and also tabulates which tools will be most appropriate during each stage of a CQI effort. Remember, however, that at most stages any one of the previously introduced tools may again apply. Also included in the ensuing discussion are several analytical techniques that can be employed during any stage of the CQI process.

Process Stage 1—Describe Process and Identify Sources of Variation

Brainstorming: A Useful Technique

Brainstorming is a team process that is useful throughout many parts of the CQI process. It will help solidify working relationships within a team, while at the same time, it will reveal useful information. While useful throughout the project, it is especially helpful during some of the beginning stages when the team is trying to describe the process. Brainstorming

Table 4–1 CQI Process Stages and Quality Tools

Tools	CQI Process Stages			
	Describe process and identify sources of variation	Conduct in-depth analyses to clarify knowledge and present results	Weigh alternatives and make choices	Measure improvements and monitor progress
Flow diagrams or charts	Key tool here	Revisit and update		Keep current
Cause-and-effect diagrams	Key tool here, especially after brainstorming	Stratify for detail		
Checksheets		Use to collect process data		Use to collect process data
Pareto diagrams or charts		Key tool here to stratify causes	Key to deciding on vital few	Use to show change
Frequency distributions (histograms)		Helpful in presentation		Helpful in monitoring
Run charts		Important to relate data temporally to changes		Key to knowing whether improvement has been associated with change
Regression analysis			Useful for testing hypotheses	
Control charts				Key to seeing whether the process is or remains under control

is not a statistical tool, but it is a technique that is often useful during continuous improvement projects.

Brainstorming is when a group of individuals gets together and comes up with as many ideas as they can pertaining to a specific task or problem.

To employ brainstorming, it is best to bring the whole team together specifically for that purpose. The facilitator must define what it is the group is going to brainstorm about, for example, the causes of variation, the potential effects of the variation, changes that might be made, or alternative methods for getting something done. It is important to stick to the stated topic (it is amazingly easy to get off track!). Additionally, you should split the brainstorming session into different sections—at certain times the team should throw out as many ideas as possible without passing judgment on any of the suggestions. It is valuable to add to the list those ideas that seem the craziest or least feasible. They may contain the kernel of a creative idea that can be modified. Later, the team can go back and evaluate the list and cull out the inappropriate suggestions. It is best to work in a room with a blackboard or a flip chart for making lists.

Tool 1—Flowcharts or Diagrams

One of the most powerful tools that CQI teams have is the preparation of *flowcharts* of both administrative and clinical processes. Also known as *process flow diagrams*, these are pictorial representations of how the system works. Simply, they trace the steps that the "object" of a process goes through from start to finish. The object may be a vial of blood in laboratory tests, a piece of paper in medical records, or a patient in a specialty clinic.

To develop a flow diagram, the group should start by:

1. defining the basic stages of a process
2. further defining the process, breaking each stage down into specific steps needed to complete the process
3. following the object through the process a number of times to verify the process by observation
4. discussing the process representation with the project team and reaching consensus on the underlying process

Flow diagrams can be as simple or as complex as you wish. The team should agree on what level of detail is suitable for the specific process and the desired performance shift. Surprisingly, the continuous improvement team is likely to find that the existing process owners and users do not share a common understanding of how the current system works. Quite heated arguments are likely to ensue until they talk it out. With an accurate, shared representation of how the system works, the team is then able to consider how to improve it.

The first step is to bring together the people involved in all stages of the process being studied, so that the information accurately represents current practice. An independent facilitator may need to be present to keep any one group member from having undue influence and to mediate arguments about what is or should be happening. If the group is not used to drawing up flowcharts, the facilitator can also help explain the notations or symbols that are customarily used. Figure 4–2 illustrates these various symbols. An activity is represented by a rectangle, a decision node by a diamond, a wait or an inventory by a triangle, a document by a symbol that looks like a rectangle with a curve on the bottom, a file by a large circle, and a continuation of the flow to another sheet by a small circle.

Visibility of the process is very important, even to individuals who are not team members. For example, we have used the technique of putting the flowchart on a large poster board or a wall using Post-it notes for both the

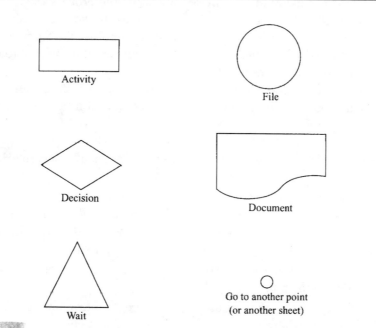

Figure 4–2 Flowchart Symbols. These symbols are commonly used to create flowcharts describing a process. Arrows are used to connect the symbols, indicating the order in which the steps take place.

activities and the decision nodes and leaving it up in clinical work areas, so that everyone has an opportunity to access it. People in the work areas and on the team should have adequate time to consider the current process representation to see whether or not it is accurate and to think about possible improvements. Where possible the motto is "No surprises!"

The poster board should be available in multiple sheets, so that new ramifications and permutations can be added to the permanent records, a requirement that often rules out transparencies or chalkboards. The latter does have the advantage of erasability, which is important early on. Do not let the obsessive members of the committee get caught up in neatening the artwork. There will always be changes. Save the neatening until the final presentation.

Information that could be added to the flowchart would be flow rates and flow times. For example, Figure 4–3 shows the flow rates in a university student health clinic with data on the average number of patients arriving each day and the percentages flowing to the various servers. Also given are the average waiting times and processing times at each stage of the process. A team is not likely to have these data when the process flowcharting is initiated, but may choose to collect them and add them later, should they appear useful for further analysis. It can be useful for the team to stop and think about which of these additional measures will be helpful to them as they are creating the flowchart.

Once agreement is reached on the representation of the current process, the team and the onlookers can begin to ask questions about that process, including:

- Who are the customers? How would they like to be served? How well are they being served now?
- Are there performance gaps or perceived opportunities for improvement driving the selection of this process? What are the data on performance? How good are they? Do they need to be validated?
- Have we identified all the relevant stages of the process? Are the "owners" of each stage represented on our team? If not, what do we do to bring them in?
- What are the inputs required and where do they come from? Are the inputs constraining the process or not? Which ones?
- Are there equipment or regulatory constraints forcing this approach? Is there historical interpersonal or political baggage behind this pro-

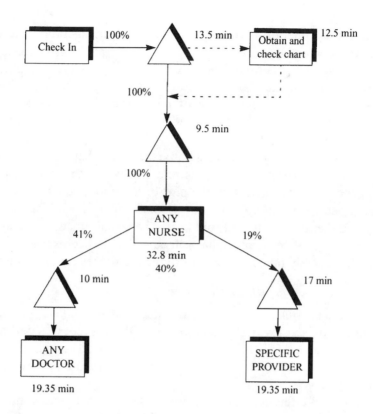

Figure 4–3 Example of a Flowchart Developed from the Process of Patients Going through a Walk-in Clinic. The average times and patient volumes are noted on this example.

cess choice? This is often the case in health care where people have been blamed for problems and have set up elaborate and expensive process embellishments so that unpleasant experiences won't ever happen again.

- What measurements are we currently collecting about this process? Are they the right ones for the issues already raised? How might we go about adding the right measures?

Experts warn against asking too many "Why?" questions at this point, because they may be threatening to the professional and personal egos of some participants. Let the whys and wherefores emerge as people loosen up and trust each other rather than forcing the issue immediately. Avoid making the model of discourse like the grand rounds procedure with its inherent power plays.

The potential benefits of flowcharting are considerable. Staff get to know the process much better. The results can be used as a training aid. People begin to take ownership of the process by participating in this activity and, most important, the possibilities for improvement become clear almost immediately.

Flowcharting should also bring home the need to have internal suppliers, external suppliers, and users (customers) involved in the process. Then one can generate more interest on the part of these individuals in joining the team process when they see the careful and impartial work already underway and their own potential role in it. The visual process analysis is one way to show your customers that you have their concerns at heart and that you are sincerely interested in improving the process in their interests.

Tool 2—Cause-and-Effect Diagrams

Cause-and-Effect Diagrams, also called Ishikawa or *fishbone* diagrams, are one of the most widely used tools of CQI. This tool was developed by Kaoru Ishikawa (University of Tokyo) for use at Kawasaki Steel Works in 1943 to sort and interrelate the multiple causes of process variation (Ishikawa 1987).

Cause-and-effect diagrams are most useful after the team has already described the process and is ready to identify the sources of variation. There is likely to be evidence of variation in the identified problem (either real or anticipated). Additional causes may be revealed either through the flowcharting process or during brainstorming.

Cause-and-effect diagrams are a schematic means of relating the causes of variation to the effect of variation on the process. If you ignore the words on the diagram, the picture looks like the skeleton of a fish, thus the name *fishbone* diagrams.

This tool is especially suited for team situations and is quite useful in making sense out of a set of brainstorming session results. It can be taught easily and quickly, allowing the group to sort ideas into useful categories for further investigation.

Sarazen (1990) suggests that there are three types of cause-and-effect diagrams:

1. cause enumeration
2. dispersion analysis

3. production process classification

Cause Enumeration. The most commonly used type of cause-and-effect diagram is the cause enumeration, which starts with a brainstorming session around an identified performance gap. If the group has trouble categorizing and sorting the possible causes into those categories, an *affinity diagramming* technique can be used to help with the sorting. In the affinity diagramming process, each cause is put on separate cards or on Post-it™ notes, and the group moves them around until the groupings (classifications) are satisfactory. Then one can begin the diagramming with the classifications already in hand. Figure 4–4 shows an affinity diagram resulting from a brainstorming session about ways to improve the process of cardiology consults to surgeons.

Figure 4–5 shows the multilayered process of making a fishbone diagram. Step 1 of the diagram starts by putting the identified performance gap in a box at the right and a big arrow leading to it, which represents the overall causation. Step 2 involves drawing spines from that big arrow to represent main causes, namely major classifications of causes such as labor, materials, and equipment. Then Step 3 adds along each major spine the specific causes, which also may occur at multiple levels down to two, three, or four levels. Sometimes it is useful to draw the diagram in two stages, one showing the main causes and then a separate chart with a spine representing the main cause and its associated levels.

Figure 4–6 shows a process flowchart for patients flowing into and completing experimental cancer treatment protocols (Hynes et al. 1992). On the right side are the various possible losses of patients to the protocol groups, which can be interpreted as quality failures. For each flow loss there is an Ishikawa or fishbone diagram showing the main causes of patient loss and the possible causal components of each main cause, as shown in Figure 4–7 (Hynes et al. 1992). This type of analysis was very useful in specifying research data needs and statistical hypotheses for studying the effectiveness of this process.

The first pass at a cause-and-effect diagram may still not be enough to understand the specific cause of an error and to quantify it. Therefore, it may be necessary to stratify cause-and-effect diagrams further to achieve finer gradations of error causes. Increasing the level of detail about causes can help with identifying specific corrective actions.

Dispersion Analysis. This approach starts with a known set of unsatisfactory variations and begins immediately to identify the causes of an

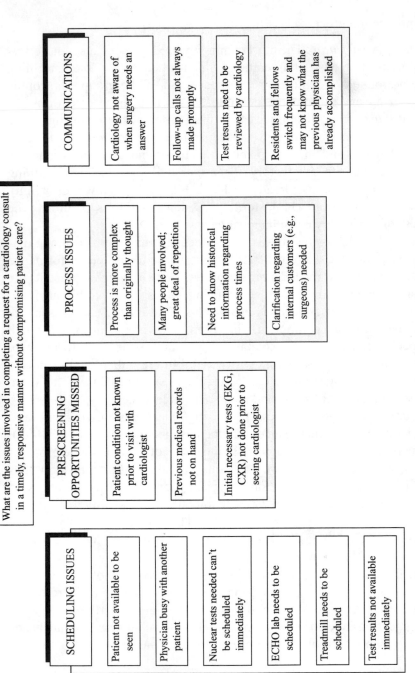

Figure 4-4 A Sample Affinity Diagram, Compiled from a Brainstorming Session on Ways To Improve the Process of Cardiology Consults to Surgeons

Step 1: Draw spine

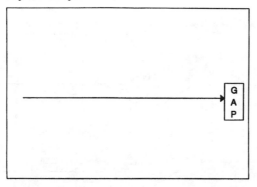

Step 2: Add main causes

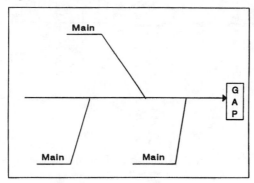

Step 3: Add specific causes

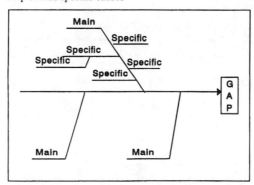

Figure 4–5 Multilayered Process of Developing a Fishbone Chart. First the overall problem is defined, then the main causes of the problem are defined. Often these main causes are segmented into those initiated by methods, materials, machines, or manpower. In the third step, these main causes are detailed with specifics.

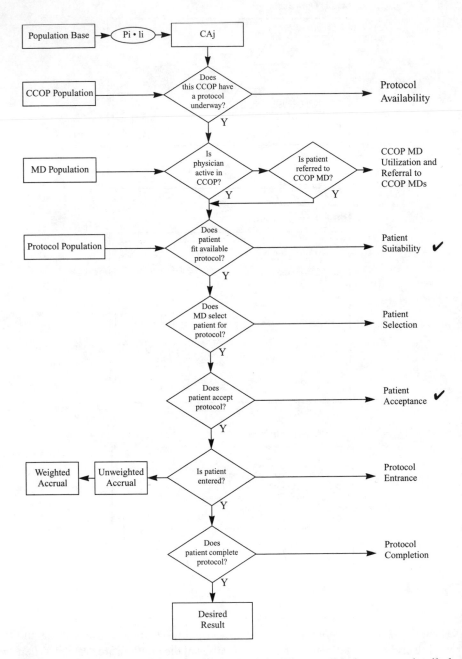

Figure 4–6 Flowchart of Cancer Clinical Trials. The possible losses are detailed on the flowchart in conjunction with the stages of the process. The two losses noted with a checkmark are detailed in Figures 4–7a and b.

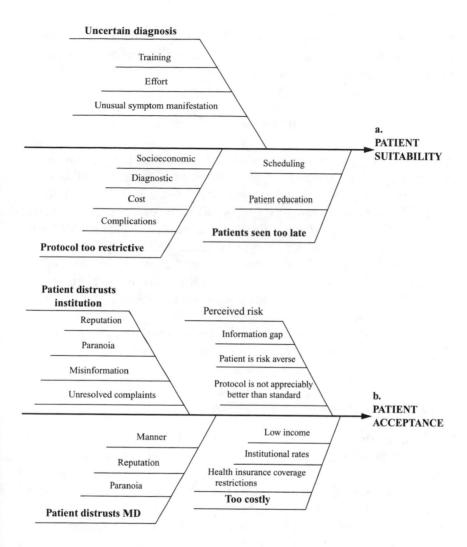

Figure 4–7 Cause-and-Effect Chart of Clinical Trials. Top: Detail of fishbone chart on patients who (a) may not fit the desired protocol and (b) patients who do not accept the desired protocol, and thus do not meet the desired result from the flowchart in Figure 4–6.

effect. The problem statement defines the effect and the team can begin by identifying the main causes and then the multilevel contributors to each gap in process performance. Sometimes brainstorming takes place around the contributing causes to each main cause. It is important in this process to keep relating various causes to each other. Note that various specific causes can appear more than once in association with various main causes. For example, patient ability to pay can affect patient failure to comply as well as the lack of availability of resources to service patients.

Process Classification. In the industrial setting it may be effective to identify variation (and causes of variation) to various process steps in a given flow. This may be more effective in the manufacturing setting where process stages are fixed and the need is to identify the causes of variation in specific process stages and organizational units. In health care that is basically what the teams are trying to avoid in order to get collective ownership of processes. One objective is to get health care professionals and administrators to look at bigger systems, ones that go beyond their narrow areas of specialization. Even when the causes are beyond the control or even intervention of the team, it is worthwhile to acknowledge their existence and impact. If, however, one cannot get a high degree of group commitment and participation to study the overall process, the process classification approach might be a useful interim alternative. Figure 4–8 shows a process classification of the information collected in a study of a cardiology consult process.

Purposes of Cause-and-Effect Exercises

While the fishbone diagram is a useful tool, it is important to keep in mind that the ultimate goal is to develop a common understanding of a process and a sense of collective ownership of it. The objective is not to place blame, but rather to understand the process as it is and how it might be improved. The outcome of this stage of CQI is a decision about what to measure to confirm the team's hypotheses about causation. In addition, the team is also beginning to build a consensus about the relative importance of a particular type of causation, which helps indicate where it wishes to put its available measurement resources.

Group facilitation is important at this stage of the process. Someone has to deflect the tendency to be judgmental of others and to get the group to withhold judgment and look for data to determine what are special effects and what are normal process variations. Some of that deflection can take place by allowing people time to discuss the work informally and to discuss and review the terminology and categories used. The desired outcome should be a decision about what actions to take next to confirm

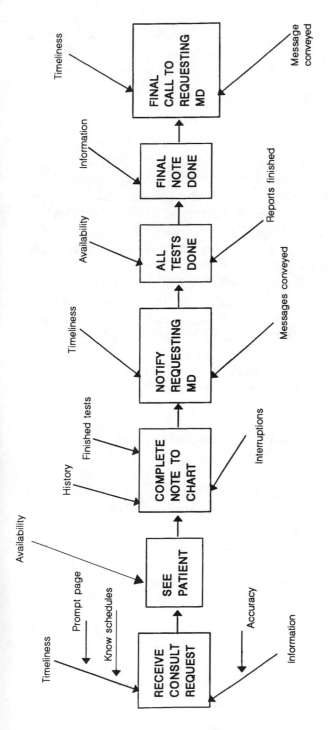

Figure 4–8 A Process Classification Diagram for a Cardiology Consult Process. The main steps of the process are detailed along the main spine of the diagram. The things that might influence the quality of each step are listed on the arrows directed toward them.

these hypotheses about causation, together with a strong common will to implement these measures.

Multivoting

Only a few hypotheses can be tested at one time. Therefore, it may become necessary to narrow down the options without discouraging specific team members who espouse specific hypotheses. Gaucher and Coffey (1993) recommend multivoting as a procedure to reduce the larger set to a few hypotheses. They warn against trying to reduce choices to a single hypothesis at this stage because of the risk to the team's sense of consensus. They also warn that one has to avoid overaggregating concepts during this weeding-out process.

During multivoting, each team member may at first vote for as many items as he or she wishes. The votes are added up, and those with few votes are eliminated. After the first round, each team member is given a number of votes equal to half the number of alternatives remaining in that round, and the voting is repeated. This process is repeated to reduce the list to between three and five items. Multivoting can be used at any process stage to reach consensus on a reduced set of alternatives.

Process Stage 2—Perform In-Depth Analyses To Clarify Knowledge and Present the Results

At this point the team's findings on causality are essentially the results of hypothesis-generating exercises. Those hypotheses must then be tested by collecting and analyzing data in as controlled a way as possible. As indicated in Table 4–1, *checksheets* and *Pareto diagrams* are important tools to use during this stage. Frequency distributions *(histograms)* are helpful in presenting the results. *Run charts* help present the data in order of event occurrence and can be used later to monitor improvements.

Tool 3—Checksheets

The simplest form of measurement is to count events, usually the frequency of activities or of outcomes, and to classify the observations using a *checksheet*. A checksheet is a matrix in which an observer records the number (frequency) of events. In the CQI context this is usually an array in which the anticipated causes of a specific type of defect are in the left-hand boxes and counts of their frequency in the central column. Table 4–2 shows one such checksheet resulting from a study of the reasons why linens are discarded.

An obvious concern of the investigator is seeing to it that the frequencies are representative of the process being observed. The data must be carefully sampled from the ongoing process to meet this goal. This can be done by randomly selecting the times to observe the process, by systematically sampling at equal intervals, or by making observations on every nth member of a population passing through a process. In some situations it may be desirable to take a stratified random sample, making sure that specific segments of the population are sampled adequately. Once this information has been collected, it needs to be presented to the group to analyze. The simplest form of presentation is the *histogram*. (See Tool 5.)

Tool 4—Pareto Diagram

A Pareto diagram is a vertical bar chart with the bars arranged from the longest first on the left and moving successively toward the shortest. Each bar represents the frequency of a specific cause of an error. The data come from a cause-and-effect diagram and a checksheet identifying the fre-

Table 4–2 Checklist for Linen Discards

| | | | | | | | Week of _____ | |
Reason for discard	Mon	Tue	Wed	Thu	Fri	Sat	Sun	Total
Large tear	卌	I		II	III		I	12
Small holes			IIII	I	II	I		8
Permanently soiled	II	II	I	卌 II	I	II	I	16
Discolored	II	I		I				4
Threadbare	卌 III	卌	II	III	I		I	20
Total	17	9	7	14	7	3	3	60

quency of a quality failure due to a specified cause. The causes would have already been developed using the procedure for doing a cause-and-effect diagram. The arrangement of the vertical bars gives a visual indication of the relative frequency of each source of error.

The diagram is named after the seventeenth-century Italian economist, Vilfredo Pareto. When he studied the distribution of wealth, he observed that the majority of the wealth had been distributed among a small proportion of the population (Pareto's law). Juran (1988) applied this concept to quality causes, observing that the "vital few" causes account for most of the defects, while others, the "useful many," account for a much smaller proportion of the defects. He noted that these vital few causes are likely to constitute the areas of highest payback to management. The objective of the Pareto diagram is to highlight these vital few. Concentrating on the high-volume causes should have the largest potential for reducing process variation.

On the same Pareto diagram one also develops a cumulative probability distribution incorporating all the proportions of the observations to the left of and including the bar. It is common to display the frequency scale on the left-hand Y axis and the percentage scale on the right-hand edge. Figure 4–9 shows a Pareto chart developed from data shown in the checklist in Table 4–2. Note that there is no X axis as such, because it is a bar chart.

Just because a cause is identified as having the greatest frequency does not necessarily mean that it should be worked on first. It must also be tractable and not cost more to change than it is worth. It is likely, however, that the first cause to be studied in detail will be among the left-most group. Remember that each Pareto chart focuses on one specific error, making the effect of reducing the frequency identical for each alternative cause. Therefore, the choice boils down to significance (frequency) and cost of modification. Another consideration is to further stratify the causes as was indicated for the cause-and-effect diagrams. Segregating the errors that have large frequencies can help identify potential improvements.

Tool 5—Histogram

Once this information has been collected, it needs to be presented to the group to evaluate. Pareto diagrams can be presented exactly as they are. For checklist data, the simplest form of presentation is the *histogram*. A histogram is a bar chart representing the frequency distribution of a set of data. The bars are arrayed on the X axis representing equal and adjacent

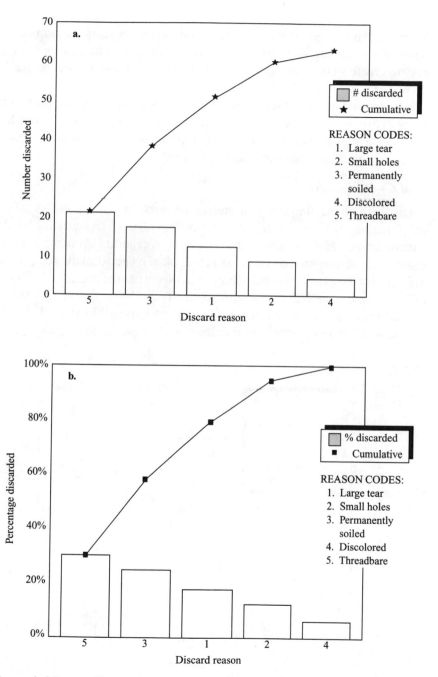

Figure 4–9 Pareto Charts of Data from Checksheet in Table 4–1, in (a) Raw Data Format and (b) Percentage Format

intervals. The length of the bar against Y axis represents the number of observations falling into that interval. With the data from a checklist, it is easy to create a histogram using any microcomputer spreadsheet or graphics package.

A histogram presents the measurements in a way that displays the nature of the distribution. Successive histograms indicate whether or not there has been a change in the variability of a process. Figure 4–10 shows a histogram based on the checksheets in Table 4–2.

Tool 6—Run Chart

Displays of the frequency of causes of error or checksheet values is enlightening, but cannot indicate trends or other characteristics of the phenomenon being observed that change over time. Another way of displaying the variation of a process is to look at its performance over time. This allows the experienced observer to (1) see what the temporal behavior of the process is, and (2) establish the time of process performance changes so that they can be linked to the time of other possibly related events. Figure 4–11 shows a series of run charts and some diagnostic interpreta-

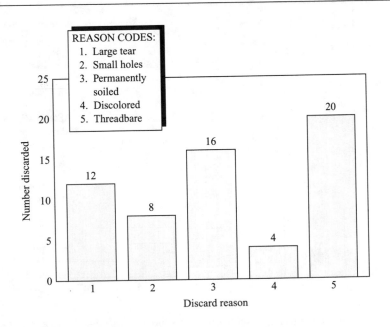

Figure 4–10 Histogram of Data from Checksheet in Table 4–2

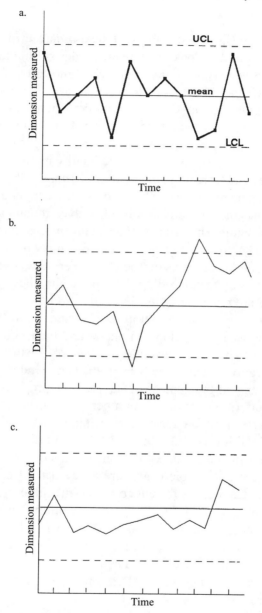

Figure 4–11 Three Examples of Run Charts. In (a), the data are considered to be under control—the points are apparently randomly distributed on either side of the mean, and do not go outside of the control limits. In (b), there are extreme values (outside the control limits), and thus the process is not in control. Another thing to beware is too many observations on one side of the mean. In (c), there are too many values in a row (>8) below the mean.

tions of those data. Since the effects of health care errors tend to be asymmetrical, it is best to look at one-sided rules of thumb for process control. A process is considered under control if most of the observations are near the centerline, if there are few points near the extreme values (above the mean plus or minus three standard deviations), and there are no runs (more than eight consecutive observations to one side of the mean). Like histograms, run charts are very easy to create on the computer.

Run charts are frequently used late in the quality improvement process to answer the question, "Are we doing better?" To answer that question one must be able to compare where one has been with where one is. There are numerous examples of run charts in this book, even though almost all are labeled as control charts. This is due to the fact that most software packages take a data set and automatically calculate and display the three standard deviation upper and lower limits on the chart. Very few teams, however, have gotten all the way to controlling the process that they are observing, so that the charts are really being used as run charts.

The industrial quality control literature talks about two types of measures that can be used to develop run charts and their cousins—control charts. Measures can be either *attributes* or *variables*. "Attribute data arise from (1) classification of items, such as products or services, into categories; from (2) counts of the number of items or the proportion in a given category; and from (3) counts of the number of occurrences per unit. . . . Important attributes (are): fraction defective, number of defects, number of defects per unit" (Gitlow et al. 1989, 78, 79, 144). Variables are measured directly or based on direct measures only and do not result from a classification scheme. Variable charts are a key part of continuous improvement as the team seeks to reduce variation, come up with a more robust design process, or make the process conform more closely to customer preferences. Charts often present the variable mean (X-bar), process range (R) and/or standard deviation (s) for a specific process parameter. One might almost go as far as to argue that unless one is following run charts of key parameters, one is not really focused on continuous improvement.

Process Capability Analysis

Given the availability of data at this point, it may be useful to try to characterize the process capability. This method of analysis is not included as one of the eight tools examined in this chapter, but it provides a check on the data that have been collected and the underlying assumptions of the statistical tools used. Process capability analysis allows one to determine the process mean and standard deviation and its closeness to the usual normality assumption of much of applied statistics.

The first step is to plot the data. If the plot (histogram) does not appear to support the normal assumptions, then a statistical consult is necessary before proceeding further. At this point it is also useful to consider whether or not you have enough observations to characterize the process and whether they are sufficiently random and representative. The sample sizes needed are surprisingly large. If a variable is to be looked at over time, then the first set of observations should include 50 samples of three to five observations each and in subsequent time periods 25 samples with three to five observations each. If the measure is an attribute rather than a variable, the sample should be even larger. Distinguishing between attributes and variables is often difficult in health care. The proportion of patients admitted due to a single diagnosis and dying from a single cause would be a causal variable in quality improvement terms. The proportion of patients admitted under a diagnosis-related group (DRG) and dying of any cause would be an attribute and would require roughly 10 times more observations in each sample.

Once the stable, natural process has been characterized, it is then important to compare its distribution with the specifications that it is trying to meet. Figure 4–12 shows two processes, one within specifications and one with a problem maintaining quality. Figure 4–13 shows the losses associated with the ability of a process to hold closeness to a desired value. This model demonstrates the potential benefit to reducing process variation.

Process Stage 3—Weigh Alternatives and Make Choices

Now the analysis turns toward collecting data on the chosen causes and on selecting alternative ways of reducing their frequency. In this stage, one is likely to turn first to more detailed flow diagrams. The team begins to examine the process in sufficient depth to find out what part of the process produces the error. At this point the group is often deciding whether or not the error being studied is due to common cause or to special cause.

Tool 7—Regression Analysis

At this point one is likely to look at the relationship between specific events and the occurrence that one is focusing on. This can usually be

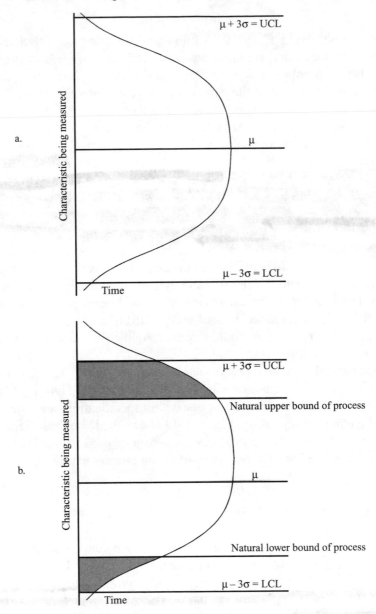

Figure 4–12 Process Performance vs. Process Limits: (a) A process that does not have difficulty maintaining quality will have normally distributed observations over time. (b) A process that has difficulty maintaining quality may still have normally distributed observations over time but may have control limits outside the natural bounds of the process and a mean that is not at the center of the normal curve. The shaded areas in this diagram represent the areas out of specification.

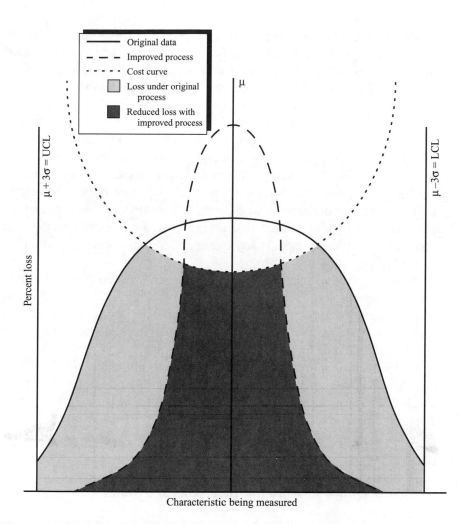

Figure 4–13 Impact of Reduction of Variance on Losses. The cost curve (noted) determines the losses associated with a process. When the variation is reduced, the amount of the losses decreases.

tested statistically by some form of correlational modeling. For example, in 1980 Gardner and McLaughlin developed a regression model to forecast the utilization of perishable blood products in a large hospital. They developed a forecast model that predicted the demand for these products quite effectively based on hospital census and some seasonal patterns. The staff reported, however, that one of the attending (faculty) physicians utilized these products much more than the other three. Since the attending physicians rotated through the service, it was possible to assign 0-1 dummy variables to account for which of the four was on duty. The model indicated that there was not a significant difference in utilization among the four attending physicians. Whatever the staff had to say about that one attending was not borne out by the data.

Getting negative findings is not a bad outcome in CQI. That eliminates one alternative and allows the team to focus on other alternatives. It is not unusual either. A significant percentage of teams report that their first impressions of the causes of problems were inappropriate. If they had not conducted analyses or experiments to check out those hypotheses early, they would have continued to work in an unfruitful area. This is one of the advantages of CQI methods. The team is able to use scientific methods of analysis to verify and support any changes that they would like to make, instead of guessing what to do.

Why is it that so many strongly held hypotheses do not prove out? Organizations usually act on their existing hypotheses. If the ones commonly held to be important had been the right ones, the performance gap would have been narrowing over time and that area would not have been a prominent candidate for attack. Areas that stay problem areas tend to linger as problems precisely because management has not been operating with the right hypotheses and has been concentrating its efforts on the wrong ones. Therefore, one of the roles of CQI teams is to test the current hypotheses and, when they fail, suggest new, more effective ones. Regression analysis provides one way of looking for unknown or underrated associations.

Process Stage 4—Measure Improvements and Monitor Progress

Once the experiments have been run and effective ways of avoiding the root causes of variation have been established, the changes will in all probability be implemented. Such changes may be effective temporarily, but then the system may slip back into its old ways. A system of measuring and monitoring must be put into place to find out whether or not these improvements are actually being captured and whether or not the new process is under control. *Control charts*—similar to run charts—are the most helpful tool for this stage.

Tool 8—Control Charts

Control charts are a popular form of presentation means for quality improvement teams. You can see them in Figure 3.6, Holston Valley

Hospital and Medical Center (Case 3) and in Exhibit 4.6, the West Florida Regional Medical Center (Case 4). Yet most often these are really run charts with the addition of notation indicating the control limits of plus or minus three standard deviations (commonly referred to as "3-sigma"). These control limits are referred to as the upper control limit (UCL), which is three standard deviations above the mean, and the lower control limit (LCL), which is three standard deviations below the mean. To use a control chart, the team would have to ensure that the process is free of special causes of variation at the time the control limits were set. It would then follow the charts to see (1) whether special causes were again creeping in, or (2) whether the underlying processes has changed. Because these charts are actually run charts, the most common form is the X-bar chart. This is a plot of the sample mean (X-bar) of the observations. In the run chart most often used in health care, the sample size per observation is usually one. This assumes that there is no sampling error and that all observations are accurate. This can become an important issue in health care where observations can vary so much. Taking blood pressure is a good example. A given patient's blood pressure will vary slightly depending on who is taking it. It will vary even more if different cuffs and measuring equipment are used. It will vary even further depending on the emotional state of the patient at the time of the measurement. All these sampling variations would have to be taken into account in a study of the effectiveness of certain hypertension procedures or drugs before the effects of the intervention could be quantified.

Control charts can be configured using the simple statistics that you calculate for the data collected, such as the mean, standard deviation, and range. There are control charts used for *variable data*, such as time or distance, and control charts used for *attribute data*, such as mortality rate or whether or not treatment is adequate or timely. For variable data, we will consider both X-bar charts and R-charts. For attribute data we consider the p-chart.

Consider a study that looks at patients who have an acute myocardial infarction (MI) and the time that it takes to administer thrombolytic therapy (known as the door-to-needle time). An actual CQI project was done on this clinical procedure at Soroka Medical Center in Beer-Sheeva, Israel (Alemi et al. 1998). Here we consider how they might have configured their data into control charts to display the time. The tabular data are presented in Table 4–3.

The first example is an X-bar chart shown in Figure 4–14. Suppose that each day for a month, the hospital observed five randomly selected cases

Table 4–3 Acute Myocardial Infarction: Door-to-Needle Time

n=5	MEAN	Range	$\overline{X}$ Chart UCL	Center	LCL	R Chart UCL	Center	LCL
1	52.1	29.32	65.56	56.13	46.70	61.99	16.34	0.00
2	47.7	29.73	65.56	56.13	46.70	61.99	17.21	0.00
3	62.7	2.77	65.56	56.13	46.70	61.99	17.21	0.00
4	42.2	19.00	65.56	56.13	46.70	61.99	17.21	0.00
5	63.1	10.33	65.56	56.13	46.70	61.99	17.21	0.00
6	60.2	18.40	65.56	56.13	46.70	61.99	17.21	0.00
7	57.7	9.38	65.56	56.13	46.70	61.99	17.21	0.00
8	56.4	25.43	65.56	56.13	46.70	61.99	17.21	0.00
9	43.9	15.89	65.56	56.13	46.70	61.99	17.21	0.00
10	54.8	18.74	65.56	56.13	46.70	61.99	17.21	0.00
11	59.4	27.65	65.56	56.13	46.70	61.99	17.21	0.00
12	62.6	2.96	65.56	56.13	46.70	61.99	17.21	0.00
13	57.7	15.76	65.56	56.13	46.70	61.99	17.21	0.00
14	54.8	9.12	65.56	56.13	46.70	61.99	17.21	0.00
15	59.4	23.88	65.56	56.13	46.70	61.99	17.21	0.00
16	42.6	3.61	65.56	56.13	46.70	61.99	17.21	0.00
17	41.5	10.13	65.56	56.13	46.70	61.99	17.21	0.00
18	59.8	15.84	65.56	56.13	46.70	61.99	17.21	0.00
19	60.2	18.40	65.56	56.13	46.70	61.99	17.21	0.00
20	57.2	9.38	65.56	56.13	46.70	61.99	17.21	0.00
21	47.8	25.43	65.56	56.13	46.70	61.99	17.21	0.00
22	57.7	7.22	65.56	56.13	46.70	61.99	17.21	0.00
23	58.1	24.43	65.56	56.13	46.70	61.99	17.21	0.00
24	60.2	15.97	65.56	56.13	46.70	61.99	17.21	0.00
25	51.4	13.86	65.56	56.13	46.70	61.99	17.21	0.00
26	49.8	7.34	65.56	56.13	46.70	61.99	17.21	0.00
27	60.2	2.28	65.56	56.13	46.70	61.99	17.21	0.00
28	63.1	28.82	65.56	56.13	46.70	61.99	17.21	0.00
29	59.2	29.98	65.56	56.13	46.70	61.99	17.21	0.00
30	80.2	19.24	65.56	56.13	46.70	61.99	17.21	0.00
Sample Mean	56.1	16.34						

of acute MI and noted the time until thrombolytic therapy was begun. The data would include the mean time for each of the 30 days that were sampled and the range of the times for each day. Armed with this information, the CQI team could create a control chart using the following formulas:

UCL: $\overline{\overline{X}} + A_2 \times \overline{R}$
Center Line: $\overline{\overline{X}}$
LCL: $\overline{\overline{X}} - A_2 \times \overline{R}$

Where X double bar is the mean of all the sample means, R-bar is the mean of all the sample ranges, and A_2 is an estimate of three standard deviations that is dependent upon the sample size and can be looked up in a control chart table (see Table 4–4).

For our example, the mean of all the sample means (X-double bar) is 56.1 minutes and the mean of the ranges (R-bar) is 16.34 minutes. Using the control chart table, and considering our sample size of 5, we note that A_2 is 0.577. Thus, we calculate the UCL to be 65.56 minutes and the LCL to be 46.70 minutes.

The X-bar chart is created by plotting the UCL, the center line, the LCL and the mean of each group of samples on the chart. The completed control chart is given in Figure 4–14.

R-charts can be used to observe and control. Similar to the X-chart, the R-chart uses a formula and a table to look up the associated factors given the sample size. The formulas for an R-chart are:

UCL: $\overline{R} \times D_4$
Center Line: $\overline{R}$
LCL: $\overline{R} \times D_3$

Using the same illustrative data, with an R-bar of 16.34 and a sample size of 5, we can look up D_4 and D_3 to be 2.114 and 0.0, respectively. The calculations indicate that the UCL is 61.99 and the LCL is 0. The R-chart is created in the same manner as the X-chart, by plotting the UCL, the center line, the LCL and the range of each group of observations. It is common to display this type of control chart directly under the X-bar control chart so that the means values and the dispersion can be viewed simultaneously. Figure 4–15 displays an R-chart.

Table 4–4 Factors to Determine Control Chart Limits

Sample Size	A_2	D_2	D_4
4	0.729	0	2.282
5	0.577	0	2.115
6	0.483	0	2.004
7	0.419	0.076	1.924
8	0.373	0.136	1.864
9	0.337	0.184	1.816
10	0.309	0.223	1.777
15	0.246	0.347	1.647
20	0.180	0.414	1.586

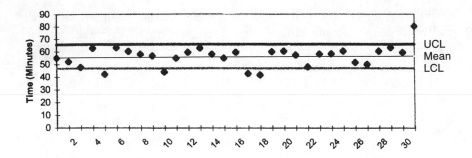

Figure 4-14 X-Bar Chart—Door-to-Needle Time

The other frequently used control chart is the *p*-chart, an attribute chart which shows the proportion of cases in which a given error or set of errors occurs. A mortality rate would be a natural set of data for a *p*-chart. There are two states: defective and not defective, dead or alive. To illustrate the *p*-chart, we are going to consider how an interdisciplinary CQI team investigated sedation during surgery. At one hospital, they use a grading scheme for conscious sedation, recording their impressions of the effect of sedation on the patients (5=in pain, 4=talking, 3=awake, 2=asleep, 1=not breathing). They considered that levels 1, 4, and 5 were not acceptable and could be avoided. Although they did not report the use of a *p*-chart for these data, one could be used that combines the adequate (2, 3) and inadequate (1, 4, 5) sedation levels into two groups. Then, the proportion of inadequate sedation could be monitored and assessed using control charts. As an

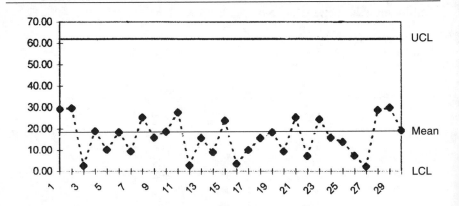

Figure 4–15 R Chart—Door-to-Needle Time

example, consider that they recorded the sedation levels of nine patients each day for 30 days. On average, inadequate sedation was seen in 4.8% of patients. This is all the information that is needed to create the control chart.

The distribution of p, the proportion defective, is binomial and easy to use. The corresponding control charts are easy to develop. The standard deviation can be calculated once you know the average proportion in all the samples and the sample size by using the following equation:

$$S_p = \sqrt{(\overline{p}(1-\overline{p})/n)}.$$

Then, we calculate three standard deviation control limits by using these equations:

UCL: $\overline{p} + 3 * s_p$
Center Line: $\overline{p}$
LCL: $\overline{p} - 3 * s_p$

In the same manner as the X-chart and R-chart, the UCL, center line, LCL, and individual data points are plotted to create the control chart. Figure 4–16 shows such a p-chart.

The major difference between the p-chart and the others is that the plot is done using attribute data rather than causal variables (and thus simple statistics cannot be calculated, only proportions.) It is important in setting up these charts to start with a historical proportion, such as the previous

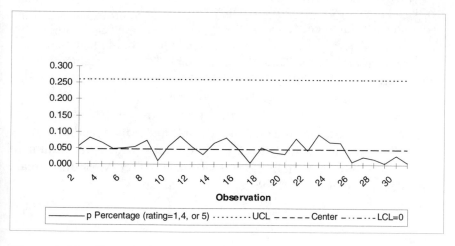

Figure 4–16 p Chart: Sedation during Surgery

mortality rates. Then you can keep track of the proportion dying over the intervention period and after and compare results.

The p-chart plots the proportion that you are measuring for each group of observations on the Y axis with a midline indicating the historical proportion. At the very least, the team can monitor that the proportion does not get worse. Then you can conclude that your efforts have improved the process without adversely affecting the outcome of the process and you may find evidence that it improves.

Continuing the Improvement

A process that is under control and showing that the latest set of changes has been effective is not the team's final objective. The next step is to return to the *Plan* stage of the PDCA cycle and determine whether or not it would be worthwhile to try to improve this process further. If so, the team should return to its Pareto analysis and cause-and-effect diagrams to develop further hypotheses for testing and implementation.

CONCLUSION

This chapter has outlined a process that is typical of how the TQM/CQI model is implemented by a team. Many of the seven tools and some others are used to help the team move along with its task. CQI participants often encounter measurement tools very early in their training programs and may assume that they are the essence of the approach. Management must continue to argue that measurement is but one of the core elements of the CQI philosophy, while still remaining flexible about which tools to use and when to use them in the process. These tools are not sophisticated, although some team members may be a little put off by their statistical nature. Used appropriately, under the guidance of a flexible and skilled facilitator, they will help teams implement the CQI philosophy with a maximum of effectiveness and a minimum of interpersonal conflict. Most of them are illustrated in one or more of the case studies in Part V.

CHAPTER 5

Measuring Consumer Satisfaction

Lucy A. Savitz

The assessment of consumer satisfaction, which reflects perceived quality, is an important part of total quality management/continuous quality improvement (TQM/CQI). These measurement efforts provide health service organizations operating in highly competitive markets with the opportunities to assess the needs of key stakeholders. Further, measurement of consumer satisfaction provides a comprehensive, systematic, and patient-centered approach for analyzing, implementing, monitoring, and improving both the perceived and clinical quality aspects of care (Ford et al. 1997).

This chapter provides an overview of key issues and methods related to the measurement of consumer satisfaction. The rationale for measurement is discussed and followed by a series of issues: measurement, data capture, timing, and functional responsibility. An example applying patient satisfaction measures as part of the Balanced Score Card is presented; and finally, the chapter concludes with a brief overview of the special issue of severity (or risk) adjustment of reported consumer satisfaction measures.

DEFINING CONSUMER SATISFACTION

From a marketing perspective, we typically view parties to an exchange of goods and/or services as the context for dis/satisfaction measures. The expectancy disconfirmation model used to explain postpurchase satisfaction suggests that consumer satisfaction can be defined simply as:

> . . . the evaluation rendered that the experience was at least as
> good as it was supposed to be.
>
> —H.K. Hunt (1977)

Postpurchase satisfaction is classically derived by the relationship be-tween the consumer's expectations and the product's (or service's) per-ceived performance (LaBarbara and Mazursky 1983). If the rendered service or product meets or exceeds expectations, then the consumer is satisfied; if the rendered service or product does not meet expectations, then the consumer is dissatisfied. Thus, it is critical to understand as much about the consumer decision process as possible in order to assess postpurchase behavior adequately, particularly reported measures of satisfaction. This entire process can be quite complex, depending on the type of health care service being offered.

Kotler and Armstrong (1993) depict the Buyer-Decision Process as a series of five sequential steps, moving from left to right. This is graphically displayed in Figure 5–1.

Here postpurchase behavior is directly preceded by four steps that shape the expectations against which satisfaction will ultimately be assessed. Further, the extent to which consumers spend time moving through these steps is largely associated with the nature of the health care problem being addressed in terms of key attributes of the health care concern such as complexity, amount of patient discomfort, degree of patient involvement, and urgency. For instance, a mother recognizing that a healthy child is in immediate need of a routine sports physical to comply with a school requirement might skip the information search step, and turn to the telephone directory to identify the closest "doc-in-the-box" with walk-in appointments. Once the most convenient and timely provider is identified, the purchase decision is made with relatively little investment in the choice. Walking out of the physician's office within 30 minutes and having paid a minimal fee to secure a completed form so that her son could sign up for a team sport may leave both mother and son quite satisfied with the medical encounter. This example can contrast sharply with patients seek-

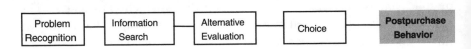

Figure 5–1 Buyer-Decision Process

ing higher order services or services where the physician-patient relationship is extended over a protracted period of time (e.g., organ transplantation, cancer treatment, prenatal care and delivery, nursing home care). In the case of nursing home care, the patient may have little or no involvement in the decision-making process while holding personal attitudes that make such placement less than desirable (Dolinsky 1997).

Application of this marketing model to health care is further complicated by the fact that "choice" is often severely limited as a result of managed care limitations constraining patient choice and/or physician referral options. Acknowledging the complexity in ascertaining consumer satisfaction related to a particular market exchange of goods and services, Mowen (1990) presented a revised definition: "Consumer satisfaction/dissatisfaction (CS/D) consists of the general feelings that a consumer has developed about a product or service after its purchase. As such, satisfaction is a type of consumer attitude. Feelings of CS/D may result from expectancy disconfirmation *(agreement between expectations and actual experience)* as well as from other processes such as equity, attribution, performance evaluation, and affect formation."(294)

The complexity of patient perceptions and attitudes together with sometimes limited cognitive ability to process the nature of their own health care situation serves to further complicate the decision process beyond attributes of patients' immediate health concern. Expectations are also shaped by a variety of inputs such as personal experiences as well as those of family and friends, physician recommendations, and directed advertising campaigns.

Who Is the Consumer?

The consumer, in general, can be viewed as the party using the provided service and/or product of the exchange. From a health care perspective, the consumer is typically assumed to be the patient/enrollee in the direct exchange of health care services; and it is this perspective that serves as the basis for the majority of discussion in this chapter. Nevertheless, measures of consumer satisfaction may broadly target measures for patient/family, practitioner, staff, and contract service administrators (Joint Commission on Accreditation of Healthcare Organizations 1998). Examples of other consumers beyond the basic patient-provider exchange are illustrated below:

- Physicians as consumers:
  1. Community doctors referring patients to a tertiary care center are consumers of that center.
  2. Physicians sending specimens to labs for testing and/or ordering scans from radiology centers are consumers of those ancillary services.
- Facilities as consumers:
  1. Hospitals outsourcing equipment, maintenance, dietary, and laundry services are consumers of those intermediaries.
  2. Hospitals purchasing information systems to monitor the quality process are consumers of those vendors.
- Insurers/managed care organizations (MCOs) as consumers:
  1. Insurers outsourcing claims processing functions are consumers of the third-party administrators.
  2. MCOs contracting with physicians, pharmacies, clinics, hospitals, and home health agencies to provide a continuum of care for their health insurance benefits are consumers of the providers and facilities.
- Government agencies as consumers:
  1. The Health Care Financing Administration (HCFA) contracting with insurers to provide Medicare and Medicaid risk coverage for eligible beneficiaries is a consumer for the MCOs.
  2. State and/or federal prisons contracting with health care facilities and providers for services for the incarcerated population are consumers of these facilities and providers.

Beyond these other parties to an exchange of health care services, it is also important to note the role of others such as health care workers, suppliers, communities, and families. In particular, families can act as a key agent in the market exchange for health care services and have often reported either directly or indirectly as proxies concerning patient satisfaction (Schweikhart et al. 1993). Also, women are widely acknowledged in the marketing community as the primary health care brokers for their families. This suggests that measurement of consumer satisfaction may be elicited in certain cases from either patient proxies and/or agents of the actual consumer. Further, research suggests that friends and family of patients, acting as their advocates, may be a harder group to satisfy than the patients themselves (Strasser and Davis 1991). In considering the various consumers of health care, it is important to recognize that patients, providers, and payers define quality differently. These differences result in different expectations of the health care system and, thus, differing measures of satisfaction in evaluation of quality (McGlynn 1997).

WHY MEASURE CONSUMER SATISFACTION?

Consumer satisfaction provides a useful outcome measure for quality of care offered by a health care organization. Patient perceptions of quality of care are reflected in reported satisfaction measures. Ford et al. (1997) review the literature that reports some of the benefits of measuring patient/enrollee satisfaction, including: increased profitability, increased market share, improved patient retention, improved collections, increased patient referrals, improved patient compliance, continuity of care, reduced hospitalization and length of stay, increased willingness to recommend the organization to family and friends, and reduced risk of malpractice. Satisfaction measures together with clinical outcomes and cost data are increasingly used by employers as part of their value-based purchasing of health care benefits, by insurers in contracting for network services, and by potential partners in establishing health care alliances and systems (Woodbury et al. 1997).

The two major sources of future utilization of health care are new customers and repeat customers. Intercorrelations of quality, satisfaction, and loyalty based on a study by Steiber (1988) are depicted in Figure 5–2.

While the direct link between patient satisfaction and market share driven by repeat utilization can be most readily made, positive intermedi-

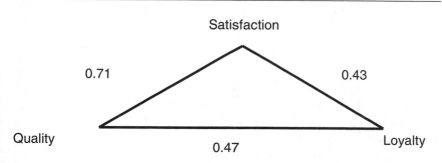

Figure 5–2 Intercorrelations of Quality, Satisfaction, and Loyalty

ary influences on compliance and provider change are key with respect to health care behaviors, and loyalty and word-of-mouth advertising are related to reputation. For instance, word-of-mouth advertising has been shown to account for a significant proportion of future encounters whereby satisfied customers tell others about their experiences and refer them accordingly (Savitz 1994; Kotler and Armstrong 1993; Davies and Ware 1988).

External reporting and accreditation requirements of the Joint Commission on Accreditation of Health Care Organizations, including its Oryx/Oryx Plus indicators (Joint Commission 1998) and the National Committee on Quality Assurance's (NCQA) HEDIS measures (National Committee on Quality Assurance 1998) have heightened the importance of patient satisfaction measures, moving them from internal to external performance monitoring and quality indicators. The Health Care Advisory Board (1993) itemized the most frequently used quality indicators for community report cards as:

- Clinical outcomes
- Patient satisfaction
- Frequency of procedure
- Charge by diagnosis-related group (DRG)

Finally, application of CQI principles in health care organizations has led to the integration of patient/enrollee satisfaction measures that can be used in identifying improvement opportunities in the key components of care—structure, process, and outcome—as described by Donabedian (1982).

MEASURING SATISFACTION

Aside from a general understanding that consumer satisfaction is maximized to the extent that consumer expectations are met in the health care market exchange, relatively little is known about how particular aspects of care relate to generalized statements. Most studies focus either on specific levels of care (e.g., outpatient clinics, hospitals) or on types of services (e.g., obstetrical services).

For example, Zifko-Baliga and Kampf (1997) found that patients used more than 500 criteria to evaluate hospital quality. Personal choice has emerged as a significant factor in predicting enrollee satisfaction. In a study done by researchers at Kaiser Permanente, 10,000 adults enrolled in a large group-model HMO in northern California in 1995 and 1996 were surveyed. They were asked to rate their care using the following nine satisfaction measures: (1) time usually spent with physician, (2) explanation of diagnosis and treatment, (3) technical skill of physician, (4) personal manner of physician, (5) use of latest technology, (6) focus on prevention, (7) concern for emotional well being, (8) their overall satisfaction, and (9) whether they would recommend their physician to others. For each of the nine satisfaction measures, respondents who had chosen their own physician were between 16 percent to 26 percent more likely than those who had been assigned a personal physician to report their health care as very good or excellent (Schmittdiel et al. 1997). Findings such as these are important to communicate to practitioners to increase their understanding of the exchange process and to evaluate appropriate satisfaction measures. Nevertheless, continued efforts to understand patient expectations are key in maximizing consumer satisfaction.

In 1993, the American College of Physicians (ACP) conducted a follow-up study (based on previous work by Fletcher et al. 1983) that used a series of focus groups with patients and physicians to understand the relative importance of measures of satisfaction in office-based medical care as part of the Patient Centered-Care Project. The critical steps suggested in this study are depicted in Figure 5–3.

ACP researchers completed a comparative analysis of physicians' and patients' importance rankings for 125 attributes of the medical care encounter. They found major discrepancies throughout the list, examples of which are provided in the partial list shown in Table 5–1.

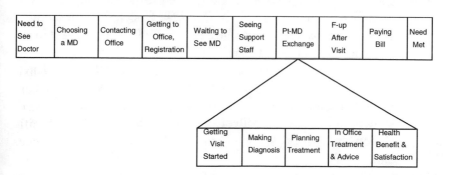

Figure 5-3 ACP, the Patient Centered-Care Project, Steps in Office-Based Medical Care

Table 5–1 Discrepancies in Patient/Physician Rankings of Medical Care Attributes

Patient Rank	MD Rank	Difference	Questions How important is it that:
26	113	(87)	the physician explains the results of any evaluation by a consulting specialist to the patients?
80	10	(70)	the physician discusses important information about patients' health in a private place?
12	81	(69)	the physician explains the purpose of each medicine prescribed in a way patients understand?
23	79	(56)	the physician clearly explains the possible side effects of medicines?
5	58	(53)	the physician gives patients solid facts about the likely benefits and risks of treatment?
11	64	(53)	the physician tells patients how to take medicines in a way that patients understand?

The ACP study underscores the critical need to measure consumer satisfaction using data from those who utilize the services rather than simply assuming that as providers we understand what patients want and what will ultimately satisfy their expectations. Clearly, practitioner understanding of patient expectations is incomplete.

DATA CAPTURE

In general, patient/enrollee satisfaction measures are among the most readily available outcome measures. As discussed, accreditation requirements and marketing efforts have already been established to collect these measures without the burden of purchasing new and/or reprogramming existing systems to generate such quality measures as is the experience with clinical quality measures. It is also important, however, to address issues involved in data capture with respect to how the data will be collected, when they should be collected, and which functional area will have the responsibility for data capture and reporting.

Alternative Modalities

There are multiple modalities available to health services researchers in collecting patient satisfaction data, which can then be translated into information for CQI purposes. Alternative modalities have important advantages and disadvantages that must be considered together with the data required in determining how to proceed.

Flood et al. (1997) provide a comprehensive comparison of advantages and disadvantages associated with various qualitative and quantitative modalities for measuring consumer satisfaction. While a detailed specification of how to capture satisfaction measures using these alternative modalities exceeds the scope of this particular chapter, an itemized list of these methods with a brief description is presented below.

Qualitative Modalities

- Management observation: formal observation and documentation of the patient care process
- Employee feedback programs: formal employee feedback on all aspects of the patient care process
- Work teams and quality circles: continuous employee input through teams
- Focus groups: homogeneous groups of consumers who are brought together and whose input is facilitated in an open-ended forum
- Mystery shoppers: an observational technique that provides a snapshot of the service experience from a user perspective

Quantitative Modalities

- Comment cards: voluntary patient/enrollee ratings of service quality
- Mail survey: questionnaires mailed to users for completion and return (Figure 5–4 shows one such questionnaire)
- Point-of-service interviews: self-administered or interviewer-administered questionnaires usually completed following service delivery at the delivery site
- Telephone interviews: personal interviews with users over the telephone by trained interviewers

(*Note:* Readers are urged to consult specific books that have been written on each of these alternative modalities, or specialized consulting groups, and/or survey research organizations in developing measurement tools in their own organizations.)

Critical considerations in comparing these optional measurement modalities involve expense, timeliness of feedback, required staff competencies to develop and administer the measurement instrument, desired depth

OUTPATIENT SERVICES: THE PATIENT'S VIEWPOINT

No. 2 pencil only

Please rate your hospital visit in each of the areas listed below in terms of whether it was excellent, very good, good, fair, or poor. Please mark only one answer for each statement.

Correct mark / Incorrect mark

Rating columns: Excellent, Very Good, Good, Fair, Poor, Does Not Apply

GETTING TO THE HOSPITAL

1. DIRECTIONS FROM YOUR DOCTOR'S OFFICE: Clearness and completeness of directions to the hospital you may have gotten from your doctor's office.
2. DIRECTIONS FROM THE HOSPITAL: Clearness and completeness of directions to the hospital you may have gotten from the hospital staff.
3. SIGNS: How clear and correct the signs were that directed you to the hospital.

PARKING

4. PARKING FACILITIES OR SERVICES: How easy they were to use and how well they met your needs.

REGISTRATION

5. WAITING TIME: Length of time you spent waiting to register AFTER you arrived at registration.
6. PERSONAL MANNER: Respect, friendliness, and courtesy shown by registration staff.
7. EFFICIENCY: How smoothly registration procedures ran.
8. INFORMATION: Clearness and completeness of explanations given by registration staff.

YOUR TESTS: Please answer the same questions for EVERY department you went to.

9. WAITING TIME: Length of time you spent waiting for your test.
   in X-RAY / in LABORATORY / in NUCLEAR MEDICINE / in MAMMOGRAPHY / in EKG / in OTHER SERVICES

10. Information from your DOCTOR'S OFFICE: How well your doctor's office staff described what it would be like to have these tests.
   in X-RAY / in LABORATORY / in NUCLEAR MEDICINE / in MAMMOGRAPHY / in EKG / in OTHER SERVICES

11. Information from HOSPITAL STAFF: Clearness and completeness of explanations given DURING your test.
   in X-RAY / in LABORATORY / in NUCLEAR MEDICINE / in MAMMOGRAPHY / in EKG / in OTHER SERVICES

12. PERSONAL MANNER: Respect, friendliness, and courtesy shown by the staff.
   in X-RAY / in LABORATORY / in NUCLEAR MEDICINE / in MAMMOGRAPHY / in EKG / in OTHER SERVICES

continues

Figure 5–4 Outpatient Services: The Patient's Viewpoint

Figure 5–4 continued

		Excel-lent	Very Good	Good	Fair	Poor	Does Not Apply
13. EFFICIENCY: How smoothly procedures ran	in X-RAY .... ➡	○	○	○	○	○	○
	in LABORATORY .... ➡	○	○	○	○	○	○
	in NUCLEAR MEDICINE.... ➡	○	○	○	○	○	○
	in MAMMOGRAPHY....... ➡	○	○	○	○	○	○
	in EKG .... ➡	○	○	○	○	○	○
	in OTHER SERVICES ...... ➡	○	○	○	○	○	○
14. YOUR PERSONAL NEEDS: Courtesy, interest, attention, and support shown for your privacy and comfort.	in X-RAY .... ➡	○	○	○	○	○	○
	in LABORATORY .... ➡	○	○	○	○	○	○
	in NUCLEAR MEDICINE.... ➡	○	○	○	○	○	○
	in MAMMOGRAPHY....... ➡	○	○	○	○	○	○
	in EKG .... ➡	○	○	○	○	○	○
	in OTHER SERVICES ...... ➡	○	○	○	○	○	○

THE FACILITIES

15. GETTING AROUND IN THE HOSPITAL: Helpfulness of signs, directions, volunteers.	➡	○	○	○	○	○	○
16. HOSPITAL BUILDING: How would you rate the hospital building overall?	➡	○	○	○	○	○	○
17. EQUIPMENT: Having the latest equipment and technology.	➡	○	○	○	○	○	○

OVERALL SATISFACTION WITH THE HOSPITAL

18. The care I received was so good that I have bragged about it to family and friends.	➡ ○ Strongly agree	○ Somewhat disagree
	➡ ○ Somewhat agree	○ Strongly disagree
19. The prices were reasonable for the care I received.	➡ ○ Strongly agree	○ Somewhat disagree
	➡ ○ Somewhat agree	○ Strongly disagree

YOUR OVERALL HEALTH STATUS

20. In general, would you say your health is...	➡ ○ Excellent	○ Good	○ Poor
	➡ ○ Very Good	○ Fair	

FACTS ABOUT YOU

21. Please mark all the departments were you were seen today.	➡ ○ Diabetes Treatment Center	○ Radiation therapy
	➡ ○ EKG	○ CT
	➡ ○ Heart cath lab	○ MRI
	➡ ○ Mammography	○ Ultrasound
	➡ ○ Nuclear Medicine	○ X-Ray
	➡ ○ Pain clinic	○ Respiratory therapy
	➡ ○ Physical therapy	
22. What time did you arrive at the hospital?	➡ ○ 6 am–9 am	○ 12 noon–3 pm
	➡ ○ 9 am–12 noon	○ 3 pm–6 pm
23. What day of the week was your visit to the hospital?	➡ ○ Mon ○ Thurs	Sun
	➡ ○ Tues ○ Fri	
	➡ ○ Wed ○ Sat	
24. Are you (the patient) male or female?	➡ ○ Male	○ Female

25. In what year were you (the patient) born? example: 5 ⑨ ⑩ ⑳ ㉚ ㊵ ● ㊿ ⑩ ⑳ ⑨ ➡ 1958 8 ⓪ ① ② ③ ④ ⑤ ⑥ ⑦ ● ⑨ ➡	⑨ ⑩ ⑳ ㉚ ㊵ ㊿ ⑩ ⑳ ⑨ ⓪ ① ② ③ ④ ⑤ ⑥ ⑦ ⑧ ⑨	
26. Why did you choose this hospital?	➡ ○ Doctor suggested ○ Insurance or employer encouraged OR my choice based on...	
	➡ ○ prior experience ○ advertising ○ what I've heard	
27. Did anything good happen during your visit that you did not expect? If so, please tell us what it was.		
28. Did anything unpleasant happen during your visit that you did not expect? If so, please tell us what it was.		
29. Why would you return or not return to this hospital? Please give us your honest opinions.		

of understanding, and complexity of the data capture effort. Work teams and quality circles have become a well-established part of CQI efforts, providing useful and timely consumer satisfaction information that is nonepisodic; however, this particular method does not offer information that is necessarily generalizable or comprehensive. Comment cards are the least expensive and complex service evaluation technique; however, the results are often biased with respect to the type of consumers who are inclined to respond and the type of information that is typically provided. In general, any modality offers only a snapshot of the service experience and must be replicated over time in order to provide feedback useful to the CQI process. While more extensive methods require relatively greater resource commitment in terms of staff time and/or financial expenditure, these methods tend to provide satisfaction measures that are more generalizable and representative of users.

Tenner and DeToro (1992) use a two-dimensional framework for determining data capture techniques for various desired levels of understanding about consumers' service experiences. Their framework illustrates the relationship between the approach (reactive vs. proactive) to understanding consumer needs and expectations as well as the attained level of consumer understanding (high vs. low). The three identified levels, as indicated in Figure 5–5, are:

- Level One: reactive approach by management and level of customer understanding is low. Comment cards and management observation would be included at this level.
- Level Two: proactive approach by management with a much greater level of customer understanding. Focus groups, quality circles, and mystery shoppers would be included at this level.
- Level Three: proactive approach by management to yield a generalizable understanding of consumer expectations. Interviews and surveys would be included at this level.

Although this structured approach is useful in categorizing available modalities in terms of level of consumer understanding, there are often benefits from utilizing techniques from each level at the same time (Macintyre and Kleman 1994). In some cases, a combination of approaches may be used to collect the appropriate type and amount of information for feedback as part of CQI.

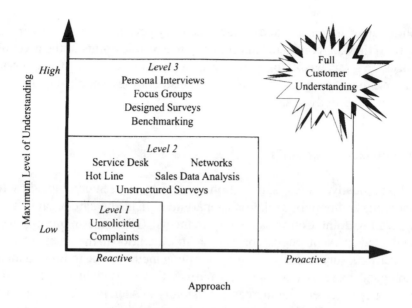

Figure 5–5 Mechanisms for Understanding Customers

A clear understanding of organizational capabilities and commitment together with the intended purpose of satisfaction measures is necessary in order to select the modality to be used. Selection of the appropriate data capture modality involves learning more about information-gathering techniques and choosing the right technique for the target group and desired depth of information sought. Trade-offs between budgetary constraints and methodological rigor are often central selection criteria.

Timing

Little attention has been paid to the appropriate timing of patient/enrollee survey administration and/or interviewing in the data collection process. The majority of marketing efforts has led to collection at either point-of-service and/or short-term, non-service-specific follow-up following discharge or encounter via mail or telephone. As we begin to use such data as part of the CQI process, consideration should be given to the appropriate timing of such data collection efforts. For instance, it may make sense to query emergency room visits at point-of-service; however, follow-up of services with extended recovery periods may be more meaningful if they are conducted at clinically reasonable points in the recovery process (e.g., six weeks following care for hip replacements). Thus, service and/or procedure-specific follow-up considerations should be incorporated into the study design.

Functional Responsibility

Traditionally, patient satisfaction surveys have been conducted by the marketing and/or public relations departments in health care organizations in meeting Joint Commission requirements. Often these surveys were conducted on a semi-regular basis with little attention to the science of item consistency, survey design, and/or sampling methods due to limited methodological expertise. Strategic initiatives tied to sustained competitive excellence together with increasing visibility of such information through such formats as HEDIS reporting has led health service organizations to address empirical validity concerns. Increasingly, this functional responsibility has been outsourced to survey research firms that do have the expertise and capacity to sample statistically valid samples of patient populations in a timely manner. As interest grows in integrating information from patient satisfaction surveys into the CQI process, the functional responsibility within health services organizations appears to be shifting with quality departments or units taking over responsibility for periodic patient satisfaction surveys. As such, additional relevant content issues (e.g., number of disability days, measures of health status such as SF-12/36), collection of comparative base-line data, sampling design, and sample selection considerations can be incorporated.

USING PATIENT SATISFACTION MEASURES

Once valid and reliable consumer satisfaction measures have been produced, they become a valuable component of the feedback loop in the CQI process. It is only through dissemination of this information that it can actually be used for performance improvement.

The Balanced Score Card (BSC) is not a new tool. Kaplan and Norton developed the premise for this approach through a series of articles that were published in the *Harvard Business Review* in the early 1990s and later compiled this work together with a more in-depth discussion of examples from the field in their book (1996). BSC is more than a measurement tool; it's a management system used to achieve long-term strategic goals by linking performance to outcomes and can be used to: (1) guide current performance through feedback and (2) target future performance improvement. The instrumentation of BSC focuses on a single strategy where multiple, relevant measures are linked together in a cause-effect network. Measures transcend the traditional financial accounting framework used to assess organizational performance, seeking to build internal assets and capabilities as well as forging the integration of strategic alliances. Leading (structure and process) and lagging (outcomes) measures or indicators are identified in four categories: financial performance, customer knowledge, internal business processes, and staff learning and growth. Customer satisfaction is typically included in the customer knowledge category. A designated group within an organization selects the indicators and disseminates periodic reports for monitoring and evaluative purposes.

Application of this innovative tool has only recently occurred in health care. Several major integrated delivery and hospital systems are currently implementing BSCs, and a national conference has been organized to demonstrate the added value of this approach in the health care industry. Examples of organizations utilizing this innovative approach as part of their strategic and CQI initiatives include Henry Ford Health System and the Duke University Health Care System.

Macdonald (1998) reported on the application of the BSC in aligning strategy and performance in long-term care at the Sisters of Charity of Ottawa Health Service. The section of their developed BSC addressing customer satisfaction is shown in Exhibit 5–1.

Severity Adjustment: Addressing a Special Issue in Measuring Consumer Satisfaction

Using performance measures to suggest improvement opportunities as part of CQI often results in internal staff criticism such as "my patients are sicker" or "my patients are different." Severity (or risk) adjustment methodologies have been used to control for explainable differences in subpopulations of patients/enrollees so that valid comparisons may be made with adjusted performance measures. These techniques are commonly applied to clinical quality measures; but Woodbury et al. (1997) explored

Exhibit 5–1 Balanced Score Card: Customer Satisfaction Objectives/Indicators

Strategic Objective	Lag Indicators	Lead Indicators
Meet clients' needs, priorities, and expectations in a manner that exemplifies the SCOHS values of respect, compassion, social justice, and community spirit.	"Overall Satisfaction"—clients and families (all programs) Satisfaction with physical, social, emotional, and spiritual care (all programs) % of patients satisfied with service in the language of their choice (all programs) % of patients who feel they are treated with respect; participate in decisions about their own care (all programs)	Volunteer hours per patient day (% variance) (Human Resources) Direct care hours worked per patient day (% variance) (Finance) Staff stability ratio (Human Resources) # and nature of projects that focus on "increasing patient, resident, or client quality of life" (all programs/departments)

the use of the patient refined-diagnosis related groups (APR-DRG) severity classification adjustment methodology with patient satisfaction measures for inpatient care at the 23-hospital, Intermountain Healthcare system based in Salt Lake City, Utah. Logistic regression was used to address the primary research question—whether severity of illness was an independent explanatory variable for differences in satisfaction among study patients.

Patient survey items used in this study included 17 items taken from a longer 72-item Inpatient Perceptions of Quality Questionnaire (Intermountain Health Care, Inc. 1993). Items included in the short-form used by Woodbury et al. (1997) are shown in Exhibit 5–2.

Trained interviewers administered questions using a telephone survey between 10 and 21 days following discharge. APR-DRG severity was not found to be a significant factor in explaining differences in inpatient satisfaction ratings; however, age and reason for admission were found to be predictive of high satisfaction for the majority (n=14) of satisfaction items. While severity adjustment was not found to be a significant factor in this particular study, variation in alternative severity (and/or risk) adjustment methods may lead to different conclusions for similar applications.

Exhibit 5–2 Patient Survey Items

Perceptions of Service Quality (scored on a scale of 1=poor to 5=excellent)

1. How well the staff worked together as a team to coordinate different aspects of your stay
2. Overall admitting procedures upon entering the hospital
3. Overall discharge procedures upon leaving the hospital
4. The cleanliness of your room
5. The quality of the food
6. Overall, the quality of care and services you received
7. The caring and concern shown to you by the nurses
8. The information provided by the nurses about your condition and care
9. The professional skills of the nurses
10. The caring and concern shown to you by the physicians
11. The information provided by the physicians about your condition and care
12. How well the physicians and nurses communicated with each other about your condition and care
13. The physician's skill in diagnosing and treating your condition

Perceptions of Clinical Quality (scored on a scale of 1=do not agree to 5=completely agree)

14. Given my condition, the medical tests and treatment I received were completely appropriate.
15. The staff did all that was possible to alleviate my pain.
16. The hospital did all that was possible to help my condition.
17. My condition has improved as much as possible as a result of my hospital stay.

Thus, this single study suggests an important line of research inquiry that can only be resolved through further assessment with alternative adjustment approaches.

The larger issue borne out by this exploratory research is that of comparability. Clearly, Woodbury et al. (1997) point out the need to stratify satisfaction measures by key attributes of the responding consumers (e.g., age, reason for admission). Other important attributes may not have been detected in this particular study. For instance, self-reported health status, educational attainment, gender, and race/ethnicity differences have been reported as important stratification variables in explaining reported differences in satisfaction measures (Linn 1975; Hsieh and Kagle 1991). It should be noted, however, that inconsistent findings for these attributes have been reported.

CONCLUSION

Efforts to adequately measure consumer satisfaction are complex. As with any evaluative (whether formative or summative) effort, the analyst must consider the ultimate application of the generated satisfaction measures. In doing so, key measures should be selected given the context of the particular health care service and/or procedure. Relevant consumers should next be identified and required input solicited. Alternative modalities for gathering data from consumers should be assessed. It is important that this choice be aligned with the intended use of this information in light of organizational constraints on resources, time, and internal capabilities. Finally, collected satisfaction measures should be applied as part of the CQI process.

CHAPTER 6

Teams at the Core of Continuous Learning

Peter J. Dean, Rebecca La Vallee, and Curtis P. McLaughlin

"A team is a small number of people with complementary skills who are committed to a common purpose, set of performance goals, and approach for which they hold themselves mutually accountable" (Katzenbach and Smith 1993, 112). Team members share leadership roles, measure their performance directly by the quality of their collective work products, and encourage open discussion and active problem solving. Teams need to focus on performance goals in an atmosphere associated with some urgency, but also spend adequate time together to develop collective values, work rules and norms, and their own behavioral interpretation.

Top management has a great deal of influence over the team's effectiveness by the way it signals the significance of the effort, provides feedback and stimuli to the members, evaluates team performance, and provides recognition and rewards (Zmud and McLaughlin 1989). Teams can make a difference by outperforming other types of work units, including individuals. "Teams outperform individuals acting alone or in a larger organizational grouping, especially when performance requires multiple skills, judgments, and experiences. Most people recognize the capabilities of teams; most have the common sense to make teams work. Nevertheless, most people overlook team opportunities for themselves" (Katzenbach and Smith 1993, 9).

This chapter focuses on teams within the continuous quality improvement (CQI) paradigm, especially teams cutting across departments, examining delivery systems, and attempting to improve organizational and caregiving processes. Forming and motivating the team is a core management process to set up the parallel organization that implements CQI. This chapter also contains information on the essential components needed to construct and maintain effective teams in an organization.

AN EXPERIENCE OF THE STAGES OF TEAM BUILDING

In 1998, 20 physicians participating in a focus group during an executive MBA course at the University of Tennessee identified the major stages of team development (Dean et al. 1998). They reported their experiences and observations after working together for 10 months in one large team and smaller subteams. They identified five major stages of team development: (1) novel politeness, (2) goal clarity, (3) vying for voice, (4) constructive communication, and (5) synergistic collaboration.

The *novel politeness* stage contained many concerns about interaction. The types of behavior during this stage that the physicians identified included tentative measuring of each other as they searched for information about each other, learning about and from each other, confusion and frustration in communication, and experiencing self-doubt along with self-confidence. This first stage of the team process had more to do with self-orientation than teamwork. A group began to form only when feedback from each other and from faculty about performance was introduced in the process.

The second stage, *goal clarity*, shifted each group member's attention from self-orientation toward an external objective. Only when feedback demonstrated the gap between the observed performance of the members and their expected performance did the team observe a change in the process. When the challenge of earning the MBA was clear, and the criteria, type, and degree of learning was realized, the group began to orient itself to the task at hand. This second stage is still orientation, but the difference is that the group as a whole has identified a direction toward success. Once the group had focused its energy and arrived at this group realization, a third stage emerged.

This third stage brought with it the necessary ingredient for any team— *vying for voice.* When the energies of the group members begin to move in the same direction, there are likely to be some exchanges among members that can be called by another name—conflict. There will be conflict with different agendas and ways of doing things and there will be bids for power over the group and within the group. It is in this third stage that diversity in thought and action originate from the group members' different views of health care. A group must persevere through this stage if it is ever to become a team.

There was a sense among these physicians that the diversity of talent in their group facilitated better decision making. The third stage is the greatest challenge for the team-to-be. The convergence of individually based norms of behavior centered around self-interest must be reconciled with the more universally accepted norms of behavior that ensure fairness, equality, and dignity to each human person.

While recognizing this third stage, the physicians also noticed that this stage never completely goes away as the team development process continues. Vying for voice is a *subprocess* within the overall process of team development and is key to the success of the team. It is well documented in the field of action learning. Marquardt and Carter (1998) and Revans (1991) have written extensively about this subprocess. It involves action learning and represents an ethical addition to the team process because each team member can voice an opinion. Each member can ask and can argue his or her opinion. Depending on the level of resolution of the conflict between self-interest norms and universal norms on different topics of study in the executive MBA, the physicians reported different outcomes.

Not surprisingly, better communication, greater respect, and sharing of information occurred when a greater number of team members reached consensus on the direction of the action to be taken. This experience can be described as a distinct fourth stage, which the physicians labeled *constructive communication*. A team exhibits true team behavior at this stage. Individual egos are still active but there is a greater awareness of a common mission. Here every individual can contribute and will be listened to irrespective of the intensity or diversity of his or her voice. The team will work through a problem until the majority of the team members have reached consensus. Working through the problem ensures optimal learning about the problem itself. As this stage becomes the team norm, moments of synergy emerge.

The fifth stage, *synergistic collaboration,* may not be a stage at all. The Tennessee physician MBAs report indicated that it came and went seemingly on its own. The longevity or brevity was not dependent on individual behavior but instead on the synchronicity of a team's behavior. In fact, one physician remarked that the harder the team tried to maintain it, the faster it was lost. The synergistic collaboration seemed almost a random reinforcement that gave credibility to the team's overall discipline, determination, and dedication to making the best decisions, not from any individual behavior. Reports of this kind of experience occurred more in subteams as opposed to the larger team of 20.

The physician MBAs identified many of the variables on teamwork that have been researched in the literature. Ann and Bob Harper, in their book entitled *Skill-Building for Self-Directed Team Members,* suggest that successful teams have a shared goal, a climate of trust and openness, honest communication, diversity valued as an asset, members who are interdependent, and consensus decision making where no one person dominates the team (1998). The Harpers wrote about turning conflict into opportunity and having adults participate in mature continuous learning. They, like the physician MBAs, recognized the effect of the group's diversity on better decision making. Diversity of opinions, ideas, and experiences are encouraged rather than the practice of "group think," where differences are viewed as a deviance from the norm. This understanding is important for the CQI process.

DIVERSITY OF TEAM MEMBERSHIP

Successful CQI requires a kind of shadow organization to operate. Suppliers of the process in question may be in one unit of the regular (formal) organization, while the customers of the process may be in a different unit. Thus, a team that comes together to work on a problem process may be diverse or multidisciplinary (sometimes referred to as cross functional) and be composed of individuals from a variety of organizational units and professional backgrounds. Indeed, the suppliers and/or customers involved may even come from outside the formal organization. It is the transient nature of these teams that makes them work and prevents their interference with the ongoing activities of the formal organization. Management must take steps, however, to ensure that the formal organization pays prompt attention to their output.

Berwick, for example, states that "teams must be created, trained, and competently led to tackle complex processes that cross customary department boundaries" (1989, 55). Professionals must come out of their individual departments and professional orientation to form multidisciplinary groups and collectively take responsibility for patient care and organizational processes. Members of multidisciplinary teams must develop common goals, engage in cooperative and coordinated activities, and take advantage of a mix of professional skills and orientations to fully utilize the CQI process. These heterogeneous groups have the potential to provide a breadth of ideas and prevent the limited mindsets that inhibit creative problem solving.

Multidisciplinary groups bring their own set of problems and limitations, however. Bettenhausen remarks that "most studies have found that diversity hinders group and organizational performance, especially in times of crisis or rapid change" (1991, 356). Malfunctions can arise from a complexity of individual member characteristics and group dynamics such as territoriality (by department or profession), role confusion, or lack of experience/training in group processes. Gaucher and Coffey (1993) observe that multidepartmental teams go through four stages, which are very similar to what our physicians described above. They are described as:

1. Form: The new group members wait for their roles to be clarified before addressing the issue at hand. The focus is on the team leader and on domineering team members.
2. Storm: There is interchange of ideas, but they are one-way, critical, and conflictful. The leader becomes less of a focus.
3. Norm: Conflict is addressed and reduced as objectives are clarified, people become comfortable with the ground rules for group behavior, and trust and common interests are developed. At this point the leadership must challenge the group to set and reach new goals and try new techniques and approaches to spur group development.
4. Perform: Team members make contributions of data, facts, and logic and are motivated by the results. Team members share leadership according to their knowledge and skills, and the task gets accomplished effectively and efficiently (235–240).

Selection of a quality improvement team member is based on the individual's professional and technical knowledge of the process being examined and ability to contribute to its improvement. The role that each individual represents, however, may be unclear. Was the team member selected as a representative of a particular department, particular profession, or position in the organizational hierarchy? These representative roles differ from the group process roles associated with effective group work and may influence the perspective from which the team member contributes and the motivation to continue participating in quality improvement team tasks. Although the representation role is played down in the literature on the CQI process, the likely case is that the individual is selected to fulfill multiple roles, some representational and some problem solving. Therefore, one of the secrets of success may lie in individuals' ability to juggle multiple roles and to signal to other team members which hat (role) they are wearing each time they offer a contribution during the flow of the meeting.

Multidisciplinary or diverse teams can be avoided early in the CQI process, but they cannot be avoided long under the CQI philosophy. In health care, multidisciplinary teams are likely to have the highest impact on process quality, costs, and patient quality perceptions. This type of team should not be avoided because of its inherent risks, even with the problems presented by using physicians as team members.

Prepare for changes in team membership due to a number of causes. One reason could be that as the definition of the task is clarified, so is the ownership. New members may have to be added to represent newly identified issues critical to the process. Team members should be representative of the issues at hand whenever possible.

Physician Participation and the Language of Teams

As Berwick described, "In hospitals, physicians both rely on and help shape almost every process pertaining to patients' experience, from support services (such as dietary and housekeeping functions) to clinical care services (such as laboratories and nursing). Few can improve without the help of the medical staff" (1989, 56). Yet physicians have not been exposed by training or experience to the type of teamwork necessary for CQI team success. In addition, a physician's sense of time urgency is often incompatible with the time-consuming group and statistical analysis processes involved in participating on a total quality management (TQM) team. Experience suggests that it is possible to gain physician participation by appealing to their:

- desire for greater control over economic stability
- desire to maintain sufficient clinical freedom to cope with the uncertainties of patient care

- sense of participation and influence in institutional development
- need for improving the diminished social value of physicians' work. (Merry 1990).

If you find people fretting about the slowness of the CQI process, you can turn to the literature on rapid improvement teams. For example, Alemi et al. (1998) offer a summary of the approaches one might use to speed up a team. One must be careful, however, to differentiate between a team that is slow and one that is stuck. If the team is stuck, teaching them to go faster will not help as much as an intervention by the facilitator or by senior management to help them get past the sticking points or concepts.

Process Owners

Important team members are the *process owners*, those who will understand the whole process as it crosses functional areas or departments and assume the responsibility to hinder or support improvement and quality efforts (or at least be candidates for that role). A process owner may reside in any department or level of the organization. These individuals become group members because of their knowledge of how the customer experiences the process. They also must possess the task-related knowledge and group skills necessary to gain the other group member's participation in analyzing and improving processes. Task-related knowledge and skills include the ability to assign and coordinate group members' tasks and activities, to facilitate group processes to reach objectives, and to maintain connections with the rest of the organization and/or environment. In addition, they must be sensitive to socioemotional responsibilities shared among group members. These skills are necessary to build group cohesion, maintain morale, and reduce interpersonal conflict throughout the process. Other roles include the responsibility for follow-up and implementation, which is the "A" of the PDCA cycle (Plan, Do, Check, Act).

TEAM CHARACTERISTICS

A quality improvement team is formed only when an opportunity for improvement is identified that is important to customers and selected as a priority issue by management. In most settings it is not possible nor practical to constitute groups based on "demographics, need, personality, or ability for particular problems, and then resort to them for new problems" (Wanous and Yautz 1986). A team should also provide diversity by selecting individuals on the basis of their professional/technical knowledge of the process being examined and their ability to contribute to its improvement, regardless of their department of origin or normal hierarchical status. Therefore, these teams represent temporary, secondary task assignments for most employees. Zmud and McLaughlin (1989) define secondary tasks as tasks that are not considered part of one's permanent job description and are not likely to be used as a component of promotion decisions. Thus, a CQI organization might overcome the secondary role and its problems by adding "contributes to process improvement" to all job descriptions and performance evaluations.

Skills and Knowledge

As discussed previously, "each group member's knowledge structure represents a fundamental element in a group's collective knowledge structure" (Walsh et al. 1988, 195). The knowledge base of the group and the skills of group members, especially those skills related to process characteristics, information management, and data manipulation, are important to the problem-solving and decision-making processes of the group.

Group Process Skills

Group process or interaction "is the way group members pool their abilities in collaborative context in order to reach the best decision" (Watson and Michaelson 1988, 495). A quality improvement team comes together to analyze a process and develop solutions or alternatives for improvement. As team members work independently, they exchange information, coordinate activities, and form interpersonal impressions of each other. The basic group process skills required include meeting skills, ability to generate ideas, and ability to reduce data to usable form. Desired interpersonal skills are listening, participation, and conflict resolution.

Organizations that have introduced TQM/CQI report that the meeting and interpersonal skills of listening and responding to others have a high payoff both inside and outside the organization. Managers often report instances of workers expressing profound thanks after practicing those skills in personal relationships at home with spouses and teenage children. Meeting skills in and of themselves also have a high payoff in productivity when meetings begin and end on time, when there is an agenda ahead of time, and when people stick to a process that they all understand, such as storyboarding.

GROUP ROLES

Accomplishing group tasks requires that certain group functions be performed and that group roles support them. Group roles are of three types: (1) group task roles, (2) group-building and maintenance roles, and (3) individual roles. Group task roles can be assumed by any group member and are focused on problem-related tasks. These roles include:

- initiator/contributor
- information seeker
- opinion seeker
- information giver
- elaborator
- coordinator
- orienter
- evaluator/critic
- energizer
- procedural technician
- recorder

Not all roles are task related. The group itself has to be developed. Therefore, group building and maintenance roles are required of individuals concerned with the effectiveness and survival of the team. Again, roles should not be restricted to any one individual. These roles are:

- encourager

- harmonizer
- compromiser
- gatekeeper and expediter
- standard setter
- group-observer and commentator
- follower

Furthermore, each individual has some potential roles to play that satisfy personal needs unrelated to group tasks and unconcerned with group development or continuity. These roles can include:

- aggressor
- blocker
- recognition seeker
- self-confessor
- player
- dominator
- help seeker
- special interest pleader

Needless to say, fulfilling some ego needs is important for motivation, but their expression has to be constrained by members' fulfilling group norms and attending to group building and maintenance needs, including their own.

Successful groups require different roles depending on the current stage of the task cycle or the level of maturity the group has reached. A high level of individual-centered role taking, as opposed to group-centered role taking, generally indicates a need for group self-assessment and further group-process training (Benne and Shcats 1948). What the group wants to avoid has been described as the garbage can decision process (Cohen et al. 1972), in which people come in and dump onto the table whatever is on top of their minds, ignoring the task for most of the meeting, and approaching it only when there is not enough time left to move it ahead sufficiently. Group members must understand that individuals may come in with a need to ventilate about something, but should be prepared then to focus them quickly on the task at hand.

Problem Solving

To take advantage of an opportunity for quality improvement or to solve a problem requires the team both to access and collect information and to assess the following:

- the problem situation—nature, seriousness, possible causes, and consequences of ineffective action
- requirements for acceptable alternatives—objectives that need to be met
- positive qualities of alternatives
- negative qualities of alternatives

In general, the greater the number and diversity of alternatives proposed and evaluated, the greater the opportunity for selection of effective solutions. Solution diversity, however, can work against successful problem solving if it leads to interpersonal conflict or decision paralysis because of lack of consensus.

Group dynamics and interpersonal relations can also influence, interfere with, or inhibit problem solving. Some of the causes outlined by Van de Ven (1974) are:

- focus effect: in a rut, group think, tunnel vision
- self-weighting effect: group members participate only to the level where they feel equally competent with other group members (called social comparison, see Turner et al. 1989)
- judgment effect: judgments are made but not expressed because they are not in agreement with those of higher status group members
- status inhibition effect: opinions are not expressed because they are not in agreement with those of higher status group members
- group pressure for conformity through implied sanctions
- influence of strong personalities on group
- overemphasis on group maintenance functions
- pressure for speedy decisions

Successful problem solving also requires the ability of the group to make decisions.

Decision Making

Efficient closure requires that the group be able to make a final recommendation effectively. Hirokawa (1988) found a positive relationship between group decision performance and the group's ability to accurately understand the problem and gauge the negative consequences of alternate choices. But individuals can arrive at different conclusions hearing the same information if their decision rule orientations are different (Beatty 1989). The key attribute of a group that allows it to become a team relates to the members' ability to self-disclose the information they know and to perceive and accept feedback about their performance in relation to that information. The feedback usually is information of which the performer is not aware.

Information

Decisions cannot be made, problems solved, or quality improved without information. Unfortunately, many researchers are pessimistic about managers' abilities to accurately read complex information environments because individuals are thought to suffer from selective perception (Walsh et al. 1988, 197). One way to surmount this problem is to pool information from all group members. Information pooling also allows each group member to have a broader understanding of work and participate in new decisions about the organization (Lawler 1988).

Communication

Hirokawa (1988) suggests that the relationship between the quality of decisions made and the communication process employed is based on three assumptions:

1. Decision-making tasks are bounded by critical requirements.
2. Meeting these requirements enhances successful decision making.
3. Group communication is the mechanism groups employ to meet these requirements (489)

Conflict Negotiation

Conflict is a natural occurrence in any group that is attempting problem solving and decision making. With respect to conflict, group leaders and members must come to understand the distinction between situational conflict and interpersonal conflict. Beckhard (1969) suggests that the successful, adaptive organization has a high level of situational conflict and a low level of interpersonal conflict. Scarce resources and organizationally challenging targets lead to situational conflict. As the environment heats up, the molecules (or actors) begin to ping off each other and the pressure builds. Situational conflict is an existential problem. The trick is to keep professionals who normally have trouble differentiating between their professional persona and their personal one aware that what is happening is situational and should not be taken personally. If people start taking situational conflict personally, the organization rapidly loses its effectiveness. Note that it is inherent in the nature of CQI to create or at least bring to light situational conflicts that team leadership must be ready to manage.

Before conflict can be managed or resolved, it is important to understand the dimensions of differentiation, clarity, and centrality. Here differentiation is the group's ability to identify distinct types (clarity) and strengths or relative importance (centrality) of points of view (Pace 1990, 83). Unfortunately, the process of differentiation tends to tag specific positions to individual group members and create the "potential for differentiation to escalate into uncontrollable conflict" (Pace 1990, 82). There are four basic dimensions of group conflict: personalized, depersonalized, competitive, and cooperative (Pace 1990, 80–81).

Pace suggests that the best decisions come out of depersonalized/cooperative personalized/competitive mixes because these dimensions allow the whole group to make the most effective use of the specialized knowledge of individual group members. This approach is recommended strongly by Deming in his book, *The New Economics for Industry, Education, Government* (1993).

> We have grown up in a climate of competition between people, teams, departments, divisions, pupils, schools, and universities. Economists have taught us that competition will solve our problems. We see now that competition can actually be destructive. It would be better if everyone could work together as a system, with the aim for all to win. What is needed is cooperation and transformation to this style of management (Deming 1993, xi).

Conflict resolution through negotiation and bargaining may take one of seven forms:

1. Simple disputes: These are limited to two people, each with full authority to reach an agreement.

2. Horizontal bargaining: Each side has a designated formal authority figure, but negotiations cannot be completed without consultation of the present informal authority figures.
3. Constituency bargaining: Negotiating individuals are serving as representatives of constituency groups.
4. Vested interests: An individual had hidden authority to allow or disallow agreement.
5. Unilateral bargaining: Cross-table agreements occur that may leave negotiators at odds with their respective teams
6. Bilateral bargaining: This involves formal problem solving.
7. Multilateral disputes: There are multiple negotiators or teams, each with multiple special interest perspectives (Gill 1987; McLaughlin 1991, 1992).

TASK

Deming stated that "a team should have an aim, a job, a goal" or a task defined by a problem statement, but not stated so specifically as to stifle initiative (1986, 90).

Type of Task

Selection of the team task is important. Quality improvement can be achieved through team effort by systematically selecting well-defined projects and assigning them to teams whose members have the knowledge of the process and the skills necessary to contribute to a successful outcome (Sahney and Warden 1991; Jackson 1992). Appropriate CQI team projects in health care organizations include patient care, administration, management processes, improved service designs, new services and process creation, and specific problem investigation (Ebel 1991). At first, the tasks will represent areas of obvious poor performance, but after initial successes, new teams will be chartered to address important processes that may not be current sources of distress but have potential for high payoffs.

TEAM MANAGEMENT

Individuals must believe that they are able to grow professionally as a result of their contributions to the group. Trade-offs must often be made regarding an individual's existing skills and his or her opportunity to develop new skills. Group members should also be able to request particular task assignments, and the group leader should periodically review what value members attach to current task assignments. Ideally, an individual's primary supervisor should attend these review meetings. In the absence of the opportunity to enhance skills, task closure remains the only intrinsic motivating force; this is a weak motivator for temporary secondary tasks and a nearly nonexistent one for permanent secondary tasks.

Maintaining Member Interest

Group members, especially those assigned minor roles, tend to experience the work of secondary groups as long periods of idleness interspersed with occasional bursts of intense effort. During periods of inactivity, a steady stream of task status information, as well as bulletins on issues affecting the group's mission, is needed to maintain member interest. Group leaders must also pay attention to nonactive members.

Maintaining Member Influence

Group performance will diminish rapidly if members believe they are without influence. This is particularly true with secondary task groups, where task assignments by themselves often generate insufficient motivation and commitment. Members must have opportunities to exert influence and then see how this influence has affected the group's processes or outcomes. For example, in a recent study of faculty administration relationships at a small liberal arts college, the faculty had adequate input to the administration's activities, because most faculty members participated on one or more standing committees. Yet morale was suffering because the president had not demonstrated the specific ways that faculty contributions through standing committees had influenced college policies and operating decisions.

Meetings that address the concerns of or allow meaningful input from only a few members should be avoided. Instead, subgroups should be created, or members should be met with outside of official group meetings. The full group should be brought together only when everyone's attendance is necessary.

Group Coordination

Group coordination is achieved by means of the good communication and mutual respect that exist in the context of a shared understanding of the group's purpose and tasks. Such coordination is best sustained via unplanned communication and informal or impromptu meetings between group members. Group coordination depends as much on the existence of well-developed personal networks as it does on task proficiency. Group leaders must spend a surprising amount of time nurturing effective networks among group members, as well as with key actors outside the group.

ORGANIZING THE ENVIRONMENT FOR TEAMS

The teams studying the organization's processes are key to CQI success, whether they operate within a function or across functions. This section will focus on the attributes of these task-oriented teams, understanding that the concepts involved are also applicable to the performance of the quality steering committee and design teams. The experience of the physician MBAs underscored many of the variables and relationships that may affect the level of quality improvement that teams achieve. Critical to these variables in the management process are what controls the selection of tasks, the agenda and assignments given to the teams, and the selection, training, and motivation of team members. Gaucher and Coffey (1993), however, report that teams can be productive only when the organizational environment is right.

Gaucher and Coffey's assertion means that teams should have adequate resources, the ability to implement decisions, the sponsorship of managers, and an effective reward and recognition system. The appropriate training materials and time for skill building must be available during team formation. A standard problem-solving process is also required to help the team stay on track. Finally, leadership commitment to support the team effort is essential for success (Gaucher and Coffey 1993, 219).

Gaucher and Coffey studied the use of cause-and-analysis on unsuccessful teams at the University of Michigan Medical Center and reported a wide range of causes for lack of success, including:

- lack of effective training, the main reason for failure
- unskilled leadership

- unclear goals, including lack of adequate customer definition
- unsupportive environment or one in which systems are unstable
- lack of reward and recognition
- jumping to a desired solution before studying root causes
- selecting a system and not a process to improve
- dysfunctional behavior by individual team members (1993, 241–242)

Gaucher and Coffey report that some teams can be put back on track by doing a CQI root cause analysis and then developing and implementing part of a series of options to address identified causes of poor team performance.

Outcome measures associated with productivity are variously defined in terms of output, performance, motivation, efficiency, effectiveness, production, profitability, cost-effectiveness, competitiveness, and work quality (Pritchard and Karasick 1973; Watson and Michaelson 1988), as well as Donabedian's seven items (1990). Group effectiveness has also been defined in terms such as a quantitative measure of productivity, satisfaction of group members, and ability of the group to survive (Ancona 1985). The CQI philosophy calls for leaving the definition of group effectiveness up to the judgment of the end users or customers of the product or services provided by the group, as well as to group members themselves. Inasmuch as CQI teams are ad hoc groups, long-term survival is not an issue. Short-term effectiveness, including survival, is, however.

Other features of supportive environments include recognition, responsiveness to the group's requests for information, resources, action legitimization of the group's task and process, and expectations of group success (Ancona 1985; Shea and Guzzo 1987; Zmud and McLaughlin 1989).

Organizational Support

Organizational support includes the involvement of organizational leaders through a regular role of participating in or monitoring of results, stating a clear mission and task, establishing team-contingent rewards, giving team performance feedback (Bettenhausen 1991; Kaluzny and McLaughlin 1992; Melum 1990), and learning within the organization that continuously improves the program. This is sometimes referred to as providing the necessary infrastructure to support the CQI teams, including resources, training, and rewards.

Resources

The organization must provide adequate resources for the group effort. The organization pays for the work time, while the group members contribute their individual knowledge and skills. The organization also provides technical information (data) to the group through facilitators, team members, and information systems and mentors both from within the organization and through outside resources. The organization must also define meaningful and tractable tasks that are of value to the participants and the organization. If presented early in the group's work, these tasks present an opportunity for team members to reduce discomfort in their units.

Training

Much group skill and knowledge is gained or enhanced through training programs that the organization provides. Training needs for TQM vary for different levels of the organization and by functional group. Organizational leaders need an understanding of fundamental concepts, strategic planning needs, and technical methods associated with team efforts. Middle managers need training to help them guide and facilitate the TQM implementation. TQM teams need training to acquire proficiency in the use of statistical tools and an understanding of group processes. Local experts/facilitators/coaches need an understanding of technical aspects of TQM principles as well as a firm grounding in organizational development (OD) concepts and practices in order to facilitate organizational change through group processes. Chapter 11 discusses the training opportunities and models that management needs to see developed to ensure that the right training takes place in the right sequence.

Organizational development (OD) interventions can be used to increase "organizational effectiveness through initiation of planned change within the organization" (Young et al. 1988, 69). They are targeted toward behavioral change in individuals or changes in organizational processes. In a sense, TQM projects are OD interventions, as are the team-building and meeting skills training programs provided for TQM group members. Porras and Hoffer (1986) reported the behaviors commonly listed by OD experts as hoped-for results of OD efforts as communicating openly, collaborating, taking responsibility, maintaining a shared vision, solving problems effectively, respecting/supporting, processing/facilitating, inquiring, and experimenting. These same behaviors markedly influence the success of TQM project groups.

Member Reward Systems

While we recognize the value of intrinsic rewards in developing motivation and commitment, member performance must also be tied to the organization's formal evaluation and reward systems. When secondary tasks contribute to organizational performance, this fact must be recognized in the assessment of employees' overall contributions. Sustained effort and commitment are unlikely if the tasks are perceived as being outside the normal reward structure.

Secondary task performance can be linked to the formal reward system in a number of ways, including the following: adding evaluations by secondary group leaders to an annual performance appraisal; having the individual's primary supervisor meet periodically with the secondary group leader; and providing group rewards.

It is also important that each member's performance be evaluated by other group members and that these comments be used in the individual's formal evaluation. This practice not only motivates effective group interaction, but also bolsters members' sense that their membership is valued.

Group Reward Systems

Secondary groups are formed to accomplish tasks best achieved by a diverse set of specialists. Interactions within the group depend on a sense of group responsibility, which in turn depends on appropriate group performance evaluation. Suggested group rewards include bonuses, other financial incentives, and less formal rewards (such as special recognition communicated throughout the organization) when important tasks are successfully completed. Such group rewards can build a sense of individual responsibility and stimulate a supportive climate within the group.

ORGANIZATIONAL LEARNING SKILLS

Kochan and Useem (1992) suggest that continued and systemic forms of change practiced by teams may be essential for organizational learning.

Yet change is not a natural state for many organizations, and it does not occur automatically in response to cues from some invisible hand. Organizations typically display enormous inertia in some areas, as well they should. Without continuity in reporting relations, completing even the most mundane task becomes prohibitively costly. Yet the costs of failing to overcome the inertia can also be the decline or end of the organization.

Kochan and Useem (1992) suggest that continuous systemic organizational change must be integrated and consistent among an organization's major components and designed for the long term to provide a more suitable foundation for cooperation, learning, and innovation. They call these organizations "transforming organizations," able to handle the pressure to change.

The systemic change that Kochan and Useem (1992) propose can take place only when the technological, organizational, and human resources are altered together, since the potential of one segment can be fully realized only when developed with all. Moreover, systemic change involves more than changes within each of these components. It challenges the underlying assumptions, tacit knowledge, and standard relationships that link these different organizational components. This challenge is especially true if health care organizations avoid risks and organize and manage from short-term, inflexible assumptions.

Learning and Change

Kochan and Useem (1992) state that learning is essential for engaging in systemic, continuous change and going beyond the isolated shifts and periodic lurching observed in so many organizations. They also suggest that the organization that has learned how to learn will master the challenges of change. They point out three mutually reinforcing features of a learning organization.

First, faster innovation and flexibility must be present so that traditional organizational forms that stress hierarchic authority, centralized control, and fixed boundaries must give way to organizational designs that rely upon work teams, decentralized decision making, and informal networks crosscutting formal boundaries. They call these *permeable boundaries* in an organization that also must foster reciprocal information sharing, shared commitment to sustained cooperation, and a common set of values.

Second, the learning organization must have a learning culture that stresses learning about the organization's components and the relationships between them, including production technologies and organization.

Third, the learning organization will learn from diversity, not simply manage it or value it. The organization will capture the innovative potential of all participants.

Kochan and Useem (1992) note that if the learning organization where CQI is practiced is to be qualitatively different from and better than traditional organizations, discovery and action cannot be limited to a privileged few at the top of the hierarchy. If everyone in the organization must be prepared for change, then everyone must also be capable of learning and be empowered to act on his or her new knowledge.

CONCLUSION

Teams are an integral part of CQI. While they are a means and not an end, they can be very effective as agents of change. CQI management must study what is known about teams and apply that to their individual processes. Management must be concerned about team composition, roles, development, and performance. Flexibility in team management is also an important learning area for CQI management. The literature on teams is extensive, but does not necessarily always offer practical advice.

The health care environment is used to teams as a way of dealing with emergencies, but not as a generalized mode of addressing day-to-day issues. The primary emphasis in health care organizations is on individualism, a physician treating a patient. Also, medical staffing is a labyrinthine hierarchy in itself, with staff and physicians separated by function, status, specialty, and training. Therefore, health care management must sell the use of teams and provide their members with both basic and advanced training in team dynamics. Facilitators must be available to help with the team process at every stage, even after training has been given. Often teams are as much a way of getting people to talk with each other and to understand each other in highly compartmentalized organizations as they are agents of change. Management remains the primary agent of change, with teams available as their collaborators and colleagues.

PART III

Implementation

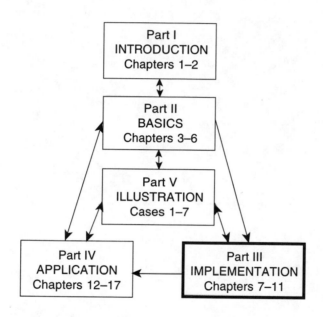

CHAPTER 7

CQI, Transformation, and the "Learning" Organization

Vaughn Upshaw, Arnold D. Kaluzny, and Curtis P. McLaughlin

Managed care has changed how we provide health care and how we manage health care organizations. While the advent of continuous quality improvement (CQI) in health care organizations was initially viewed as a panacea for many of the problems associated with quality, the realities of the managed care world have challenged many of these initial expectations of continuous improvement efforts. Consider a few of these realities (Batalden 1996a):

- "Quality" is not the only criteria by which to judge organizational performance and cost reduction is the watchword of managerial action.
- Organizations are characterized by "right sizing," "downsizing," and layoffs unprecedented in health services, with declining employee loyalty.
- Improvement initiatives are short-lived and avoid dealing with the substantive challenges facing the organization.
- "Integration" has not fulfilled expectations and there is increasing interest and experimentation in the "unbundling of provider risk" (The Advisory Board Company 1997).

Yet managed care and the emerging transformation in the delivery of health care need a continuous improvement process: a process that goes

Source: Portions of this chapter have been adapted from C.P. McLaughlin and A.D. Kaluzny, Total Quality Management Issues in Managed Care, *Journal of Healthcare Financial Management*, Vol. 24, No. 1, pp. 10–16, © Aspen Publishers, Inc.

beyond incrementally reducing variance to improve quality, but one that aggressively promotes quality of health services through organizational learning. The objective of this chapter is to assess the underlying dimensions of the transformation in health services, explore the changing roles for CQI, evaluate new approaches to transformation and organizational learning, and identify strategies for securing physician participation and leadership in organizational learning and change.

TRANSFORMING HEALTH CARE

A fundamental change accompanying the transition to managed care is that the locus of control for technological decision making in health services has moved from the individual professional to the organization (Hurley 1997). Managers assume that greater control over costs and quality will be achieved through managed care mechanisms, such as DRG (diagnosis-related group) reimbursements, capitation, or prior approvals. The dynamic nature of work processes within health care organizations, however, may or may not be consistent with the implementation or use of these managed care approaches. Given the particular nature of health care organizations, the challenge is to effectively and efficiently provide a continuum of clinical products, each with sufficient variability to adapt to the individual needs of patients and providers.

The practice and management of health services will undergo continued refinements and further codification; however, these changes will be successful only if they are accompanied by organizational learning as a way to enable the customization of care to meet the needs and expectations of providers and patients. *Organizational learning* means an institutional commitment to expand the organization's capacity to maintain or improve performance based on its own experience, utilizing the skill, insights, and knowledge of individuals within the organization and to meet the challenges of new situations (DiBella et al. 1996). Appropriately practiced in health services, CQI is one of the building blocks for institutional knowledge and learning, but will only succeed with the active participation of physicians who bring intellectual capital and leadership to facilitate learning and innovation.

Traditionally, managers merely consulted or hired a health care professional to determine whether managerial strategies would be in serious conflict with physicians' methods, norms, and values; organizational values; or the patient's interests. Health care managers were neither concerned with nor technically prepared for evaluating clinical performance. The growth of managed care, however, has required health care managers to assume greater managerial competency, responsibility for, and control over clinical issues.

Why the change? The continuous and significant introduction of science and technology into the art of medicine over the last 50 years had made possible, perhaps inevitable, a shift from the craft or guild structure of medicine toward an industrial structure. As described in Chapter 1, most sectors are in some stage of the transition to mass customization (Boynton et al. 1993). Manufacturing industries went through the first step, adopting mass production approaches in the late nineteenth and early twentieth centuries. Medicine and many other professional services have made this transition much later because of insufficient predictability of cause-and-effect and the natural variability inherent in their work processes, and because of the high degree of autonomy and highly decentralized, local organizational structures (McLaughlin 1996). The historical analogy—the craft guild—was especially applicable to physician practices, which were often referred to as a cottage industry. As with most technological change, the transition did not take place until all the factors—technical, economic, and social—were aligned.

In the 1970s and 1980s hospitals served as the industrializing institutions of health care. They amassed large amounts of capital and absorbed the emerging technologies quickly. Some even experimented with mass production, for example, the "surgicenter" focused on cataract removal (McLaughlin et al. 1995). They tended not to employ physicians, but rather operated as the physician's workplace. As hospitals increasingly began to resemble corporations, however, an uneasy truce developed between the craft orientation of the physicians and the hospitals' industrial model. Health care went through a period of rapid technological change where the increased technical capacity also meant increasing costs. Employer concerns about rising health care costs and the obvious excesses of fee-for-service medicine created a demand for managed care.

Accepting Continuous Improvement

Hospitals were once considered impersonal at best and at worst, dangerous. Organizations made little effort to promote institutional learning, and the institution had little or no control over the performance of professional personnel. Even today, hospitals find variable needs of individual patients and providers are often poorly accommodated. Information flows are fragmented and unreliable, and glaring differences in costs and outcomes are evident to those paying claims. Because of the craft nature of medicine, best practices are not easily disseminated nor widely adopted. Each provider has considerable autonomy over his or her work, often maintaining practices that are questionable or simply obsolete.

The adoption and institutionalization of CQI provided an opportunity to better manage professional personnel. The premise of continuous improvement is process dynamism and institutional learning. Teams within the institution, usually multidisciplinary teams, work cooperatively on the improvement of the institution's processes. Establishing ownership of patient-level processes that integrate professionally dominated knowledge and skills is one of CQI's objectives. One might even go so far as to classify this as capturing a competitive edge in intellectual capital. This was not a problem when the intellectual capital was assumed to be that of the professionals and not the institution. There is evidence, however, that in the future processes improvements may not be shared among the profession, once they are considered to be competitive weapons of organizations (McLaughlin and Johnson 1995).

CONTINUOUS QUALITY IMPROVEMENT AND MANAGED CARE

Managed care covers a variety of organizational forms. Some forms of managed care maintain provider autonomy—as in an independent practice association (IPA) or preferred provider organization (PPO)—but oversee care delivery processes by monitoring and comparing the results among providers on broad criteria such as cost, readmission rates, etc. Other less open systems, such as a staff model or group model HMO, give greater attention to the actual process of care applying various CQI innovations initiated by both the clinicians and corporate-level managers and staff.

Fully integrated health care delivery systems may have multiple internal perspectives seeking to improve a single treatment process. For example, epidemiological research, cost-containment, cost analysis, and care delivery units may all undertake CQI activities for a particular disease process. These four perspectives are likely to differ not only in the technology they use, but also with respect to evaluative standards, quality criteria, economic criteria, the relevant time horizon, and the relationship to the enrollee population. Although difficulties can result when these perspectives are at odds with one another, the opportunity for organizational learning greatly improves when these groups communicate with each other and share their respective views.

Continuous improvement is well aligned with many elements of managed care such as DRG reimbursement, capitation, and prior approvals. By continually seeking to reduce errors and improve processes, CQI offers an opportunity to facilitate the larger transformation of health care organizations. Under DRG reimbursement systems, institutions are paid a flat amount for a specific type of admission based on a measure of industry best practices, and it is assumed that institutions will exercise sufficient control over their processes to operate within that cost range. Under capitation, providers receive a flat monthly fee for providing a specified set of services to enrolled individuals during that period. Providers are expected to profit on the basis of their ability to appropriately manage the care for people enrolled. Other cost-containment procedures, such as prior approvals for admissions and surgical procedures, assume that employees possess sufficient technical knowledge to accept or countermand the decisions of the clinician. Prior approvals assume institutional knowledge is superior to the professional training and knowledge of providers.

Fundamental to the application of both CQI and managed care is the mutability and dynamic nature of clinical processes and the ability of both institutions and clinicians to improve their performance over time. Both CQI and managed care consistently seek to identify and implement best practices, using tools such as clinical guidelines and clinical pathways, and processes such as product and case management. Nevertheless, many clinicians perceive both CQI and managed care as a challenge to their personal and professional autonomy and financial security.

Despite physician concerns, CQI is fundamental to organizational learning. CQI allows all personnel, including providers, an opportunity to participate in shaping and transforming how the organization provides health services. It builds institutional skills needed to analyze processes, and it provides a mechanism for providers to retain their sense of autonomy and maintain control over organizational activities that affect clinical outcomes.

The critical issue currently facing managers and clinicians working within a managed care environment is how to accommodate the trade-offs between quality and cost now that early savings achieved under managed care are diminishing and health care costs are again beginning to rise. Conflicts that must be resolved include balancing quality improvement and cost control processes as well as decision-making power for upper management and operational level professionals. For these and other issues, CQI provides a mechanism by which the organization learns to effectively accommodate the quality/cost trade-off facing managers and clinicians.

Getting to Mass Customization

Patients and providers are quite variable, and both expect care that adapts to a range of conditions including differences in anatomy, physiology, cognitive style, psychological status, family setting, and economic resources. Both will evaluate their health care experiences in terms of how those needs are met. One concern is that managed care and health professionals will never agree on the role of variability in an efficient system. Management tends to follow industrial models that focus on the importance of reducing unnecessary variability rather than coping with inherent variability. Health care providers, on the other hand, use medical approaches that focus on inherent variability, often ignoring issues of unnecessary variability. Because insurers manage in the industrial model, they generally ignore or penalize inherent variability, creating potential barriers to mass customization.

The tendency of continuous improvement efforts is incrementalism—starting with the existing process and improving it, rather than radically changing the process altogether so that it better integrates new technologies, especially information technologies. As well described by Ellen Gaucher (1994): "Within health care, some of our processes are so bad that we could spend the rest of our professional careers trying to continuously improve them. We need to throw them out and begin with a clean sheet of paper and make sure we understand what the elements of each of these processes are. We need to redesign them to be effective in the long run."

The Task Ahead

Both continuous quality improvement and managed care need to recognize the inherent transitional nature of health care delivery. Continuous improvement efforts must shift their focus from simply avoiding unnecessary variation to facilitating organizational learning for mass customization as a means of providing health services. Managed care organizations must recognize that their role is not just to minimize costs but to develop the institutional knowledge that will result in the types of integrated delivery systems that can provide quality and efficient care to a defined population. Increasingly, care is being customized so that it meets and adapts to specific needs without compromising overall standards for cost and quality. The challenge for hospitals, HMOs, and other providers is to demonstrate that services are efficient and that they are improving health outcomes for individuals, enrolled populations, and in some instances, for the larger community.

Under the challenges of capitation and restricted resources, the health care industry must ensure that its services are high quality, provide access for those who need care, and limit escalating costs. To create organizations capable of meeting these demands, health care providers and managers need to balance choice, quality, and cost while maintaining values that enhance services, efficiency, and overall performance. Merely selecting the lowest cost provider that is unwilling or unable to invest in the information systems that will provide the key to mass customization is not acceptable. All stakeholders, including HMOs, hospitals, insurers, and various professional groups, must see themselves in a transition process that customizes care for the individual, while improving the health status of the population given available resources. Simultaneously, purchasers, consumers, competitors, and regulators will require information to assess the cost, quality, utilization, and availability of health services.

To meet these multiple demands, data and information systems must be flexible, expandable, available, and user friendly. Information technology must provide information that is accurate, timely, useful for decision makers at all levels, accessible, and able to accommodate the demands of providers, managers, and employees. Information systems are critical to monitoring and improving the long-term performance in an organization, so they must provide feedback that can integrated back into the system in a timely and functional manner.

Concurrent with the increased need for information in health services is the realization that organizations must reduce and reorganize staffing. Large numbers of categorically skilled employees who provide institutionally based services are no longer required. Instead, employees are needed who can perform multiple functions, work in cross-disciplinary teams, and operate in smaller units. Reducing work forces, retraining and reassigning personnel, and requiring new working relationships all contribute to compromises in morale. To make these changes successfully, clinicians and managers must foster quality work, reward loyal and high-level performance, secure commitment from employees, and build a spirit of learning while undergoing transitions.

MANAGING TRANSFORMATION AND LEARNING

Health care organizations are undergoing continuous and fundamental change. To succeed in a rapidly changing economic environment, health care organizations need to smoothly manage the transformation process and take on the challenge of becoming what Peter Senge (1990) described as "learning organizations. . . ," places where "people continually expand their capacity to create the results they truly desire, where new and expansive patterns of thinking are nurtured, where collective aspiration is set free, and where people are continually learning to learn together"(3).

As presented in Exhibit 7–1, health services are in the process of transition from a *professional model* characterized by individual responsibility, professional autonomy, and accountability to a *transformational model* characterized by shared responsibility and collaborative decision making, continuous innovation, and learning. Traditional CQI provides important skills needed to make the transition, but transformational models provide organizations the opportunity to ensure that both incremental and radical learning occur in order to meet the challenges of an uncertain and complex environment. Through organizational learning, health care organizations can better face the reality of managing costs, providing high-quality services, and improving outcomes while accommodating individual needs through case management, patient education, phone triage, and supportive patient decision making.

As presented in Exhibit 7–1, the transformational model has a number of distinguishing characteristics fundamental to CQI, as described below.

- *Leaders and employees share overall responsibility, as well as take individual responsibility.* Operating under transformational models, health care managers and clinical leaders share responsibility with other personnel for accomplishing the organizational mission. All personnel understand that they are important to the success of the

Exhibit 7–1 Emergence of Transformational Models for Organizational Performance

Professional	*TQM*	*Transformational*
Individual responsibility	Collective responsibility	Leaders and employees share overall responsibility, as well as take individual responsibility
Professional leadership	Managerial leadership	
Autonomy	Accountability	
Administrative authority	Participation	
Professional authority	Performance and process expectations	People at multiple levels assume leadership
Goal expectations	Flexible planning	
Rigid planning	Benchmarking	Outcome driven
Responses to complaints	Concurrent performance appraisal	Shared decision making
Retrospective performance appraisal	Continuous improvement	Continuous planning
Quality assurance		Future orientation
		Performance enhancement appraisals
		Continuous innovation

organization and they know what role they play in that success. Individuals, teams, units, and departments are committed to carrying out their responsibilities.

- *People at multiple levels assume leadership.* Leadership roles for making decisions and guiding change must be afforded to people working in managerial or clinical roles, line staff, and field positions. Changes and decisions designed by people in offices apart from where the work is performed usually have limited effect. For real innovation and improved performance, people working directly with problems and systems need to be involved in designing and deciding how to improve processes and quality.

- *A transformational health care organization is outcome driven.* People throughout transformational health care organizations demonstrate commitment to achieving outcomes, improving quality, and adding value. Employees, providers, and managers recognize that improving clinical and organizational outcomes means that individual expectations for quality and clinical services, such as disease treatment and management, meet or exceed standards.

- *All levels of the organization share in decision making.* It is critically important that all employees understand the core business, values, and mission of the organization so that they can participate in the decisions that affect it. Straight talk about what is occurring in the environment, how the organization is positioned to respond, and what changes are needed must be modeled and supported by managers and leaders. Employees need to understand their roles in helping the organization succeed, but they also need to define their roles and how they will contribute.

- *Continuous planning occurs throughout the organization.* People must be motivated to make change, and able to participate meaningfully in the change process. In general, participation will be more effective when the issues and changes are not routine (Schwarz 1989). Transformational change in organizations prepares people to participate in planning and to anticipate the next steps in an evolutionary change process. When the organization is undergoing regular and dynamic change, people from across the organization must be informed and involved in deciding what changes should be made, in what order, and by what methods. Through functional and cross-functional teams, providers and managers can involve others in mapping strategies and preparing for new challenges.

- *The organization maintains a future orientation.* Unlike what has come before, health service organizations must be defining what the future will be and setting their sights on how they will make that happen. A potential danger for the transformational organization is that it might achieve its objectives for the future and turn its attention to categorizing its accomplishments. Such a retrospective orientation will slow the organization and reduce people's motivation to stay ahead of the trends. Transforming leadership continually brings forward the vision of the future organization and indicates how the organization can get from where it is in the present to where it wants to be in the future.

- *Performance enhancement appraisals are routine practice.* In addition to assessing and rewarding employees for performance improvements, transformational organizations commit real resources and support structures to recognizing creativity and innovation. We need to look beyond improving how we get things done, to question and explore new ways of doing what needs to be done. Employees need to know that they will be rewarded for going outside of the traditional structures to redesign and recreate the organization. Such changes will improve more than employee performance, they will increase employee dedication and contributions to the organization's future success. Commitment is greater in organizations that are actively managing change, obviously uncomfortable with the status quo, and creating a new standard for performance (Pascale et al. 1997).

- *The organization is committed to continuous innovation.* To excel in the future, health service organizations will need to establish systems that recognize and reward individual efforts that surpass expectations. Transformational models provide support for people to demonstrate creativity and innovation that extend beyond standard performance. Clear systems for highlighting outstanding performance and contributions of providers, administrators, and employees can energize others and provide standards against which to assess poor performance (Pascale et al. 1997).

PHYSICIAN LEADERS AND TRANSFORMATION

There are multiple roles for physicians in leading and managing within transforming organizations. Physicians may be designers of change, developing incentives, exploring opportunities, and gathering resources to promote transitions. Physicians may also serve in stewardship roles to ensure that there is a broad commitment to organizational learning, or they may contribute by performing in teaching roles where they demonstrate vision and values related to the work of the organization (Barnsley et al. 1998).

To secure physician leadership, it is important to identify what will make it attractive for physicians to participate in planning and leading organizational change and then to provide them opportunities to exercise leadership within the transformational organization. It will be important, for instance, for physicians see that they have a central role in making and controlling key decisions that affect the provision of health services. It is also important for physicians to help identify where targeted cost savings can occur which will enhance efficiencies without compromising patient care. Physicians and managers both want to see the organization enhance its performance, but physicians have a particularly important role in designating common measures for preventive care activities and setting targets for meeting primary care goals. Other areas of interest to physician leaders include improving patient satisfaction, utilization rates, and resource consumption.

Physicians have central roles in helping define what the overall goals should be with regard to health status and quality outcomes. To foster participation in the design, planning, and implementation of transformational strategies, physicians need to understand how their participation will contribute to the change process. They should have access to trained facilitators who can support their efforts, and the organization should provide physicians with opportunities to develop their leadership competencies.

Organizational strategies can complement physician roles to improve quality and cost of clinical care if they are well designed. Ensuring that the organization's incentive structures and strategies are consistent and complementary can have a significant influence on physician performance. One organization, for example, treating both capitated and fee-for-service clients, was successful in controlling costs by providing the same incentives to physicians regardless of the patients' source of reimbursement (Flood 1998).

Beyond the physicians' role in the provision of care, there are additional areas in which physicians have an interest. For example, providers are concerned with issues such as market growth, percent of revenue allocated to medical costs, administrative costs, and financial returns. These factors directly influence organizational decision making and clinical activities. As a result, all participants need to know that their interests are being protected as the organization develops strategies for enhancing growth and reducing costs.

To secure a shared vision around which to align strategies for improving organizational performance, managers, providers, and employees must participate in developing a common view of the future, clarifying the values associated with the core business, and articulating shared beliefs about how to achieve high-quality health care at reasonable cost. The successful health care organizations will be those able to make the transition from focusing exclusively on standardization of all processes, to reducing instances of *poor* care for individuals.

Strategies for Learning

To develop an organizational culture that promotes learning and teaching, managers and physicians need key strategies that support such activity. Because people generally act as if their beliefs are the "truth," and that this truth is obvious and based upon real data, organizational leaders need techniques that help people learn how to achieve desired results. Figure 7–1 presents the *ladder of inference* (Argyris 1990) and illustrates why most people do not recognize that beliefs and truth are not the same thing. Further, this model demonstrates why it is important to clarify perceptions, check perceptions against facts, and assess the influence of cultural beliefs and attitudes (Senge et al. 1996).

As illustrated in this diagram, the world of observable data is not perceived in the same way by all observers. Individuals independently select the data perceived to be important, add their own cultural and personal meanings, make assumptions and draw independent conclusions, adopt their own beliefs, and then, finally, take action based upon these beliefs. When working in teams, all members may have access to the same data, but every member may act differently in response to the same information.

The *ladder of inference* can improve communication in three ways: (1) By becoming aware of one's own thinking and reasoning, an individual learns to be more *reflective*. (2) Once a person has reflected upon his or her own thoughts and reasoning, then that individual can better *advocate* his or her position to others. (3) As individuals better understand how to reflect upon and advocate for their own positions, they are also better able to *inquire* into the thinking and reasoning of other members of the team. In combination, the skills of reflection, advocacy, and inquiry are important communication skills that facilitate team and organizational learning. To improve learning within the organization, manager and physician leaders can stimulate communication in a number of ways. They can:

- *Test assumptions by gathering facts.* Once people describe their beliefs then others can ask them to provide evidence for their conclu-

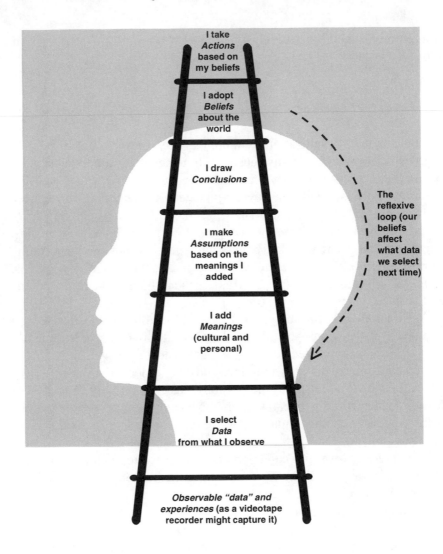

Figure 7–1 The Ladder of Inference

sions. Often people reach conclusions based partly on evidence and partly on assumptions. Only by having open discussions where people can explain what facts they used and how they reached their conclusions is it possible to learn what data they selected, what data they ignored, and what data are missing.

- *Engage people in discussion of what they assume to be true.* Physicians and other clinicians need to listen to others' views of reality. All people witnessing the same event do not necessarily have the same understanding of what has occurred. Differences emerge based upon our own experiences, biases, and beliefs. Therefore the physician and other clinicians must invite others to share their views of the situation and seek to understand what others believe to be true.

- *Prepare people for teaching and learning.* Not all people are equally able or prepared to learn the same things at the same time. Research has shown that learning occurs more readily when the message is delivered in a way appropriate to the level of the learner (Hersey and Blanchard 1984). Managers and clinicians must be able to recognize levels of readiness for learners and apply appropriate methods for teaching and coaching.

- *Integrate learning and teaching focus.* Do physicians and other clinicians ensure that everyone in the organization is supported in his or her efforts to teach and learn? To build a learning organization, managers and clinicians must be sure that policies and practices are aligned with incentives for people to acquire, develop, and practice their skills. For example, if the policies support learning but incentives only reward work, people will chose to work instead of attending workshops or seminars that enhance their learning. Managers must ensure that their expectations for performance are reinforced by the incentives within the system.

- *Develop a teachable point of view.* Physicians and other clinicians need to tell their own stories, which illustrate core values, beliefs, and expectations. What are the key experiences that have shaped your own life? How do these experiences continue to guide your own work? When leaders develop a teachable point of view they engage people's imaginations and encourage commitment. By telling their own stories leaders provide real and honest examples of success, failure, and learning while communicating values, behaviors, and skills which are important to the organization.

- *Be a role model.* Leaders who demonstrate a positive attitude toward achievement encourage commitment and performance from those around them. Leaders can increase participation in decision making as employees gain familiarity with the organization's mission, values, and goals. As people gain ownership of the organization's mission, leaders must provide them with ongoing opportunities for participation in shaping the organization's future. Through greater participation and ownership, leaders create an environment where big ideas can lead to big accomplishments.

Central to applying these strategies is ensuring that managers and clinicians communicate in ways that others within the organization understand. Through storytelling and shared participation, leaders work with others in building "mental models" that incorporate the vision of the organization that they want to create. Developing common models requires more than creating a desirable vision for the future, however. Before people can build new organizational patterns, they must have a clear understanding of what is not working, why it isn't working, and how it needs to change.

A common understanding depends upon different groups within the organization learning and becoming familiar with complementary values and norms which collectively contribute to the organization's vision. The key is to build a shared mental model while accommodating different viewpoints and expectations that arise based upon people's varying roles and responsibilities. Clinical leaders, for example, need the flexibility to develop expectations for the organization that respond to improving care for individuals, while management needs mental models that represent improving organizational efficiencies. Using scientific evidence from clinical applications and research, clinicians can accumulate the necessary information they need to motivate changes in the provision of care. Similarly, managers can improve organizational processes by gaining cooperation from clinicians in designing, implementing, and evaluating organizational changes using relevant evidence and proven methods of improvement.

In health services delivery, rapid change and competitive markets frequently require organizational responses and innovations that are more dramatic than what can be accomplished through incremental quality improvement efforts. Making big changes and fostering a climate of innovation only occurs when people understand their roles, apply CQI tools, have the flexibility to make key decisions that affect their work, and are accountable for their service to customers. Managers and clinicians must articulate expectations for quality and service, but then give people the opportunity to meet these expectations in a manner consistent with the needs of the situation. An individual with multiple complex health problems cannot be successfully managed in a single 10-minute office visit; thus clinicians and managers need to have both the flexibility to develop and tailor cost-efficient options for managing complex patients and incentives that reward appropriate customization.

Using data and evidence that demonstrate why changes are needed helps keep expectations realistic and focuses people on the key issues that will have the greatest effect. To gain commitment, physicians and other clinicians need to provide concrete evidence for their points of view. Leaders can reduce assumptions about what they mean by giving specific examples and illustrations of what is not working and how it could change.

Learning to provide specific information about what needs to be accomplished, supported by evidence, will facilitate others' acceptance. By communicating how change will be accomplished using concrete and measurable terms, leaders can stimulate others to find ways to make the vision a reality. Leaders must demonstrate the same kind of energy, commitment, high standards, continuous learning, and willingness to share information that they expect from those around them.

By sharing stories, modeling commitment, and listening to others, it is possible to move organizations toward deeper learning. It will not happen without commitment from all participants, however. And pursuing a comprehensive organizational priority on learning demands a substantial commitment of the leader's time and attention. The reward for such commitment is a greater capacity to grow leadership within the organization (Tichy 1997).

Individuals respond to a crisis by changing their behaviors, yet when there is no perceived crisis, little change occurs. What is needed is a way for health care leaders to communicate a sense of crisis—not to create panic, but to create a sense of urgency, a need to make change in order that the organization, the patient, the community, and the system survive and thrive. Managers, physicians, and other key personnel must help others recognize that the traditional treatments will not cure chronic organizational problems. Just as chronic health problems grow more severe the longer they remain undiagnosed and untreated, many of our current organizational problems will not be cured if treated incrementally. The organizations that will survive will be those that institute revolutionary strategies and foster opportunities for quantum ideas to emerge (Tichy 1997).

Managers and clinicians alike need to find ways to expose chronic, underlying organizational issues that are amenable to correction and invite participation in figuring out how to correct these problems. In many instances, changing long-standing problems will need new approaches and greater organizational flexibility. Building an innovative culture will only occur if employees are rewarded and recognized for their contributions to resolving organizational problems. Leaders need to commit themselves and their organizations to employee training and development that promotes innovation and change, learning and teaching (Barnsley et al. 1998).

Strategies for Physician Involvement

Within the health care organization, physician participation and involvement in organizational change and transformation is imperative. In order to secure participation from physician leaders, there are numerous strategies managers can employ, such as:

- *Provide information about organizational goals and objectives.* Disseminating information that describes the organization's interest in change and improvement allows physician leaders to consider the impact on their work and patients. Providing explicit information about the goals that are to be accomplished is essential to gaining buy-in and participation from others. In addition, the organization must make sure that incentives for participation are clear and available. Another key component of information sharing is to outline the outcomes that are expected as a result of the effort. People are more likely to participate in planning and implementing strategies when they understand what final results are expected.
- *Align leadership styles and tasks.* By attending departmental meetings, board meetings, intraorganizational meetings, and practice meetings, managers can observe physician interactions and identify clinical leaders who have the skills and recognition needed to persuade others for the need to change. Different leadership styles are needed for different types of issues. By observing how physicians interact with one another and learning who the opinion leaders are for various issues, managers can better match physician leaders to the tasks that need to be accomplished.
- *Use data and partnerships.* Physicians, because of special expertise or commitment, have particular issues upon which they want to focus. By

inviting physicians to take leadership on a specific issue, administrators can gain clinical participation in improving key parts of the system. Physicians' medical training prepares them to use scientific evidence as a basis for decision making; thus they are particularly well suited to using data to identify solutions for organizational problems. Physician leaders are also instrumental in gaining the support of their peers in organizational change. The traditional "separate but equal" hierarchies that characterize health care decision-making structures persist in keeping medical and administrative decisions apart. To overcome such artificial boundaries, health care leaders must seek out physicians who are willing to partner with administrators at multiple levels in leading organizational change.

• *Minimize boundaries.* Physician participation in organizational decision making occurs only if the incentives across the organization are aligned to support their contributions outside of clinical areas. Physicians and administrators need to know that the organization values and rewards participation in activities that foster team decision making. Further, the organization's policies must promote integrating information from multiple sources that collectively contribute to good clinical and management decisions (Barnsley et al. 1998).

Ultimately, successful health care organizations will be those that learn to communicate across formal and informal boundaries. Boundaries may be ideological, vertical, horizontal, geographic, external, or a result of time (Barnsley et al. 1998). Regardless of the type of boundary, these restrictions create limits on what our health care organizations might become. The goal is to become "boundaryless" in seeking options to improve health care.

CONCLUSION

This chapter examined some of the underlying changes occurring in the health care industry and an analysis of how these changes are transforming the business of health care. Understanding the nature of the changes in the health care industry serves as a platform for assessing the changing roles for CQI within health care organizations. New approaches to transform CQI are presented so that it better attends to both incremental and radical changes that are needed for organizational learning. This chapter empha-sized the development of organizational structures and processes that promote mass customization and challenges health service providers and organizations to look beyond traditional roles and methods for ways to improve services for individual customers. Professional managers and clinicians are both involved in leading health care organizations, and both must adopt strategies for securing physician participation and leadership in organizational learning and change.

CHAPTER 8

The Process of Implementation

Lucy R. Fischer, Leif I. Solberg, and Thomas E. Kottke

While many organizations have implemented continuous quality improvement (CQI), few have assessed the process and the factors that influence that process:

- How does change in the health care environment affect a quality improvement (QI) process?
- How does clinic organization influence a QI process?
- What is the impact of a QI process on clinic organization?

The following analysis is part of a larger study presented in Chapter 13 by Solberg, Kottke, and Brekke. Below is a description of the quality improvement initiative entitled Project IMPROVE and an analysis of selected clinics relevant to understanding the implementation process and some of the factors that influence that process.

PROJECT IMPROVE

IMPROVE (Improving Prevention through Organization, Vision, and Empowerment) was a four-year study that began in July 1993 and was designed to test the hypothesis that primary care clinics can increase their preventive service delivery rates by learning and applying CQI concepts to the development of prevention systems. The 44 primary care clinics

Source: L. Fischer et al., Quality Improvement in Primary Care Clinics, © *JCAHO Journal on Quality Improvement*, 24:7, Oakbrook Terrace, IL: Joint Commission on Accreditation of Healthcare Organizations, 1998, 361–370. Adapted with permission.

volunteering to participate in the project were randomly divided into 22 comparison sites (that is, left alone) and 22 sites that received an intervention from the IMPROVE project beginning in September 1994.

The intervention consisted of a program of leadership facilitation, training, consultation, and networking. Each of these program elements was designed to facilitate a CQI process focused on eight adult preventive services: (1) mammograms, (2) breast examinations, (3) Papanicolaou (Pap) smears, (4) tobacco use, (5) hypertension, (6) hypercholesterolemia, and (7) influenza and (8) pneumonia shots. These systems generally consisted of methods for consistently identifying the prevention needs of individual patients as they visited the clinic, reminding clinicians about which preventive services each patient needed, and ensuring that those needs were met in a comprehensive way.

Two persons (a team leader and a facilitator) from each clinic were invited to participate in six group training sessions that lasted four hours each and were conducted during a six-month period. The training consisted of a series of modules to teach the skills and tasks needed to implement an improvement process and develop systematic prevention processes.

During the training process, each team leader and facilitator met biweekly with an interdisciplinary team within their own clinic to define their goals and current process, gather and analyze data on needs and problems, develop and implement systems to increase preventive service delivery rates, and evaluate the systems' effectiveness. Throughout a 21-month period, both the clinic and team leaders had access to regular consultation with IMPROVE trainers. In addition, bimonthly networking sessions for team leaders and facilitators offered opportunities to share ideas, materials, and experiences with other clinics participating in the intervention.

The intervention was designed as a training-consultation model that any external organization, such as an HMO or a preferred provider organization, could implement to help clinics improve their preventive service delivery rates. Each clinic team, although offered substantial information and advice through Project IMPROVE, made its own decisions about how to proceed and what specific form of prevention system to implement (Solberg et al. 1995; Solberg et al. 1996; Solberg et al. 1997d).

Case Studies

Case studies were conducted in a sample of 6 of the 22 clinics participating in the intervention arm of the IMPROVE trial. The case studies' purpose was to provide a qualitative analysis of *the process* of developing and implementing a CQI process in primary care clinics.

Sample

A stratified random sample of intervention clinics was selected for in-depth case studies: three large clinics (employing eight or more physicians) and three small clinics (employing seven or fewer physicians). When one clinic from each size category declined to participate as a case study site because of concern about time demands, two additional names were drawn randomly from the remaining clinics. Characteristics of the six case study clinics are shown in Table 8–1. Project IMPROVE was initiated in September 1994. The case study interviews were conducted from January through June 1996, approximately 16 months later, at a time when most of the clinics had already implemented systems for improving prevention services.

Data

The case study data consisted of results of open-ended interviews with "informants" and observations of CQI team meetings. The informants included two to four members of each CQI team plus other nonteam members knowledgeable about the project. Altogether, 30 interviews were conducted with clinic staff, and five team meetings were observed from January through June 1996. Detailed notes were transcribed for each interview and meeting observation. The interviews, each approximately

Table 8–1 Characteristics of Six Case Study Clinics

Clinic	Primary Care Physician (FTE*)	Staff	Patients/ Week	Year Founded
A	1.2	103	1,500	1965
B	1.1	64	1,250	1929
C	1.0	177	1,266	1975
D	4.0	19	missing	1964
E	1.5	7	160	1988
F	4.0	24	650	1947

Note: Data on clinics' characteristics were collected in 1994, when Project IMPROVE began.
*FTE, full-time equivalent.

30–45 minutes long, examined *the process of* participating in this QI initiative, focusing on informants' accounts of the history of the clinic's involvement in the project and their perceptions about the team experience.

In addition, IMPROVE researchers/consultants contributed to the qualitative study their accumulated documentation on the clinics and teams. Concern about intrusion and additional burden on the clinics arose because participation in Project IMPROVE required substantial amounts of clinic time. Whenever possible, data were drawn from existing IMPROVE sources to lessen some of the time involved. IMPROVE researchers also were interviewed and provided their own observations and insights for the qualitative analysis.

Analysis

The data were analyzed in five ways. First, each interview or set of observations was studied to identify themes and generate concepts. Second, data from each "case" (each clinic/team) were reviewed to assess and compare the experiences and perspectives of multiple informants. Third, all the open-ended data were coded and organized for a thematic analysis. The coding involved an iterative process: initial coding to identify themes, grouping data by themes, refining the codes, regrouping, and so forth. Throughout this process each unit of data was assigned an identifier so the context could be recalled for validation. Fourth, a conceptual framework was developed, stimulated by relevant research and theory literature. Finally, other analysts (including IMPROVE researchers) provided feedback and insights on preliminary analyses and interpretations.

Limitations

Three factors limit generalizability from the case studies. First, the 44 Project IMPROVE clinics do not constitute a nationally representative sample: They are all located in the same HMO-dominated region, within 60 miles of the Twin Cities, in the metro area and nearby towns in Minnesota and Wisconsin. Although the clinics varied in size, none is really large and none is a solo practice. Second, the case examples are not necessarily representative of the full sample of IMPROVE clinics inasmuch as they constitute a small sample selected randomly from a small pool. Finally, the interview and observation data reflect the perceptions of a limited number of informants at a particular time. Perceptions about a team process might differ not only among individuals but also over time, reflecting events and changing circumstances.

HOW DOES CHANGE IN THE HEALTH CARE ENVIRONMENT AFFECT A CQI PROCESS?

During the intervention phase of Project IMPROVE, two-thirds of the clinics were involved in some form of substantial reorganization, including mergers and acquisitions (Magnan et al. 1997). Thus, CQI was introduced to the clinics as a method for innovation within the context of turmoil and rapid change in the health care environment (Hoff and McCaffrey 1996).

As Exhibit 8–1 shows, all the smaller clinics in the case study sample allied with large conglomerates of health care organizations during the study period. In the process, each clinic essentially lost much of its independence. The mergers led to changes in staff, procedures, equipment, location, and administrative structures. For example, when Project IMPROVE was initiated Clinic D was independent and affiliated with several other clinics, all located in small towns within the same region. Soon after the project was launched, a large HMO bought out the affiliation of clinics. The HMO introduced a number of technologic improvements across clinic sites, such as a new telephone system and a personal computer with software designed to be compatible with the HMO's. The team leader commented: "It's a stressful time because of the changes in the environment. It's stressful for everyone, not just me or the providers. The positive part is that it's an opportunity. We're on the same learning curve, learning the computer and the phone, together. It's a time to problem solve and share and teach each other."

Another small clinic, Clinic E, aborted its IMPROVE project and never actually developed or implemented a comprehensive prevention system. This clinic had undergone what it described as "huge changes" in administrative organization. Before IMPROVE was launched, the clinic had belonged to a loose affiliation of small clinics. This group of clinics was bought out by a much larger health care network, which then centralized most administrative services. The physician team leader commented:

Exhibit 8–1 Overview of Project IMPROVE in the Six Case Study Clinics

Overview	Health care environment	Impact of IMPROVE
Larger clinics		
Clinic A		
The project is led by a physician team leader and a nurse facilitator, both of whom are very active in the project. Clinic has invested substantial resources in Project IMPROVE. The team has argued that the project will bring economic benefit to the clinic by increasing fee-for-service business. The clinic provides lunches during team meetings and pays all staff for time spent on the project. This team has used unusually creative efforts— such as humorous skits and bulletin boards—to publicize team activities.	No mergers during this project.	Top priority for clinic Using CQI for other projects.
Clinic B		
A physician with a strong interest in preventive services is the team leader; a nurse is the facilitator. Both have been actively engaged in the project, along with other team members. Despite major upheaval in the clinic as the result of a merger, the project has proceeded and appears to have an impact on preventive services. When the clinic demanded that Project IMPROVE be put on hold, the team refused. Their chart audits showed improvement in all their preventive services.	Merged with another clinic in town; became monopoly in small town.	Top priority for clinic; project continued despite merger. Chart audit showed improvement on all preventive services. Using CQI for other projects

continues

Exhibit 8–1 continued

Overview	Health care environment	Impact of IMPROVE
Clinic C		
Although two physicians were initially involved, by the end of the project, a nurse was both the team leader and the facilitator. The sponsor is also a team member. Team members appear to be quite committed to the project. Lack of physician leadership may make it more difficult to obtain the commitment of other physicians in the clinic. Flowcharting, a CQI method for systematically identifying problems in operations, was very difficult for this team; they felt frustrated with the amount of time this exercise required. However, it provided critical information. For example, it showed how patients were not being properly followed in their system.	Suburban clinic, trying to stay independent. Substantial turnover in management and other staff.	Created a new history and physical form. Anecdotal evidence of improved preventive services. IMPROVE team is CQI team for clinic.

Smaller clinics

Overview	Health care environment	Impact of IMPROVE
Clinic D		
The team leader is a young physician assistant who has put a lot of energy and time into the project. Her enthusiasm and commitment have been the most important factors in sustaining the project in this clinic. At the time at which the interviews were conducted, team members were concerned that the project was losing steam, and there was decreasing compliance with the prevention system they had implemented. The physician	Affiliated with a network of clinics bought out by an HMO.	Raised awareness about preventive services, but increased concern about the decreasing use of the prevention services form.

continues

Exhibit 8–1 continued

Overview	Health care environment	Impact of IMPROVE
assistant's role on the team was described, by herself and others, as useful for her career in the clinic.		Using CQI for other projects
Clinic E		
In this very small clinic, a physician and her medical assistant are the only team members. The clinic has experienced substantial turmoil and change since Project IMPROVE began. This clinic has had only limited involvement in Project IMPROVE, in part because of the environmental factors and the clinic's small size and lack of resources. Although the team developed a prevention form to be used in the charts, they did very little implementing and more or less dropped the project: "We've put in less—and we've got less out. . . ."	Belonged to a loose network of clinics that was bought out by a larger medical organiza-tion.	Project IMPROVE aborted; did not implement comprehensive prevention system. Raised awareness about process.
Clinic F		
In this small clinic, the team consists of a nurse, a certified medical assistant, and a receptionist. They stopped having regular meetings early in the project, although they would meet in the hallways to discuss the project. They said that it did not make sense to have formal meetings in their clinic. They implemented a reminder form, after which they believed some preventive services increased in	Merged with another clinic, then pulled into a large medical organizaiton.	Made CQI process more informal. Perception that preventive services improved.

continues

Exhibit 8–1 continued

Overview	Health care environment	Impact of IMPROVE
frequency. They complained that they have too few people to meet and spend time on this project. Posters on the examination room walls alert patients to preventive services.		Using CQI for other projects.

"From the point of doing our original chart audits, there have been so many external changes that they would have dwarfed anything we could have done through the IMPROVE project. . . . Our system has lost to entropy."

One of the larger clinics, Clinic B, merged with another clinic. The top management wanted to put the project "on hold" while they were in the throes of the merger. It was only through the insistence of the physician team leader and other team members that the project continued. Even so, the merger complicated the IMPROVE project. For example, the IMPROVE team had developed a system for sending reminder letters to patients who had not had recent mammograms. After the merger, the system for documenting mammograms was at risk of falling apart because staff in the radiology department had come from the other (non-IMPROVE) clinic site and did not understand the new protocol. In a general sense, team members were worried about loss of influence in their organization, which was now much larger and involved a merger of cultures. A team member complained: "With the old group, it was easy to get things set up and going. Now we have to go through committees and it takes too long. It's important to get going; the committees can be a big holdup. . . . To get that many doctors to do something will be impossible. Good ideas will be dropped, so two years of work may go down the tubes. If everybody doesn't buy in, it goes by the wayside."

The physician team leader commented, "We have good working relationships with physicians at [XYZ] Clinic, but their systems are different, so there's a lot to be worked out." The change in the workplace environment increased the stress level. The physician team leader added, "If it had been implemented at a different time than [after] the merger, it would have been better. . . . It was a little overwhelming. There were all these new forms—just learning how to use a new voice mail. And then we had to learn the flow sheets. . . ."

The relationship between environmental instability and Project IMPROVE is complex. On one level, the stress associated with environmental change and uncertainty constitutes an obstacle to QI. But from another perspective, Project IMPROVE *was a response to an environment of uncertainty.* It was designed for an environment where change not only is widespread but also may connote *desirable improvement.* In essence, many of the clinics were motivated to participate in Project IMPROVE *because* they exist in an unstable, highly competitive, and uncertain environment where change management skills could prove valuable, perhaps even necessary for survival (Flood and Fennell 1995; Tuckman 1992; Glassman 1995; Peters 1994).

Project IMPROVE offered an ideology of change and adaptation and a systematic methodology for QI. In this sense, the project provided an appealing solution to the problem of environmental uncertainty. As Flood and Fennell (1995) have stated:

> The adoption of expensive cost systems and CQI techniques can be explained as an example of mimetic pressure, the pressure to mimic seemingly successful organizations. This pressure stems from the need to "do something" when conditions become uncertain. When successful adaptation is not well understood, an easy path is to copy or mimic what other organizations have done, particularly those which appear to be doing well. . . . New forms of management are adopted, not because they are known to help the organization, but because they reflect current norms and beliefs about what modern managers do (16).

The project successfully recruited primary care clinics (for the scientific trial) on the basis of the perceived potency of process improvement methodology. When asked why his clinic agreed to be part of Project IMPROVE, a physician at Clinic D said, "We jumped at the chance. It is exciting to improve care to patients; this includes preventive services." All the clinics made a business decision in committing staff time to Project

IMPROVE. Participation offered a potential competitive advantage associated with being an early adopter of process improvement in the region (Solberg et al. 1997).

HOW DOES CLINIC ORGANIZATION INFLUENCE A QI PROCESS?

A recent study of QI in hospitals reported that larger hospitals, tending to be more hierarchical, are less effective in implementing QI efforts than smaller hospitals (Carman et al. 1996; Peters 1994). Our qualitative analysis of Project IMPROVE also suggests that clinic size is an important factor in shaping a QI process. In contrast to the hospital QI study, however, the three larger clinics in our case study sample appeared to absorb the process improvement initiative with the most ease, whereas the QI process seemed to overwhelm the three small clinics. The study settings are different, of course—hospitals versus primary care clinics—so these observations are not necessarily mutually contradictory. Moreover, both our qualitative study of IMPROVE and results from the hospital QI survey underscore the importance of organizational features. Social theorists and management consultants have argued that organizations need to be adaptive and flexible to survive in a rapidly changing environment (Kaluzny et al. 1992; Solberg et al. 1995; Felkins et al. 1993; Tornatzky et al. 1980; Glassman 1995; Peters 1994). The implication is clear—the ability to adapt is, at least in part, related to organization factors.

Our analysis suggests that clinic size is associated with two underlying factors: access to resources and cultural compatibility. The relative lack of resources in the smallest clinics made the QI process more difficult. In addition, the formal QI process, as developed by Project IMPROVE, seemed inept and awkward in the small clinics.

A number of studies have found that access to "slack resources" is a key predictor of ability to innovate (Damanpour 1991). The case examples illustrate how having relatively easy access to funds and personnel time can facilitate a change process, whereas, conversely, lack of available funds (worrying about survival) is a serious impediment.

One of the large clinics, Clinic A, invested substantial resources in the IMPROVE initiative. For example, this was the only site (out of the six case study clinics) that provided lunch for members during their noon meetings to compensate team members for giving up their lunch hour. The clinic administration also allocated paid coverage for time staff spent away from their departments working on the IMPROVE team. Moreover, the clinic hired a chart auditor to identify needed prevention services of scheduled patients as part of the new prevention system. Its investment was, in large part, motivated by an expectation that in a fee-for-service context, augmenting preventive services would generate increased revenues: "We estimated the clinic could earn up to $1.6 million more." The decision to hire an additional clerical person was based on this calculation. "It was unusual that they approved [hiring the chart auditor]. . . . At the meeting one of the doctors [not on the team] said: 'Is there any question about this?' and the whole thing took three minutes to approve."

Clinics B and C, the other large clinics, were somewhat more cautious about direct monetary expenditures for IMPROVE. Even so, they brought substantial resources to the project: meeting time for 6 to 10 clinic employees, supplies, and expertise (for example, experience with chart audits and research). Although the larger clinics, including Clinic A, were concerned about the project's cost, they were able to invest in their future, knowing that monies spent on the project would eventually increase revenues.

In contrast, the smaller clinics (D, E, and F) were more constrained in their ability to invest in future potential earnings. The team leader at Clinic D lamented, "Size is the major issue. There is no one to relieve people to [work on the team]." In general, resources were tight. The clinic did not have appropriate meeting space (team members had to use a meeting room in an adjacent building), and it lacked equipment and special expertise. The clinic had only one transcriptionist, who did almost all the typing and copying for the team, taking her hours away from her regular job. Because no funds were available to cover staff for their time on the team, some of the cost for doing the project was borne by team members contributing their own time. This was especially true of the team leader, who contributed a large number of hours of her own time. She reported that her husband also spent about 30 hours working at home with her on a spreadsheet: "It's hard not to be envious of larger clinics—all the resources they have, like an IS [Information Services] department that can help them collect and analyze data. We don't even have a PC, and where we do have some equipment, we don't have the skills."

The team leaders at Clinic E, which terminated its IMPROVE initiative, blamed the project's failure on their clinic's size and lack of resources: "It's harder in a small clinic. . . . We have two and a half doctors and about seven or eight employees. We're small and still getting off the ground

. . . the clinic started about eight and a half years ago. We don't even have time for cleaning or stocking. . . .We have no administration time in our schedules, so everything we do comes out of clinic time, our working time."

Theoretically, small size should facilitate innovation. Compared with large clinics, a small clinic might have a more cohesive staff and fewer bureaucratic hurdles, as Shortell and colleagues concluded in their study of QI in hospitals (Shortell et al. 1995). Even so, a QI process requires an investment in infrastructure, and to a large degree entails a fixed cost, irrespective of clinic size. Thus, the cost is likely to be especially burdensome for small clinics with little capital.

Clinic size is also related to another factor: the compatibility of a particular culture and specific change process. In his classic book, *Diffusion of Innovations*, Rogers (1995) argued that innovation is most likely to be accepted when it is consistent with the experience and values of a culture. The larger clinics were organized into departments or units. The IMPROVE project recommendation that teams be composed of representatives from a cross section of units or personnel positions made sense within this type of organization. Moreover, these clinics frequently organized committees to address various problems or tasks. Committee work is always expensive and takes time away from revenue-generating activities. Even so, the formal structure of IMPROVE was compatible with these clinics' tradition and experience.

In contrast, the team leaders in the smallest clinics, Clinic E and F, complained that Project IMPROVE did not fit well within their organizations; they had only a handful of staff who interacted with one another informally virtually everyday, so that the formal meeting process seemed awkward and inappropriate. A physician in Clinic E asserted, "It's difficult to make something that will work in all sites."

WHAT IS THE IMPACT OF A QI PROCESS ON CLINIC ORGANIZATION?

Project IMPROVE introduced a new paradigm to primary care clinics in a double sense: the CQI approach and the focus on prevention systems. CQI, offering a systematic change process and emphasizing continuous improvement rather than a one time "fix," is intended to change the perception about management. Furthermore, it undermines the traditional hierarchical method of decision making and introduces a more interpersonally complex operational method. Concurrently, IMPROVE created a new paradigm for preventative services—not only emphasizing the importance of prevention but also encouraging clinics to integrate prevention into routine medical care.

In his book *The Structure of Scientific Revolutions,* Thomas Kuhn (1962) described the concept of paradigm shift in science: "Led by new paradigm . . . It is rather as if the professional community had been suddenly transported to another planet where familiar objects are seen in a different light" (110). For clinic IMPROVE leaders and team members alike, acceptance of the IMPROVE paradigm entailed a conversion experience expressed in several ways. First, faith in the project was emphasized: "People on the committee truly believe in this." Second, an insistence on the uniqueness of this commitment—that IMPROVE is qualitatively different from other committees—was evident. Third, the ideology was suggested by a shared language code associated with IMPROVE concepts. For example, team members insisted that quick solutions to problem solving are "just Band-Aids." Another example is the fact that a number of informants at different sites repeated the phrase, "Titles are dropped at the door."

Although case study observations suggested that the physician title tended to be used in team meetings, it appeared that the ideology of equal participation was an accepted and shared concept. A number of theorists have discussed the importance of perception, belief, or faith in adopting innovation. Faith in a new paradigm is a critical factor because the change process is difficult and expensive. In all the case study clinics, expressions of faith in their new CQI paradigm were heard. In this sense, Project IMPROVE appears to have had a qualitative impact on each of the clinics.

Diffusion of an administrative innovation, such as a QI process or a prevention system, however, is much more difficult than a technologic or material innovation (Rogers 1995; Kaluzny et al. 1992). Whereas the relative advantage of the latter tends to be clear, administrative change is often complex and difficult to understand. Our case studies illustrate the difficulty and tenuousness of administrative innovation. For example, the CQI process was often slow and time-consuming. A member of the team in Clinic A commented, "We never made fast progress. . . . The whole process is tedious. As individuals we would like to see things solved quickly. I felt frustrated when some doctors were asking, 'What are we accomplishing?' and I couldn't produce anything just yet." The project in that clinic seemed to operate in stops and starts, going for long periods with no team meetings. Although a productive meeting was observed in January 1996, the team had not met since October 1995 (they were waiting to hire a chart auditor who would play a key role in the project).

A related problem was the time needed to implement the prevention system. A nurse in Clinic C said, "We room six patients an hour. If a nurse adds additional questions and it takes one minute more, for 36 patients, that's an additional half hour. So that's a problem." Most of the clinics indicated that they were not able to implement their new prevention system at all times and with all patients. A nurse at Clinic F commented, "There are days when scheduling is horrid and we just don't use the IMPROVE form. Our doctors are overwhelmed since Dr. I's heart attack. . . . [On some days] I get yelled at if I try to get them to counsel about prevention services."

Time was also a factor in the issue of clinics' innovative systems over time. The concern of team members at Clinic D about recidivism, for example, was evident in comments such as "now people are backing off from using [the prevention tool] that was being filled out here and there. A lot of stuff isn't being done."

Finally, getting buy-in from other staff at the clinic was, at best, a formidable challenge. All the case study teams confronted substantial resistance from some individuals or groups within the clinics. In most of the clinics, a process of rejection and negotiation helped other staff feel empowered in the change process. For example, when physicians and nurses were uncomfortable using a prevention form developed by the team, they were given an opportunity to revise it. This feedback mechanism helped other staff to feel empowered in the change process. The teams used various "trickle in" methods for communicating with other clinic staff and implementing a change process. For example, Clinic B's team initially attempted to put prevention stickers on every chart that came through the clinic. After it became apparent that this effort was too burdensome, the team designated no more than six new charts a day per clinician for the new prevention system. In effect, they succeeded in "breaking down" a complex system so that dissemination became more feasible and palatable (Rogers 1995).

Despite these difficulties, our qualitative analysis indicates that Project IMPROVE had two substantive impacts on the clinics. First, the project enhanced awareness about preventive services, for both the patients and the professional staff. The increased emphasis on prevention was noticeable on entering the clinics, most of which displayed postures and brochures on improvement in their preventive services. A member of Clinic

B's team remarked, "The patients are getting more educated. . . . I sit by the lab control desk, so I overhear more people scheduling protocols. And I've seen a lot of patients in the lobby reading the boards." (A more quantitative analysis of the impact on preventive services will be reported in Chapter 13.)

Second, one of the findings noted in the case studies was that in all these clinics, the CQI method was being applied to other problems and issues. A team member from Clinic A, for example, reported, "Now they're beginning to talk about a process for Peds [Pediatrics]—the Peds doctors are interested. It's exciting that Peds found out what we're doing and wants to be part of it." Similarly, a team member at Clinic B commented, "It taught us a lot about CQI, how useful it is. . . . We have some spin-off projects now, like in UC [Urgent Care]. It takes it out of the personality conflicts, gives us a problem-solving approach." All the clinics had examples of applying the change concepts and methods to other areas and needs.

CONCLUSION

An Unstable and Uncertain Environment

Our case study analysis suggests that environmental change has a paradoxical effect. Environmental instability complicates an improvement process, yet the changing environment also forces changes to be made and stimulates improvement. To survive in an uncertain, unstable, and highly competitive environment, an organization needs to change and adapt. Thus, the application of QI methods is essentially a way to respond to an environment of "perpetual revolution" (Peters 1994).

One implication is that environmental change is not necessarily a sole reason to delay QI efforts. To the contrary, leaders in HMOs or other change agents in regions wrestling with change might want to encourage QI in medical clinics as an appropriate and potentially rewarding response to competition and change. Of course, an organization in chaos, uncertain of its very survival, might be unable to launch an orderly improvement process. So a balance between sufficient strength and stability to sustain operations, and environmental competition and change to motivate improvement, is necessary.

Organization and Culture

Our case studies of the smallest clinics suggest that an elaborate change process may be too costly for clinics with few resources. Although the improvement process and change concepts were useful, in the very smallest clinics a large team structure was awkward and seemed to be incompatible with the organization structure and culture. The lesson learned was that one format does not fit all situations. Thus, the CQI process needs to be flexible, adaptable, and variable.

The QI Process and the Impact on Clinics

A QI approach in medical clinics appears to have a number of qualitative benefits that are difficult to quantify. For example, the approach creates a cross-departmental functioning team useful for addressing various organizational problems and tasks. All the case study clinics found the CQI process useful and applied it to other problems and tasks, thus creating an apparent ongoing diffusion of the change process. Moreover, involvement in a QI effort raises awareness about important issues in providing health care. Participation in Project IMPROVE increased the focus on preventive services, with discussions in staff meetings, posters in lobbies and examination rooms, and educational materials all emphasizing the importance of these services. Finally, another significant benefit of the project was an enhanced awareness about the importance of, and techniques for, improvement. In effect, the IMPROVE teams, by all their activities in the clinics, increased sensitivity about specific needs for change and also promoted the concept that clinics can and should improve their systems of care.

CHAPTER 9

Information Management and Technology for CQI

David C. Kibbe

As health care organizations supplement a decade of experience with continuous quality improvement (CQI) with a rigorous population-based approach to performance improvements fueled by the managed care environment, their leaders must anticipate the need for a strategy to manage emerging data and information. This chapter is intended to help health care leaders visualize the role of information technology in their performance improvement strategy, regardless of the size of the organization or its mission. The chapter presents a framework for the management of informational resources along the continuum from data collection, to information and knowledge management, to decision making. It also describes how recent advances in information technology (IT), including the Internet and World Wide Web, make it possible to support and enhance health care CQI efforts given the right mixture of leadership, training, technological expertise, and financial investment.

The health care information technology industry is very large and growing, both in terms of the numbers of products and the resources expended on them annually by health care organizations. Table 9–1 is a list of the top 25 health care information systems companies ranked by 1997 revenues, a group whose sales of software and information systems amounted to $5.3 billion in just that single year (*Healthcare Informatics* 1998). As an indication of the size of this industry's segment devoted to quality and performance, The Joint Commission on Accreditation of Healthcare Organizations (Joint Commission), at the time of this writing, had selected more than 125 vendors' outcomes and performance measurement information systems as meeting accreditation requirements for the Joint Commission's Oryx initiative (Joint Commission 1998).

Table 9–1 1997 Revenues for Top 25 U.S. Information System Vendors

Company	Location	Revenue $M
HBOC	Atlanta	$ 1,203
SMS	Malvern, PA	$ 896
Science Applications International Corp. (SAIC)	San Diego	$ 351
IDX Systems Corp.	Burlington, VT	$ 251
Cerner Corp.	Kansas City, MO	$ 245
Medic Computer Systems, Inc.	Raleigh, NC	$ 245
Lanier Worldwide, Inc.	Atlanta	$ 198
Medical Information Technology (MEDITECH)	Westwood, MA	$ 194
Per-Se Technologies	Atlanta	$ 182
National Data Corporation-NDC Health Information Services	Atlanta	$ 176
CSC Healthcare	Southfield, MI	$ 150
ENVOY Corporation	Nashville, TN	$ 114
PeopleSoft, Inc.	Pleasanton, CA	$ 113
Sunquest Information Systems, Inc.	Tucson, AZ	$ 102
Physician Computer Network	Morris Plains, NJ	$ 100
Eclipsys Corp.	Delray Beach, FL	$ 99
3M Health Information Systems	Murray, UT	$ 90
Health Management Systems, Inc.	New York City	$ 90
Companion Technologies	Columbia, SC	$ 89
HCIA, Inc.	Baltimore	$ 83
Synertech	Harrisburg, PA	$ 79
Medical Manager Corp.	Tampa, FL	$ 78
SAS Institute	Cary, NC	$ 69
Protocol Systems	Beaverton, OR	$ 64
Geac Computer Corporation, Ltd.	Markham, Ontario, Canada	$ 57

It would be mistake, however, to think that CQI in health care requires expensive, sophisticated software programs. There is available a large selection of easy-to-use general purpose personal computer (PC) applications for collection, storage, and analysis of data, capable of meeting many of the needs of quality improvement teams and quality managers. This chapter concentrates less on the choices of particular software programs or vendors' products than on the underlying components and functions that are most usefully applied to the study of health care processes, to understanding the causes of variation in process outcomes, and to the efforts to make improvements. This approach emphasizes the underlying concepts involved, while simultaneously immunizing the content against the swirling winds of technological change, mergers and acquisitions in the IT industry, and new product developments!

Information technologies do not in and of themselves solve many quality problems. More sophisticated information technology, which brings greater access to more data, more information, and more advanced decision aids, does not guarantee better decisions or better decision makers. We live in a world enamored of technological solutions and bedazzled by the progress we've made in getting machines to operate at faster speeds across farther and farther reaches. In fact, despite enormous promise and hype from the media, software vendors, and consultants, modern information systems may in fact *detract* from a health care organization's overall ability to improve performance. Today's frantic and increasingly impersonal electronic world, replete with fax machines, voice and e-mail, has as much potential to create confusion in an organization's processes—and disorientation or even alienation among an organization's members, who are urged to "adopt and adapt"—as it has potential to improve productivity, enhance quality, or bring clarity to complex decisions.

The approach to information management and technology's role in quality improvement efforts, therefore, calls for a balance between skills, methods, and technologies, together with some skepticism about what can be accomplished through the application of systems from software vendors.

A FRAMEWORK FOR CQI INFORMATION MANAGEMENT: THE DATA-TO-DECISION CYCLE

Information Management Under QA and CQI

CQI challenges many of the assumptions held by both traditional quality assurance (QA) and health care information services (IS) bureaucracies regarding health care information and its uses. There are important differences between QA and CQI regarding the kind and scope of data to be collected, who collects the data, and where the data are used to make improvements in quality. Because of these differences, the shift from QA to CQI calls for an entirely new approach to the management of health care quality-related data and information.

In the traditional hospital clinical QA program, data flow in a convergent path from patient charts located on the hospital wards, through staff reviewers from the QA department, to centralized peer review committees. QA data are usually collected by hand, and analysis is limited to simple counts and percentages. Reviewers screen cases for adverse occurrences, tally events, and report summary information. Data may not be displayed, nor widely disseminated. In fact, clinicians receive feedback from this process only when their performance is unacceptable. Finally, any action to address problems or make improvements must originate from the central peer review committees. Utilization review data are often collected by the same reviewers for a different set of peer review committees.

Information management systems in hospitals have been driven by the requirements of administrative and financial functions, such as billing, purchasing, payroll, and accounting, not by the needs of quality improvement. Typically, a central IS department staffed by systems analysts and managers maintains computers and data systems to serve these administrative functions. IS-supported hospital data management systems are not linked to quality-related data collection efforts except to supply quality analysts with patient identification information, diagnostic codes, and length of stay data. In effect, administrative data management and clinical quality improvement have remained separate domains, with distinct information needs and uses. The common thread linking administrative data management and traditional QA activities is that they both exhibit a convergent flow of data whose endpoint is upper management. Convergent data flow, storage, analysis, and usage are the sine qua non of *centralized data management*.

CQI Calls for Decentralized Management of Data, Information, and Knowledge

In contrast to QA, one of CQI's central requirements is that cross-disciplinary teams composed of managers *and* front-line employees participate in the collection and analysis of process- and outcomes-related data, as well as in the decisions about what data should be collected and what actions should be taken to bring about improvements. The scope of the information that could be relevant to such teams is very broad: It routinely includes both clinical and administrative data captured from multiple sources inside and even outside the organization. For example, a CQI team charged with improving the emergency room evaluation of patients with chest pain would gather information directly from patients and other customers; from the current medical literature; from suppliers of medical and diagnostic equipment; from data systems containing financial, scheduling, and demographic information; and from patient charts, among other sources. Furthermore, CQI team members commonly analyze the data and take action at the local level and share data with other teams. This combination of activities that improvement teams perform can be termed *decentralized data management*.

Dispersed and decentralized data traffic of this sort lends itself to personal computing and other network technologies (e.g. groupware and e-mail). In fact, health care organizations implementing CQI have found that quality improvement teams spontaneously reach for desktop software to aid them in handling their data management needs. Decentralization also requires wide dissemination of new skills in the management of data, information, and knowledge to adequately support organizationwide CQI. When these skills are merely an afterthought, as they often are, problems quickly arise that can place the entire CQI initiative in jeopardy.

> Two years into the adoption of a CQI program, the leadership at Alpha Medical Center felt optimistic about their progress. Every employee had received basic training in the principles and methods of quality improvement. A quality management department had been established to coordinate CQI activities. Most important, they had initiated more than 30 CQI projects, ranging from improvements in the hospital paging systems to benchmarking the preoperative cardiology consultation process. A number of significant cost savings and quality improvements could be documented.
>
> Unfortunately, the hospital CQI program had rapidly acquired almost as many approaches to managing data and information, and as many computer software packages, as it had CQI teams. Several teams chose special purpose, personal computer-based quality control software to help them draw graphs and charts, but used other software to gather and analyze data. Some teams used software that was based in a departmental minicomputer and required special programming to use. A few teams refused to take advantage of the risk adjustment software purchased by the IS department for the quality management department, saying that

the physicians on their teams did not trust the methodology to be reliable. Two teams farmed out all their graphical display work to the hospital medical arts department while sending their data management problems to the IS staff. Still others opted to hand-draw most of their charts and graphs. The result after two years: a Tower of Babel consisting of many languages and many methods for handling quality-related data and information. Software incompatibility caused duplication of efforts when teams tried to share data sets and had to re-enter information, made training and support by IS staff almost impossible, and left everyone wishing they had planned this aspect of the CQI initiative more carefully from the start. Now the center is about to launch a CQI project team to improve the support of CQI itself!

The organization depicted here is not incompetent, nor should its members reject CQI when they encounter these kinds of problems. Rather, they need to recognize that CQI in complex organizations is a data- and information-intensive enterprise, and that it is dynamic. If successful, CQI increases the demands within the organization for access to data, information, and knowledge from a whole new set of "customers" with a whole new set of questions they'd like answered. As this phenomenon, seen over and over within health care organizations that have adopted CQI, occurs, organizational leaders must be ready to guide the organization to a new level of expertise with information management and technology.

A framework presented in this chapter is called the Data-to-Decision cycle. It recognizes that both centralized and decentralized data management needs exist in complex organizations such as hospitals and provider networks. The Data-to-Decision cycle, however, offers all organizational members a framework for understanding how information management and technology that they use is capable of promoting the best possible performance of the organization as a whole.

The Data-to-Decision Cycle

The Data-to-Decision cycle is illustrated in Figure 9–1. The cycle describes how *data* are transformed to *information*, how *information* becomes *knowledge*, and how *knowledge* supports *decisions* and actions for improved performance. The cycle suggests that in the ideal setting data collection efforts occur as the routine delivery of health care occurs, and that our performance improvement decisions determine what data are to be

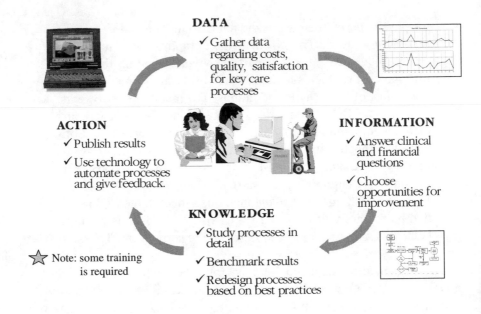

DATA
- ✓ Gather data regarding costs, quality, satisfaction for key care processes

INFORMATION
- ✓ Answer clinical and financial questions
- ✓ Choose opportunities for improvement

KNOWLEDGE
- ✓ Study processes in detail
- ✓ Benchmark results
- ✓ Redesign processes based on best practices

ACTION
- ✓ Publish results
- ✓ Use technology to automate processes and give feedback.

☆ Note: some training is required

Figure 9–1 The Data-to-Action Cycle

collected in the future, thus improving the feedback between data and decisions.

The cycle uses terms that are commonly used as synonyms: *data, information*, and *knowledge*. Information management for CQI, however, requires that these terms be defined more precisely, and the distinctions between them be clarified.

Data are facts. Data elements by themselves have no meaning: They are simply isolated facts. For example, in Figure 9–2 we see that in the month of April there were 14 medication errors reported from nursing unit 12BG. Management at the data level is concerned with the problems relating to the accuracy of the facts, their accessibility, their formatting or organization, and their storage. Data that are accurate and structured properly can be retrieved easily and combined with other data elements in a relational database for purposes of analysis. Conversely, data of poor quality, or stored in nonstandard formats, may be next to impossible to find, and therefore useless for performance improvement work.

Information is data that has become meaningful. Data assembled to answer someone's question becomes information. At the information level, management deals with proper framing of questions, identifying

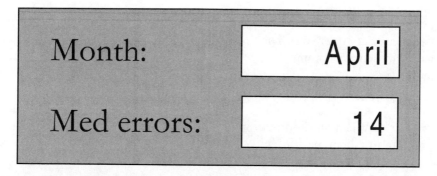

Figure 9–2 Data on April Medication Errors for Unit 12BG

sources of data necessary to answer the questions, selecting and combining views of data to provide answers, and communicating these to people who want them to aid decisions. In Figure 9–3 enough data have been collected, assembled, and displayed to provide information about the behavior of the medication delivery processes on unit 12BG, and to answer the question, "What was the average monthly number of medication errors?" One very practical example of a common problem in information management involves the identification of *denominators* when rates or percentages are needed. A denominator requires that the question, "How large is the whole

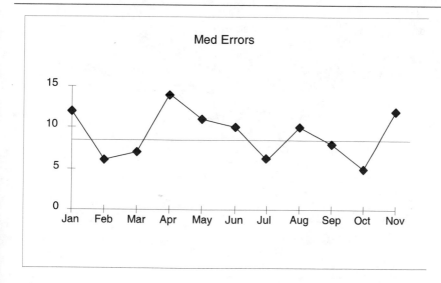

Figure 9–3 Information on Medication Errors for the Year

population from which the numerator was selected?" be answered. If the data necessary to answer that question have not been collected, or are not accessible from computing systems, then that question will go unanswered.

Knowledge implies prediction. Management uses information to predict, and as much as possible, to control the future performance of care processes. When our information is robust and plentiful enough to permit predictions about performance, individuals and organizations possess knowledge that can be used to intervene or prevent intervention, as required. In Figure 9–4, statistical process control methods have been applied to the information about medication errors on unit 12BG to answer the questions: "Is the behavior of the process predictable? Should we intervene? and What kind of intervention is required?" Statistical process control techniques can provide knowledge about the causes of variation in a process. Other methods of interpreting and synthesizing information may provide knowledge about the appropriateness of specific treatments for individual patients or populations, or may identify patients at risk.

Decisions lead to action or inaction. Feedback about the likely results of our actions, which is based on knowledge of processes and systems, is the best possible motivation for improvement. Some organizations threaten

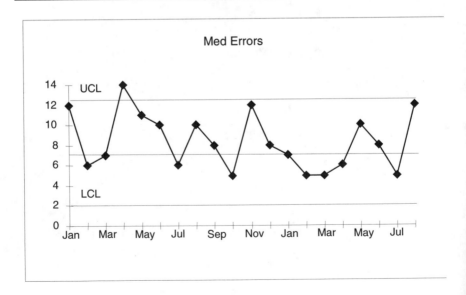

Figure 9–4 Knowledge about the Medication Error Process

and punish individuals who are "noncompliant"; however, it is preferable to seek improvement based on knowledge and collaboration based on shared goals and on an appeal to evidence. In Figure 9–5 a quality improvement team has used data, information, and knowledge of the medication delivery process to make specific decisions about how to improve the processes. The subsequent data collection efforts shown here illustrate that the desired results (e.g., consistently fewer medication errors), have been achieved.

Over the years a number of other frameworks have been developed for describing the taxonomy of health care information systems, including those that divide systems into layers differentiated by financial or clinical orientation, and more technical schemata that are based on models in which there are conceptual, logical, and physical categories (Tan 1995). These can be useful models and the reader is encouraged to learn more about them. For the quality improvement audience, however, the Data-to-Decision cycle has the advantage of focusing squarely upon the ultimate goal to improve decisions that affect patient care, while providing a conceptual model that will guide further discussion and learning about CQI data, information, and knowledge management tasks. This frame-

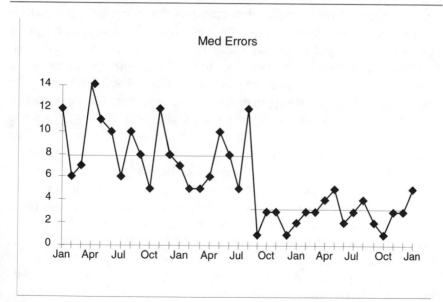

Figure 9–5 Decisions Have Been Taken To Improve the Medication Delivery Process

work will also lead us in a systematic discussion of the technological components that can be of assistance to CQI. Finally, the Data-to-Decision cycle points directly to the issues of data management and data quality as a place to begin any discussion of information systems related to quality improvement.

DATA QUALITY CONCEPTS, ISSUES, AND TECHNOLOGIES

The Dimensions of Data Quality

One of CQI's most basic tenets is that management decisions be based on data, not opinions or hunches. Health care data, however, may not always be, and often are not, of very good quality. And if the underlying data are unreliable, how good are the decisions based on that data likely to be?

Regardless of the information system(s) used, data quality is of paramount importance to quality improvement efforts. Electronic medical records, decision support systems, survey reporting systems, executive information systems, cost accounting systems, and quality management/ performance systems all utilize data elements that come from somewhere to be stored in electronic databases. For example, the data most hospitals collect for profiling and administrative analysis come from HCFA's UB-92 (universal billing form, 1992 version) claims form produced when patients are discharged from the hospital. The UB-92 form provides demographic data about the patient (birth date, sex, race, discharge status), codes for several diagnoses and procedures, and total charges aggregated by type of service, such as pharmacy, laboratory, and radiology. The claims data contain no clinical results, nor do they include any measures of the patient's satisfaction or functional status before or after treatment.

How good is the quality of claims data? Not very. Investigators have consistently found serious quality problems in large federal and insurance claims databases, including error rates and rates of discrepancy between similar databases of between 10 percent and 30 percent (Fisher et al. 1992; Whittle et al. 1991; Roos et al. 1991). In a study of almost 13,000 patients hospitalized for cardiac catheterization, the authors found that "claims data failed to identify more than one-half of patients with prognostically important conditions." The authors concluded that, "insurance claims data lack important diagnostic and prognostic information when compared with concurrently collected clinical data in the study of ischemic heart disease" (Jollis et al. 1993, 845).

Data Modeling for Electronic Data Collection in Databases

To get a better understanding of the dimensions of data quality, we have to consider how data exist in electronic format within computer systems. Databases store data in a controlled, orderly fashion. The first step in any database design is to decide what data elements will be included, how they are related to one another, what values are permissible, and how the data will be represented or viewed according to certain rules.

A *data model* interprets the real world. It seeks to describe or capture the real world in a structure that will support specific goals for storage, access, and analysis. The basic unit of this structure is termed the data *view*, composed of *entity, attribute,* and *value* (e, a, v). For example, the entity *employee* could contain the attributes *name, address,* and *date of birth.* Each of these attributes has many possible *values,* for example *Tom Jones, 123 Broad Street,* and *5/10/1950.* It is important to recognize that any data collection involves *choices* about how the entities, attributes, and values are set up, and these choices may greatly affect what happens (or can't happen) with the data later on. For example, we may choose to create a single attribute called *telephone number* for each employee-entity, or we might choose to create two attributes, one called *home telephone* and the other *business telephone.* Similarly, we could choose to collect the date information in the format *dd/mm/yy* instead of *dd/mm/yyyy* (more about this choice later). Finally, data have *representations* that involve how values are exported and displayed during analysis or reporting. For example, the choice as to how to represent null values is an important one in the design of data collection systems. Will an empty data field represent the *absence* of a value, because for example a reply was not applicable, or will it represent that a datum is *missing*? A general schema for data modeling is shown in Figure 9–6.

Data quality is directly related to these categories of *view, value,* and *representation* in electronic databases. The ideal data view will be relevant (capture only the data needed by the application), possess clarity of definition (avoid confusion between entities), be comprehensive (include all the attributes necessary to describe the entity), attain appropriate granularity (get the right level of detail), and be precise about the domain

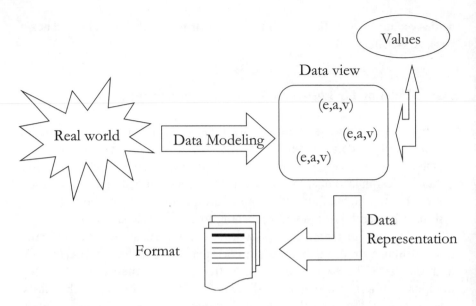

Figure 9–6 Data Modeling Results in Views, Values, and Representations

(allow for all the right possible values). The data values should be accurate (not misspelled or incorrect), complete (not missing components), current (up-to-date), and consistent (the same in different places). The data representations should be portable (able to be exported from the database), precise as to format, able to express null values, and efficient in use of storage space. See Table 9–2 below for an example.

The Year 2000 Problem: A Data Quality Problem of Special Concern to CQI

The Year 2000 Problem, also known as the Millennium Bug and Y2K, is a data quality problem of special concern to those involved in CQI. In the halcyon days when "computer" referred to a sheet metal and Plexiglas behemoth kept in an air-conditioned room crunching zillions of financial transactions with programs written in COBOL, storing data on punch cards, tapes, or "diskpacks" was cumbersome and expensive. So, to economize, programmers decided to record only the last two digits of the year: 1968 became just 68. By itself that wouldn't matter, except that

Table 9–2 Data View, Value, and Representation

Data Model Component	Example	Ideal Characteristics
Data View	Triplet: entity, attribute, value (e, a, v), as in (employee, first name, John)	Relevant, clearly defined, comprehensive, appropriate level of detail (granularity), allow for all possible values
Data Value	The telphone number 919-929-5993, the date May 10, 1950	Accurate, complete, current, consistent
Data Representation	Data formats, expression of null value (e.g., none vs. not known vs. zero)	Exportable from one database to another, precise as to format, efficient use of memory

computers do lots of arithmetic with those dates. For example, a program might subtract the year of your birth (let's say it's '48) from the then-current year ('68) to get your then-current age (20). The problem, of course, occurs on January 1, 2000 when the now-current year becomes 0, and the age calculation yields –48!

From the previous discussion, readers should now recognize that the Year 2000 Problem is a data quality problem that arises from faulty database design, in particular, a *data view* problem. The two-digit date field did not allow for sufficient *granularity* of data about dates. It is also a *domain* problem because not all possible values are permitted.

The unique exposure to Y2K in health care derives from three conditions: (1) health care technical devices, computers, and information systems that utilize dates are ubiquitous, and we depend on them for critical, life-sustaining tasks, (2) many health care processes are interdisciplinary, interdepartmental, or depend on coordinated efforts among multiple caregivers, but, (3) computing devices and systems in health care tend to be somewhat independent and isolated from one another, like islands, the so-called "Archipelago effect."

Quality managers use data and information sets that may pass through several applications, or layers of software, before they reach them. It is not uncommon for utilization and quality data to pass from a hospital's general ledger system, to a coding system, to the cost accounting system, to an external entity for risk adjustment, and, finally, to the quality manager.

This passage exposes data to several different vendors' hardware and software and the software interfaces between them. It increases the likelihood that a Y2K problem in a data collection, storage, or transfer process in a computer or program along the way will have its ill effect, and thus increase the overall data error rates. Furthermore, individual case, procedure, or patient data errors may be hard to spot in a large data set. At best there will be empty data fields, at worst erroneous values. Y2K could turn a good data set into hamburger.

The Y2K problem may not be all bad news. As a result of the widespread attention paid to this trivial yet far-reaching data quality problem, the concept of "computer continuity" may become firmly established. To the extent that health care professionals and their organizations focus attention on the strategic importance of their information systems' interdependence, and on the relationship of this interdependence to quality of care issues such as error reduction, it will be for the good of both the organizations and the individuals served by them. Merely the attention being given to data quality—to the processes involved in collecting, storing, analyzing, and accessing data—is, to my mind, an important positive. Health care organizations that commit to a serious review of their information systems' integrity with an eye toward finding Y2K problems are likely to find and solve many other problems along the way, provided they put their best people on it.

Medical Vocabularies and Standardized Data Definitions

The Y2K problem is directing a great deal of attention to database views as a source of data quality errors, but probably the single most important element to ensuring data quality in health care is the use of standardized vocabularies to describe patient care. To put the problem succinctly, there is no "universal language" to describe medical care. Two equally competent nurses or physicians might describe the same patient and his or her degree of severity of symptoms in very different terms.

Medical vocabularies have been developed, of course, but they serve specific and limited purposes. The ICD-9-CM (International Classification of Diseases, Ninth Edition, Clinical Modification) has become the *de facto* standard in the U.S. for coding inpatient and outpatient diagnoses. The International Classification of Diseases (ICD) was developed by the World Health Organization primarily to collect health statistics, not to support detailed clinical descriptions. The ICD-9-CM (1977) added the "Clinical Modifications" extensions to the basic ICD, but the ICD-9-CM still cannot express the detailed granularity needed for today's complex diagnoses. For example, the same ICD-9-CM code "600" would appear as the primary diagnosis for two men undergoing the same procedure to remove prostatic tissue, even if one of the men had twice as much tissue removed as the other and suffered significant bleeding during the operation while the other did not. Because the ICD-9-CM was intended only to classify diseases for aggregate statistical purposes, it cannot describe important aspects of the patient's history or physical exam.

The American Medical Association's Current Procedural Terminology, Fourth Edition (CPT-4), has become the standard coding system for billable physician and hospital outpatient procedures. Like the ICD coding system, the CPT system has no descriptors of patient attributes. Furthermore, there is no compatibility or interpreting between the ICD and CPT coding systems. They remain distinct coding systems for claims and billing purposes only.

The Systematized Nomenclature of Medicine (SNOMEDIII) was developed by the College of American Pathologists to include clinical concepts lacking in ICD-9-CM, and to encode concepts of the history and physical exam, as well as laboratory studies, diagnoses, and procedures. The SNOMED system has not gained widespread use, however, in part because there are multiple ways one can link numerical codes to represent essentially the same entity. For example, the entity "acute appendicitis" can be represented as any of the following:

1. D5–46210: acute appendicitis, not otherwise specified
2. D5–46100: appendicitis, not otherwise specified
   G–A231: acute
3. M–41000: acute inflammation, not otherwise specified
   G–C006: in
   T–59200: appendix, not otherwise specified
   Key: D=diagnosis axis, G=general axis, M=morphology axis, T=topology axis (Horn et al. 1994)

Medical Subject Headings (MeSH) were developed by the National Library of Medicine (NLM) to index biomedical literature. MeSH serves well the needs for indexing articles from the literature, but was not designed to describe procedures and patient attributes such as history and physical findings.

A host of other institutions have developed proprietary vocabularies to serve the needs of their specific information management systems. Among them are the following:

- The Medical Record (TMR) at Duke University
- The HELP System at LDS Hospital
- The STOR system at the University of California at San Francisco
- The READ Codes developed in Great Britain and endorsed by the Conference of Royal Medical Colleges

Given the diversity of proprietary coding systems, the NLM has inaugurated a project to map the terms in the widely used vocabularies ICD-9-CM, CPT-4, SNOMED, and MeSH. The project, known as the Unified Medical Language System (UMLS), has created a *metathesaurus* that helps health professionals and researchers retrieve and integrate electronic biomedical information from a variety of sources. It can be used to overcome variations in the way similar concepts are expressed in different sources. This makes it easier for users to link information from patient record systems, bibliographic databases, factual databases, expert systems, etc. It is a very valuable resource for solving the most difficult problem in exchanging health care information: the multiplicity of coding systems in use today. One online use of the UMLS is the Medical World Search site (www.mwsearch.com). When you search the World Wide Web for a medical concept, the Medical World Search uses the UMLS to include synonyms in the query. The UMLS is not itself a standard coding system, however; it is a cross-referenced collection of standards and other data and knowledge sources.

Still Needed: New Vocabularies To Capture the Patient's Experience

So far, we have been considering vocabularies that originated with the medical profession or as a result of researchers' needs to describe the patient's condition. Paul Ellwood, MD, who coined the term "outcomes management" described this new field as "a technology of patient experience," and he placed great emphasis on the need for a "patient-understood" language of outcomes (Ellwood 1988). None of the vocabularies mentioned so far meet this definition, but there have been recent attempts to construct data sets and measurement tools that are more patient experience oriented. A prime example is the SF-36, or Health Status Questionnaire, Short Form 36, used to measure patient perception of physical and mental well-being, which was first developed by Dr. John E. Ware, Jr., as part of the Medical Outcomes Study in the late 1980s (Ware 1989). The SF-36 is administered by the Medical Outcomes Trust. Other health status survey instruments, such as the Outcomes Assessment and Information Set (OASIS) used by Medicare for outcomes study for long-term care patients, are gaining popularity among health care quality improvement profession-als in a wide variety of settings and institutions, precisely because they get closer to the patient's experience.

Practitioners of CQI in health care organizations constantly face the challenges that disparate medical vocabularies pose to the quality of the data used to compile reports and analyses. The ambiguity and vague terminology inherent in standard coding systems makes it possible for physicians, practices, and departments whose clinical or financial perfor-mance is being examined to question whether the comparisons made are fair, or to assert that "apples are being compared to oranges." Leaders of these efforts need to understand that until a comprehensive dictionary of valid terms to be used in information systems to support CQI is produced, these problems will persist at the data quality level and are not solvable via more complex or expensive information technology. While efforts can and should be made to code patients correctly and consistently across the organization—for example by encouraging physician order entry to have physicians participate more directly in the structured data process—the lack of uniform descriptors for the patients' experiences in care processes will likely affect CQI efforts in health care for a long time to come.

Applying CQI to the Improvement of Data Quality in Health Care Organizations

A potentially fruitful area for the application of quality improvement methodology in health care is the improvement of data quality. Improve-ments in data quality should theoretically lead to improvements in deci-sions by favorably impacting the reliability of information and increasing the trust that is necessary for interdisciplinary teams to work well together. Not much attention has been paid to improving data quality among CQI practitioners in health care. Given the obvious importance of data quality to the analyses and studies that underlie CQI activities in health care, it is a curious omission, one that may in part be due to lack of technical and data management familiarity on the part of most health care professionals engaged in CQI. Even more significant a reason may be that information systems designed for health care have not been designed with enough regard given to the processes that will use them. Finally, it must be acknowledged that technology continues to explode, and merely keeping up with it is a huge task.

Data-generating processes can be studied and improved, however, using the same basic principles employed to improve any health care process. It is beyond the scope of this chapter to go into detail regarding data quality improvement methods and examples of their application. But the basic approach is one that considers the customer's data quality requirements, studies the current data generating processes for causes of variation in specific quality or performance attributes, acts to change processes in a systematic fashion, and then holds the gains while ascertaining and antici- pating new customer requirements. Data-intensive processes can be de- scribed in terms of the Data Life Cycle (Redman 1992), a version of which is illustrated in Figure 9–7. Typically, the data life cycle includes stages

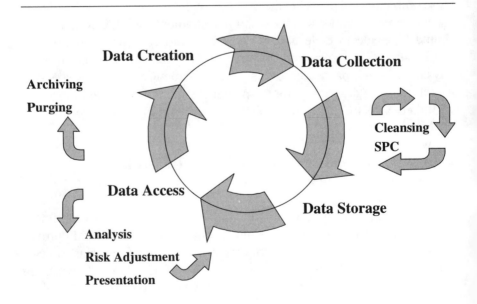

Figure 9–7 The Data Life Cycle

during which data are created, collected, stored, and accessed. In most situations, data may also be manipulated, cleansed, or used in a variety of ways and returned to storage. Occasionally, data are retired, and this may occur through archiving or actual destruction of the data.

If these data processes are described and their performance measured, then statistical process control (SPC) methods can provide the technical horsepower to manage them and improve their performance. That this has not occurred on any large scale in health care organizations to date is not the fault of technical know-how, but rather through lack of will and cultural consensus that the dividends returned will be large enough to warrant the expenditure in effort and dollars.

Data Quality Improvement through Error Checking and Validation

Increasingly more information systems are able to assist efforts to improve data quality by checking for data entry errors and performing range validation. In most cases, this "artificial intelligence" is really a set of simple rules that are coded into the application, making it impossible or very difficult for the end-user or data enterer to send bad data to the software application. As data entry in health care increases, this feature of information systems becomes more valuable as a means of decreasing costly errors that can lead to re-work or unreliable information.

Figure 9–8 illustrates error checking and range validation in progress in a Web-based case management information system designed for a pediatric individual practice association (IPA). Javascript™ code written into the HTML (hypertext markup language) form viewed on the Web browser software Microsoft® Internet Explorer automatically checks to see that the dates entered are consistent with rules in the program. In this case, the data enterer has mistakenly entered the admission data as 9/30/1948 instead of 9/30/1998. The rules in this application are that date of birth must *precede* the date of admission, and since this rule was violated, the program returns the error message seen here telling the data enterer to check for data inconsistencies. Note that this online error checking is occurring on the client's computer, that is, on the data enterer's computer, and not in the database computer itself. No communication need take place between the client software and the remote database server for this error checking to occur, thus saving both time and network traffic.

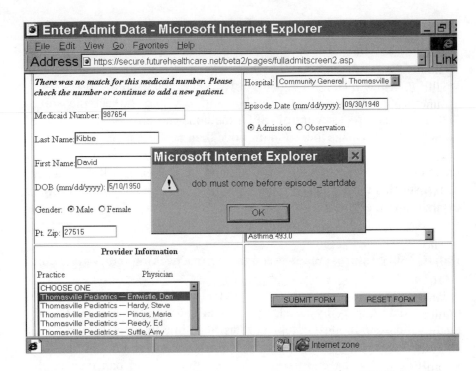

Figure 9–8 Error Checking Done by Javascript Code in an HTML Document. When the data enterer hit the "submit form" button, the application noted that the patient's date of birth (DOB) was *after* the admit date, and prompts the data enterer to check for errors in the date fields. Here, the admit data should have been 1998, not 1948.

INFORMATION MANAGEMENT ISSUES, CONCEPTS, AND TECHNOLOGIES

Information management involves the skills, methods, and technological tools required to answer questions from available sources of data, and to communicate information in a timely manner to those in need of answers. CQI in health care has grown increasingly dependent on communication networks or channels that enable health care professionals in distributed locations to share information and simultaneously access information stored in electronic databases. Also gaining importance is the capability to merge information from disparate electronic databases (e.g. inpatient and outpatient) into single data repositories that permit complex analysis linking clinical and administrative output and permitting flexibility in the definition of what constitutes a patient care episode across the continuum of time and geography. These needs have placed extraordinary demands upon information managers and the technologies available. Health care professionals involved in CQI need to possess a thorough grounding in information management in order to be good customers of their IS department colleagues and to have reasonable expectations about getting their needs for information met.

Relational Database Technology Is at the Foundation of the Data-to-Information Conversion

Those interested in health care CQI have come to recognize that many of their work environments are "data rich but information poor." By this, they mean they are in the uncomfortable position of being aware that data which (actually or potentially) hold answers to their questions are stored electronically somewhere in the enterprise, but significant barriers exist to getting the data out and manipulating them in order to arrive at desired analyses. In some cases, this is a purely technical barrier, in others it can be a combination of technical difficulty, cost, and simple lack of will.

Here is an example of the kinds of technical barriers that can be encountered. At the time of this writing the author is engaged in a project to assist policymakers in a state Medicaid program develop care management programs in local community provider networks. Quite naturally, the program's leaders want to analyze historical claims data for the population involved to determine factors such as rates of hospitalization, emergency room use, and specialty referrals. They want to look at these data by aggregating them into groups by locale (counties, practices, and providers), and by diseases and conditions. This information could then inform them where the greatest opportunities for quality improvement lie, a prerequisite step to targeting care management interventions.

The databases in which these data are stored are virtually incapable of yielding up such information, however, except through intense programming that is both time consuming and very expensive. Why is this the case? The simplest answer is that the databases that store the claims data are not relational databases. They use an older database technology that was designed to perform repetitive transactions in very large volumes at high speed, not for easy querying, aggregating, or analyzing the data stored. To be available for transformation into information, the data within these older databases must be exported to newer, relational database systems, often known as data warehouses, or the old systems need to be converted entirely to relational database systems capable of supporting both transactions and data manipulation for reporting and analysis. This conversion process is a daunting one.

Fortunately, almost all new information management systems used in health care organizations employ relational database technology, including those used in general ledger systems, laboratory and pharmacy systems, cost accounting systems, and performance measurement systems. Relational database technology is at the heart of information system applications that are built on databases from popular vendors such as Oracle®, Sybase®, and SQL Server®, as well as the popular desktop programs Microsoft® Access and File Manager. While not a panacea for all the problems of transforming data into information, the almost universal adoption of relational database technology and the standard query language (SQL) which is a common feature, has made it much easier for analysts to manipulate data for reports and to merge data from one database into another in order to answer complex questions about performance and outcomes.

The basics of relational database technology are straightforward. All relational databases organize data in tables that store data belonging to specific entities. A table for the entity "patient" would have places to store the attributes first name, last name, Social Security number, etc. A table for "lab tests" would likely store the test name, the data obtained, and the result. Because each table is independent of the others, new data (e.g. new patients, new tests) can be added almost indefinitely, and new tables can be added as the need arises for new entities to be included. This arrangement is both flexible and expandable, therefore cost-effective.

Of course, what we usually want to get out of the database involves knowing how the data in the tables are *related*. For example, we want to know the test result for a particular patient, or all the test results for a particular patient for a specified date range. Relationships between entities can be one to one, as in the relationship "case number: patient last name," or one to many as in "case number: laboratory tests." These relationships are mediated or controlled by *keys* that permit all lab tests for a particular patient to be assembled and reported to a computer screen or printer, as illustrated in Figure 9–9. The key number in this case is the Social Security number. Standard query language (SQL) provides for standard definition

Patients		
ID	Last Name	Date of Birth
105-58-1866	Jones	4/20/78
472-10-3959	Smith	7/17/84
889-75-1865	Williams	3/14/67
833-68-1345	Freidlander	8/28/44
614-41-0798	Statler	5/6/40
356-02-0128	Eddings	7/3/53
601-20-8124	Blondel	1/23/53
339-42-9100	Elfish	6/17/81
346-06-9595	Adelberg	6/10/54
010-22-4893	Calvander	7/11/55
662-35-1882	Delbert	7/26/60
087-11-6498	Gump	10/19/88

Lab Tests		
SSN	Test	Date of Test
346-06-9595	CBC	3/16/94
833-68-1345	HGB	3/8/94
346-06-9595	HGB	3/7/94
833-68-1345	HGB	3/2/94
105-58-1866	LYTES	3/1/94
346-06-9595	LYTES	2/27/94
105-58-1866	HGB	2/27/94
105-58-1866	CBC	2/22/94
105-58-1866	HGB	2/21/94
833-68-1345	CBC	2/20/94
105-58-1866	HGB	2/18/94
346-06-9595	LYTES	2/17/94

Key Values Are Unique

Figure 9–9 Relational Databases Permit One-to-Many Relationships To Be Mediated by Keys

of various commands to perform relational operations, and is used by all commercial vendors to provide connectivity between systems.

Interface Standards Are Key to Communications between Medical Information Systems

SQL is an example of an "interface standard" that permits communication between information systems. Standards in general are essential to provide computer "interoperability," which is the ability to access information and manage it independent of the types of computing devices storing the underlying data. Prior to the establishment of interface standards, organizations were burdened with many point-to-point applications existing on mainframe computers. During the 1970s and 1980s, the adoption of new, network-based, client-server health care applications made it necessary to link these point-to-point applications with systems outside the mainframe. Interfaces required an enormous amount of time to build, test, and install, and they typically required a separate interface to be built for each application. Interface standards ameliorate this maintenance nightmare. Standards are also required because data are distributed throughout numerous databases, controlled by different groups and with different rules for access. There must also be standards to ensure the security and confidentiality of data that identify patients.

Every reader has direct experience with the World Wide Web and the use of the Internet to access documents, and therefore has experienced the power of interface standards. The Internet uses a set of standards for data communication known as IP/TCP, or Internet protocol/transfer control protocol, which have been essential to the creation of a worldwide network: Users can access the same documents whether their computers are running on Windows™, UNIX®, or Apple® operating systems! Hypertext markup language, HTML, the language in which all World Wide Web documents are written, is another standard at use on the information highway.

There are a number of messaging standards specific to health care with which health care CQI professionals should be familiar.

- HL7. Short for Health Level 7, this system grew out of hospital information system vendors' efforts to design an open standard for transmitting clinical data. HL7 is named for the seventh, the data presentation level and highest, layer of the Open Systems Interconnection (OSI) model of the International Standards Organization (ISO). The six lower levels of the OSI, the network, hardware and software, are used to transmit the data through the network. HL7 includes standards for formatting of admission/discharge/transfer (ADT), financial order entry, clinical laboratory tests, X-ray reports, diagnostic studies, and several other areas. The current version of HL7 is known as 2.3. An enhanced version, Version 2.3.1, is scheduled for release in the first quarter of 1999. HL7 Version 3.0 is tentatively scheduled for release sometime in 2000.
- ACR-NEMA. In 1982, the American College of Radiology and the National Electronic Manufacturers' Association began developing standards for exchanging radiological images. A revised version of the standards was published in 1988. In both versions, data transfer was defined for point-to-point connections (i.e., a networked environment was not considered). ACR and NEMA have recently completed the third version of the standards, which has been renamed DICOM v3.0. DICOM stands for Digital Imaging and Communications in Medicine. The v3.0 refers to the fact that there were two prior versions of the standard.

- ANSI ASC X.12. ANSI stands for the American National Standards Institute, which has accredited an independent organization, X.12, to develop a number of messaging standards for health care provider information, benefits and eligibility information, and insurance claims forms information.
- ASTM. The oldest of the standards organizations, the American Society for Testing and Materials, has been involved in developing health care data interchange standards for many years. Relevant ASTM efforts include standards for connecting laboratory instruments to computers, standards for ADT transactions, bar codes, and medical records. ASTM E31.12 has also proposed for acceptance a number of documents, including an approach to patient identifiers, a general approach to medical records, and a Standard Description for Content and Structure of an Automated Longitudinal Health Record.

A Remaining Information Management Standards Challenge: A Patient Universal Identifier

One of the most imposing challenges to information management in health care is how to develop and gain acceptance for some standard for universally identifying patients and their data. Because patients receive care across primary, secondary, and tertiary care settings, and because numbers that identify patient records in these settings are generally assigned by detached computer databases, patients often end up with many different identification numbers.

Researchers, policymakers, and quality improvement professionals have long recognized that patients' episodes of care commonly span multiple providers, institutional settings, and occur over time. As more health care delivery activity has been pushed out of the hospital and into the ambulatory care setting, accounting for the activities and experiences of patients has become even more difficult. An episode of congestive heart failure, for example, could include visits to a primary care physician's office, diagnostic studies in an outpatient radiology center, a hospitalization for acute care, and follow-up with a visit to a cardiologist's office. Any attempt to study the processes of care throughout this sequence requires gathering data from each site, which is made very difficult, if not impossible, if each site's computer system identifies patients with its own unique identifier. Some indexing system that maps all those different numbers to each other, and provides a single unique identifier by which all parties could be assured that they were working with the data of the right patient, is a requirement for community-wide or systemwide quality improvements.

Attempts to create "master patient indexes" that would map these various identification numbers to a single universal number have been frustrated by a variety of sources, including social fears that such a system will allow unwanted intrusion into patient privacy. The Healthcare Insurance Portability and Accountability Act (HIPAA) of 1996 mandated Congress to establish a methodology for instituting a national unique patient identifier system. At the time of this writing, however, it would appear that public debate and political pressure from concerned voter groups have delayed action indefinitely.

Desktop Software Technology for Quality Improvement Data Analysis and Informational Reporting Is Now Widely Available

Microsoft® Excel, a software program that started out as a spreadsheet tool for financial modeling and analysis, has become something of a standard for health care quality improvement data and information manipulation because of its ease of use and wide range of features for converting data in rows and column format into summary tables, graphs, and charts. Numerous basic descriptive and inferential statistical operations for research and statistical process control (SPC) operations can be performed in Excel. Over the years, quality improvement experts also have developed supplementary Excel "add-in" programs that can automate common CQI data-gathering and analytical processes using Excel. One of these is QI-Tools™, an Excel add-in from Future Healthcare, Inc., downloadable free off the Internet (www.futurehealthcare.com), which automates many of the most common descriptive statistical chores used by health care data analysts, including Pareto analyses, histograms, and control charts. QI-Tools™ has become quite popular among health care quality improvers as a means to short-cut some of the labor involved in producing quality improvement and financial charts and graphs.

KNOWLEDGE MANAGEMENT AS THE NEW FRONTIER FOR CQI INFORMATION TECHNOLOGY

Knowledge can be defined in many ways, but its most essential quality is prediction. Knowledge of a drug's action, a disease's prognosis, or the outcomes of a care process means that we can predict future activity, within limits, of course. Medical knowledge is multidimensional and exists in numerous formats: as stored personal experience in the mind of a professional; as the results of clinical trials; as recorded evidence of the progression of an illness or condition; as a control chart that captures the behavior of a process that dispenses medications and produces errors. Clearly, knowledge is useful in assisting both the manager's and clinician's job of making good decisions in the interest of the patient. Knowledge tells us both when to intervene—because the probability of the intervention leading to a salutary effect is high—as well as when not to intervene— because the probability that the intervention leading to a salutary effect is low, or, equally important, is not known.

Knowledge management is a rapidly evolving, multidisciplinary field that includes (depending on whose definition is being considered) the areas of best practices and benchmarking, business communications, document management, electronic publishing, groupware software, decision-support services, statistics, organizational behavior, and systems thinking. Knowledge management focuses on the processes and the people involved in creating, sharing, and leveraging knowledge in the organization to support strategies for improving performance and meeting business objectives. And, it almost goes without saying, to be successful knowledge management depends on the quality of the underlying data and information used to create explicit knowledge "products" that, when used, can be of benefit to the organization, its members, or their customers.

The Internet Technologies Have Enabled Knowledge Management on a Universal Scale

Perhaps no other information technology has affected the quality and quantity of communications of health care data, information, and knowledge as has the Internet and its associated technologies, which include the World Wide Web, e-mail, HTML, and Java™ language, among the most noteworthy. Although these technologies are just beginning to have a direct impact on CQI in health care, there is no question that their future effect will be profound.

The establishment of a set of universal computer communications standards that permit unlimited, worldwide communications ability regardless of computer type, manufacturer, or operating system, over common carrier telephone lines, defines the Gutenberg moment of the late twentieth century. These open standards used by the Internet, intranets, extranets, and hundreds of thousands of local area networks within health care and worldwide, have freed information to travel unhindered, permitting individuals as well as organizations to extend their reach to unimaginable distances. The standards and the software applications that use them are certainly not perfect, nor do they allow for every kind of health care information to be exchanged with magical ease. But users are discovering that they are good enough for performing a surprisingly large number of useful health care tasks and hold the promise of doing many more in the very near future.

Free Access to Health Care Information, Knowledge, and Knowledge Services Is Proliferating Rapidly

No one knows precisely how many Web pages, e-mail groups, news groups, and online databases accessible through the Internet, extranets, and intranets are devoted to health care topics. But a recent query on a popular Web-based search engine for documents containing the term "health care" yielded over 28 million Web pages; for "asthma" more than 190,000 documents; for "diabetes" more than 220,000. Some of those Web sites provide information of a nature heretofore unknown, both highly interactive and customizable by the viewer, and many are from entrepreneurial for-profit companies. A few examples follow:

- *Dr. Koop's Community* is the name of Web site dedicated to offering greater consumer access to free health care information and to encouraging electronic communications among consumers and health care providers. It contains information on topics as diverse as nutrition, cancer, and addiction recovery (www.DrKoop.com).
- A company in Conway, Arkansas, called The Health Resource, Inc. will comb the medical literature and provide the customer—for a fee of $350—with a personalized list of the latest clinical trials, articles from medical journals, centers of excellence, and alternative therapies to pursue (www.thehealthresource.com).
- A Web site maintained by the publisher of *Mademoiselle* and *Glamour* magazines offers free online calculators that will compute individual ideal body weight, caloric needs, percent of body fat, and prescribe

individualized diets at the click of a mouse. All the visitor does is enter his or her statistics (www.phys.com/a_home/01home/home.htm).

- As of July 1997, the National Library of Medicine began to offer *MEDLINE*, the NLM's compendium of more than nine million references, abstracts, and related articles from 4,000 medical journals, *free* to Internet users (www.ncbi.nlm.nih.gov/PubMed/). The response has been staggering, with the NLM *MEDLINE* PubMed Web site now receiving more than one million "hits" a day. Links to *full-text* medical journals are available from some abstracts, and the list of full-text articles is growing daily.

- *Self-Help Central* is a Web site maintained by Tom Ferguson, MD, a senior associate at the Center for Clinical Computing, Harvard School of Medicine, which makes available a database of hundreds of disease and condition-specific self-help forums online, a large database of information on the diagnosis and treatment of common conditions, a link to daily health news stories, a free *MEDLINES* database search engine, and many, many more resources, free of charge (www.healthy.net/home/index.html).

- A Web site funded by the National Asthma Education Program Office of Prevention, Education, and Control National Heart, Lung and Blood Institute, National Institute of Health, contains *movie clips* illustrating the proper and improper use of hand-held inhalers and spacers (www.meddean.luc.edu/lumen/MedEd/medicine/Allergy/Asthma/asthtoc.html).

Online sources for evidence-based clinical guidelines, protocols, and other best practices are expanding rapidly, as are the forums available for sharing new knowledge as it becomes available. Examples of knowledge management resources of this kind include the following:

- The American College of Physicians(ACP) publishes *ACP Journal Club* online bimonthly (www.acponline.org). Featured articles are selected and reviewed according to explicit criteria by physicians, with emphasis on studies that warrant immediate attention by physicians attempting to keep pace with important advances in the treatment, prevention, diagnosis, causes, prognosis, or economics of disorders managed primarily by internists. The basic criteria for reviews are available at the ACP's Web site.

- *The Virtual Hospital* is a continuously updated digital health sciences library maintained by the University of Iowa and the Department of Radiology, University of Iowa's College of Medicine (www.vh.org). It contains multimedia information of use for providers, patients, and medical scientists.
- *The Cochrane Database of Systematic Reviews* is a rapidly growing collection of regularly updated, systematic reviews of the effects of health care, maintained by contributors to the Cochrane Collaboration. Cochrane reviews are reviews mainly of randomized controlled trials. Evidence is included or excluded on the basis of explicit quality criteria to minimize bias. Data are often combined statistically, with meta-analysis, to increase the power of the findings of numerous studies each too small to produce reliable results individually. The Web site contains information about how to subscribe to the Cochrane Library's services (www.update-software.com/ccweb/cochrane/cdsr/htm).

Public access to the measured performance of individual health plans, practices, and practitioners is now becoming readily accessible on World Wide Web sites, with many more in the planning stages at the time of this writing. A few examples include the following:

- The Pacific Business Group on Health maintains a Web site called *California Consumer Healthscope* (www.healthscope.org) intended to assist consumers and payers select health plans, hospitals, and practices. The site contains report cards that display measures for key outcomes in the areas of preventive care, chronic illness care, and patient satisfaction. The data is reported on practices in California, Oregon, and Washington.
- The National Committee on Quality Assurance (NCQA) publishes on its Web site (www.ncqa.org) detailed accreditation information for more than 350 managed care health plans. Accreditation is based in part on the health plans' submission of HEDIS (Health Plan Employer Data and Information Set) outcomes data sets.
- The Health Care Financing Administration's (HCFA) Nursing Home Database is now online (www.medicare.gov/nursing/home.asp). Called *Nursing Home Compare*, the database contains information on every Medicare and Medicaid certified nursing home in the country. Con-

sumers can locate nursing homes in their areas and find information about compliance with Medicare and Medicaid regulations from the Web site.

• New York State maintains a Web site that reports, in PDF format, mortality and complication rates for major cardiology procedures by hospital and by individual practitioner (www.health.state.ny.us/nysdoh/consumer/heart/homehear.htm).

Electronic publishing is beginning to offer new knowledge resource connectivity and knowledge management tools, some specific to medicine and health care. For example, a searcher using the Internet *MEDLINE* search engine PubMed will find that approximately 15 percent of the article abstract pages contain direct links to full-text versions of the article in the electronic magazine or journal cited. If the reader has reached an article in the electronic version of the *British Medical Journal* (http://www.bmj.com) he or she is offered additional online knowledge management features, such as reproduction of the article in PDF format, e-mailing the author of the article, and downloading of the citation to the popular software Citation Manager™. The reader can even choose to be notified by e-mail when a new *British Medical Journal* article cites the current article!

The Information Revolution Has Spurred Worries about the Quality of Information and Purported Knowledge Available on the Net

With good reason, many observers of the rapid pace of Internet information technology used for health care purposes have raised questions about the quality of information and knowledge available over the Internet. The problem for those seeking best practices information is, first, how to find best practices among the wealth of resources on the Internet, and then how to separate the proverbial wheat from the chaff. Quality is a critical issue any time Internet information is accessed as was recently pointed out in an editorial in the *Journal of the American Medical Association* on the subject: "At first glance, science and snake oil may not always look all that different on the Net" (Silberg et al. 1997, 1244). The Internet can facilitate information and knowledge flow, fostering realistic expectations about health care treatments and outcomes, which may enhance patient self-care and responsibility for lifestyle changes. The Internet can and does function as any other mass marketing tool, useful to those who wish merely to gain profit from the sale of drugs, treatments, or advice. But the Internet can be a menace because it permits low-quality messages to be accessed by many people who might otherwise receive better quality health information from professional sources.

At the present time, a number of organizations worldwide are addressing this important issue of ensuring the quality of health care information on the Internet, but there is no easy solution as long as the Internet remains what has made it so popular, a *public* network. It is this author's opinion that the greatest potential for improving the quality of health and health care information on the Internet may lie in greater public involvement and use of the new technologies, rather than through medical authorities' attempts to regulate or limit them. Greater public involvement with the Internet as a source of health information could give the medical community much needed assessments as to what information is truly useful in making decisions, and how desirable are particular efforts by professionals and the industry as a whole to improve quality of care and service (Robinson 1998; Kibbe 1998).

Security and Confidentiality of Patient Identifiable Data Transmitted Electronically Is an Important Social, Legal, and Technological Issue

As the Internet is used increasingly to transmit and maintain health care data, information, and knowledge, the important issue of protecting confidential patient and provider information is receiving considerable attention. No one wants the benefits of the new technologies in terms of reach and ease of communication to come at the expense of patient privacy. Yet the extent of procedural and technological protection needed for adequate guarantees of privacy is being hotly debated by politicians, ethicists, representatives of the technology industry, and just about everyone else.

Standards for the security of health information are coming soon. The Health Insurance Portability and Accountability Act (HIPAA) passed by Congress in 1996 mandated that HCFA set guidelines for the electronic transmission of health care data. In August 1998 HCFA published in the *Federal Register* its proposed standards for the security of health information and the use of electronic signatures in the health care industry. (Available at the HIPPA Administrative Web site, aspe.os.dhhs.gov/adminsimp/nprm/regindex.htm.) It is anticipated that the standards will be finalized in late 1999 or early 2000.

The proposed security and electronic signature standards have much broader applicability than any regulations so far enacted. Section 142.302 imposes a federal mandate that all health plans, clearinghouses, and providers will make appropriate provision for the security of health information. The standard's applicability is not limited to administrative transactions, but to *all* health information pertaining to an individual that is electronically maintained or communicated, including all internal organizational communications. Thus, the standards represent a clear federal intent to create a national information security standard for health information.

The proposed standards organize the security requirements that must be met into four broad categories, which include administrative procedures, physical safeguards, technical safeguards for health information maintained and stored by a health care organization, and technical safeguards for health information communicated over a network.

The standards explicitly allow for the use of open networks including the Internet and dial-up public networks, while mandating encryption when using open networks. For most organizations, the most significant challenge contained in the technical safeguards sections is the requirement for unique *individual* authentication. This implies that any individual accessing health information over a network must be individually identified and granted access either on the basis of an explicit privilege extended to that individual, or on the basis or a role occupied by that individual. So, for example, the requirement precludes the use of a personal identification number (PIN) that is shared among provider staff.

The standards also set criteria for an acceptable electronic signature. The electronic signature must ensure the identity of the signer (authentication), ensure the unaltered transmission and receipt of the message (message integrity), and prevent a signer from successfully denying the signature (nonrepudiation). The standards explicitly require that a digital signature is the only technology that satisfies these criteria. Digital signatures employ digital certificates to bind user identity to a cryptographic element called a *public key pair*. The technology generally assumes that a trusted third party creates the certificates and in so doing confirms the identity of a key holder. The collection of certificates created by these trusted third parties is known as a *public key infrastructure* (PKI).

It can be expected that standards and guidelines for the electronic maintenance and transmission of health care information will be a "moving target" in the coming months and years, influenced both by public and political opinion and by the rapidly advancing technologies in security areas. The general trend, however, is clearly toward broader use of public communications systems like the Internet, World Wide Web, and e-mail to link providers with consumers and both with ever larger stores of health care data, information, and knowledge.

INFORMATION TECHNOLOGY TO IMPROVE DECISIONS MADE BY CAREGIVERS AND PATIENTS

The ultimate purpose of using information technology to manage data, information, and knowledge is to inform the decision-making processes and improve the decisions made by patients and clinicians.

Clinical decision support systems (CDSSs), which are clinical consultation systems that use population statistics and expert knowledge to offer real-time information for clinicians, are beginning to become a reality and to prove their value (Hunt et al. 1998). For example, physicians who have direct access to information about the medical formulary at the time of ordering drugs make better prescribing decisions and reduce medication errors that often lead to adverse reactions and unnecessary use of scarce medical resources (Bates et al. 1998). There is also growing evidence that patients who are well informed tend to participate more in the decisions about their care and to be more satisfied with the outcomes than those who are less well informed (Wennberg 1995; Barry et al. 1995).

For many organizations, the trend towards supplying both providers and consumers of health care services with more and better quality information near the point of care and decision making converge in the new and rapidly growing field known as *disease management* (DM).

The "Informatics" of Disease Management

The idea of improving quality of care through preventing disease and intervening early for patients with chronic conditions such as asthma, diabetes, or congestive heart failure, is certainly not a new one. To an extent, DM is little more than a marketing or packaging device whereby familiar and often long-standing concepts are combined into a single philosophy or approach and offered as a complete package. The success of a disease management program depends on several factors: committed physicians, a staff prepared and willing to take this route, a structured process of change management, an organized approach to analysis, a well-developed quality improvement system—and information systems to support all of these.

As practiced by the large HMOs and pharmaceutical company spin-offs, DM has become a data and information intensive endeavor dependent on information technologies and management tools aimed at improving clinical decisions. These include the use of databases of enrollee and claims data for tracking large patient populations, electronic linkage with pharmacy and laboratory databases, intelligent "agents" (software) that perform risk assessment and stratify patients according to risk profiles, and communication networks that link nurse triagers and managers with patients, providers, and payers in order to monitor compliance and, in some cases, even collect key physiological data directly from the patients' homes.

A fundamental tenet of DM is that it improves care decisions by getting the right information to the right people at the right time. Or, as John Roglieri, MD, MBA of NYLCare puts it, "You have to provide intensive, multiple inputs to the patient using whatever works to enhance compliance, and be sure that the treating physicians get accurate data back" (personal communication, 4 June 1998). The entire DM process can therefore be seen as supported by a set of information management tasks using "informatics" tools to (1) identify at-risk populations, (2) assess and stratify individual risk, (3) exchange and integrate information, (4) communicate interventions, and (5) collect and study outcomes.

Identifying At-Risk Populations

Most disease management companies use health plan enrollment data to try to identify patients with diabetes or asthma, and supplement this with risk assessment surveys, usually done over the phone. Identifying at-risk populations may be more difficult than it seems, however. Tom Hagen, chief information officer of Franklin Health Systems (Upper Saddle River, New Jersey), says that one of the big problems for health systems of any kind is locating who is sick and where and when they've been treated. "You'd be surprised how little information most health plans have about their at-risk populations, particularly the very sickest. What information they do have is scattered in multiple databases at multiple caregiving sites. Even within a single health plan it is not uncommon for claims and encounter data to be submitted to and stored in separate, unique claims databases that can't talk to one another. But to manage these patients well, the value comes from integrating data about a patient's hospital, outpatient, specialty clinic, pharmacy, laboratory, etc. experience into some coherent whole that is centered on the patient" (personal communication, August 1998). He describes the process of using the software and databases to identify patterns of the highest risk patients in particular diseases as "fingerprinting."

A "Catch-22" of disease management, aimed at preventing high-risk, high-dollar episodes of caregiving such as a hospitalization, is that the claims data used to identify candidates for programs are available usually only *after* a high-risk, high-dollar episode, such as a hospitalization, occurs. Thus the greatest opportunity for savings may have already been lost. It makes sense, then, that the informatics tools of predictive modeling—a method for identifying patients *before* hospitalization—will gain greater use as disease management matures. Axonal, Inc. of Durham, North Carolina, is one of a handful of companies now developing and marketing predictive modeling software for the "front end" of disease management programs to prospectively identify at-risk patients. Based on the branch of higher mathematics known as *neural networks*, this software "learns" who will be at increased risk of utilization six months from the administration of a "test" (for example a health status survey), and, it is claimed, can increase the ability of disease managers to prevent hospitalizations in the first place by targeting educational or monitoring resources well in advance.

Stratifying Patient Population As Risk

Closely related to risk identification is risk stratification, whereby an identified population of patients with a particular disease is segmented based on risk or opportunity (or both). This is another area of rapid informatics innovation. WellMark, the Blue Cross/Blue Shield carrier in Iowa, uses risk stratification software from ThinkMed (Milwaukee, Wisconsin) to answer the questions: "How do we target interventions to the patients most in need of them?" and "How can we avoid unnecessary and inappropriate disease management investment?" The software works by extracting claims and pharmacy data, then applying a set of proprietary clinical rules developed by the physician principals of ThinkMed. These rules stratify patients within a particular disease category and flag those that are appropriate for the different levels of disease management activity (e.g. case management or education materials mailing). A number of companies are developing similar risk stratification tools for the purposes of narrowing the field of patients who are candidates for costly educational or home health interventions to only the ones most likely to benefit from it.

Exchange and Integration of Information

Data integration is needed to support disease management with online treatment advisories, automated care protocols, and routing of work flow and task assignments, and requires a data warehouse into which data collected from medical, laboratory, claims, and prescription drug encounters can be collected. At this time, only a few disease management entities possess robust data warehouses of this kind. But the companies that do have such software—for example SmithKline Beecham Healthcare Services—possess a powerful tool that gives case managers desktop access to patient-centered lab, pharmacy, and protocol information, and gives medical directors and financial managers access to cost and utilization information which is close to real time.

Communicating with the Patient or Provider for Interventional Purposes

Communication is most often carried out by telephone, or by directing the patient to visit his or her physician. For example, a disease manager can track asthma patients who discontinue regular use of peak flow meters or prescribed inhaled corticosteroids, and direct a patient whose insulin dose needs adjusting, advising them to be seen in the clinic that afternoon. But a number of companies are starting to make use of the distributed information system of the Internet and World Wide Web to facilitate patient education, gather data from patients directly, and communicate the need for changing treatment (e.g. drug dosage). CareSoft, Inc. (Mountain View, California) has developed disease management interactive software that utilizes the Internet. The Joslin Diabetes Center, Boston, Massachusetts is using the software in a two-year pilot study with the Veteran's Administration Hospital System and the Department of Defense Hospital System to determine its effectiveness in managing diabetic patients with varying levels of severity.

Outcomes Measurement and Reporting

Outcomes analysis is largely a function of having gathered good quality data on cost, quality indicators, and patient health status over time, for use in determining the effectiveness of care. For some, the most important thing is to meet accreditation reporting standards (e.g. NCQA's HEDIS), and to make the collection of data the product of the routine delivery of care, thus lowering data collection costs. For others, the major issue is being able to link processes of care with meaningful outcomes, so that the basic question "How well did this program work?" can be answered. The quality of data, their reliability, validity, and currency are all going to determine how much information can be extracted at the reporting stage.

Practice-Based Disease Management Is Growing

Disease management programs are not limited to HMOs and large health care organizations. Particularly in the last two years, DM programs have developed within smaller community-based health care systems and individual groups and practices (Kibbe 1998; Kibbe and Johnson 1998). The brief case study here illustrates how effective practice-based DM programs can be.

> Douglas Kelling, MD is an internist in Concord, North Carolina, who has developed a practice-based diabetes DM program that has made striking improvements in the care of the almost 600 patients enrolled in the program since late 1995. For example, during 1996 and 1997 there were only four patients in his practice who required hospitalization for diabetes, for a total of five hospital days. One of these was a new patient who came to his practice late one afternoon, was found to have a blood glucose of 900 mg/dl and who spent one night in the ICU on an insulin drip and was discharged home the next day to be followed by the DM program. The average hemoglobin A1C (a marker of long-term diabetes control) of patients in the DM program has decreased from 8.6 to 7.1 over this period. Also, there have been no amputations required for patients in the DM program during the past year.
>
> Dr. Kelling will tell anyone who asks that the key to this clinical success is a combination of his own commitment to "do the right thing for the patient, for the quality of care," the use of evidence-based guidelines to direct patient care processes, and the community-wide network of caregivers—clinic nurses, staff

members, home health personnel, public health nurses—that he has organized and trained to become a "system" for patient care, education, risk stratification, and intense follow-up. "We are all working off the same page, everyone knows what to do and when to do it, and nothing falls through the cracks or gets mislaid. Patients don't wait long for their visits or tests anymore, and I have much more time per patient to give each my personal attention, which is what they come to see me for" (personal communication 1998).

At the heart of Dr. Kelling's DM program is a computerized database management system written in Microsoft® Access, the desktop software program that is part of the familiar Microsoft® Office Suite, and guidelines from the American Diabetes Association (ADA). The database system tracks all important patient information for each visit, graphically and in color displays trends in key test results and physiological parameters, and alerts the physician, nurses, and staff when scheduled preventive care, screening tests, and educational sessions are due. The database requirements were set by Dr. Kelling, and changed many times over the past two years, while the actual programming for the database was done by a local consultant who had experience designing databases for the banking industry, but not for health care prior to this project.

The brief case study above epitomizes how data, information, and knowledge management, aided by current information technology, can be used to apply evidence-based principles to improve clinical and administrative decisions, in this case the decisions involving the care of diabetes patients. The skills, methods, and technologies are all available for use, but putting them together in a concerted and organized fashion is not always easy to accomplish.

CONCLUSION

The fundamental importance of data—their collection, storage, protection, analysis, and use—has emerged as one of the key characteristics of the changing health care delivery system in the United States. No matter what the health care setting or population, the dual imperatives of controlling costs and improving quality can be achieved only through managing with data, that is, through careful evaluation of how the processes of care are linked to the outcomes of health care delivery, and through the application of information systems that help achieve the best possible outcomes. This means that outcomes data collection, the assurance of health care data quality, and the methodologies for accessing health data and information when needed, have become almost overnight highly desirable capabilities—indeed, core competencies—for professionals involved in producing health care services.

As Dr. Kelling and his practice with diabetic patients demonstrates, quantifiable improvements in patient care quality do not always require that the information management skills, methods, and technologies employed in support of CQI cost millions of dollars or demand teams of highly trained information technologists. Health care providers should feel enthusiastic about the advances in the application of information technology to patient care processes. Powerful, small, and relatively inexpensive computerized systems for collecting, storing, and communicating patient health care data across local, wide-area, and global electronic networks offer the opportunity to meet or exceed patient and payer demands for information at almost every level of care delivery and point of care.

CHAPTER 10

Collaborating for Improvement in Health Professions Education

G. Ross Baker, Sherril Gelmon, Linda Headrick, Marian L. Knapp,
Linda Norman, Doris Quinn, and Duncan Neuhauser

Health care organizations today are under enormous pressure to reduce costs without compromising the quality of care they provide to patients. Health care workers face continuing demands to increase productivity and to work more closely with other service delivery personnel. The Pew Commission, in its report (1995) on revitalizing the health professions, noted that health care workers will increasingly be working in a health care system that is more managed, more accountable, and more aware of population needs. Workers must be able to use fewer resources more effectively and be more innovative. The work itself will reflect a broader definition of health, being more concerned with education, prevention, and care management; more oriented toward improving the health of the entire population; and more reliant on outcomes data and evidence. What knowledge and skills are needed to accomplish these goals? How can health professions education programs better prepare their graduates to meet these challenges?

Hospitals and other health care organizations have used the principles and tools of continual improvement to redesign services to better meet the needs of patients, provide more effective care, and reduce costs. Increasingly these ideas are seen as relevant to the educational organizations that prepare health care workers, but the implementation of continual improvement in educational environments has been slower than in practice settings. This article outlines some of the key factors that have slowed the

Source: Reprinted with permission from G. Ross Baker et al., Collaborating for Improvement in Health Professions Education, *Quality Management in Health Care*, Vol. 6, No. 2, pp. 1–11, © 1998, Aspen Publishers, Inc.

teaching and learning of continual improvement in health professions education. The approach used in a recent effort, the Interdisciplinary Professional Education Collaborative (IPEC), is discussed, and key findings from the four academic groups engaged in this effort are examined in an attempt to understand how continual improvement might be more widely used by those engaged in health professions education (Joint Commission 1996).

INTEGRATING CONTINUAL IMPROVEMENT METHODS INTO HIGHER EDUCATION

Education in continual improvement has grown slowly in health professions schools. A number of programs in health administration initiated courses in continual improvement in the late 1980s. These efforts were further disseminated by the work of an Association of University Programs in Health Administration and Pew Foundation task force that brought together key faculty, program leaders, and experts in continual improvement to share ideas about how to teach these methods in graduate and undergraduate programs in health administration (Gelmon et al. 1995).

In medicine, efforts at Case Western Reserve University and a few other schools provided early experiences in teaching medical students and residents the principles and tools of continual improvement. A 1993 survey found, however, that only 17 percent of medical schools included continual improvement ideas and methods as part of their curriculum (Headrick et al. 1995).

Nursing programs have also increasingly included continual improvement in courses on quality of care. Only a few have incorporated training in continual improvement in their curriculum, however.

Accreditation requirements in health administration education have speeded the dissemination of continual improvement methods in that discipline (Gelmon et al. 1995), but use by other health professions education programs has been primarily determined by the initiatives of individual faculty members.

Slow Diffusion of Change

Why has the dissemination of continual improvement been slower in health professions educational settings than in practice environments?

While health care organizations have adopted continual improvement methods and techniques in the last decade, colleges and universities have only begun to teach and use these ideas in the past few years. Moreover, many of these efforts have focused on improving administrative processes, not on the teaching and research efforts important to changing the skills and knowledge of physicians, nurses, managers, and other professionals. Both the nature of the changes required and the process needed to implement this change pose difficulties for educators, students, and other stakeholders who wish to integrate improvement knowledge into the curricula and work settings of higher education.

Part of the reason for the slow diffusion of continual improvement in educational curriculum stems from the nature of this innovation. Rogers notes five characteristics of innovations that influence their rate of adoption (Rogers 1995). The five characteristics are *relative advantage,* the extent to which an innovation is perceived as better than the idea it supersedes; *compatibility,* the degree to which an innovation is perceived as consistent with the existing values, past experiences, and needs of potential adopters; *complexity,* the extent to which an innovation is perceived to be difficult to understand and use; *"trialability,"* the degree with which it can be experimented on a limited basis; and *observability,* the extent to which the results are visible to others.

Different instructors vary considerably in the content they include in teaching continual improvement. These differences make it difficult to assess dissemination of continual improvement within and across health professions education. Nevertheless, one might suggest that the relative advantage of incorporating continual improvement into health professional curricula is not clearly established. Although some faculty believe that these principles and tools are valuable in creating a more effective learning environment, others are skeptical. Banta notes that many faculties in colleges and universities believe that American higher education is the best in the world, and thus it does not require change (Banta 1995). Faculties maintain they know what is best for students and how to do research, so they are not motivated to ask others how they might improve these activities. Evidence that establishes the relative advantage of the tools and methods of continual improvement in improving the quality of higher education is scant.

The values inherent in continual improvement are consistent with those often expressed in the mission and value statements of colleges and universities. Nevertheless, efforts to encourage faculty to redesign courses to meet student needs and to work together in teams to improve curricula and teaching strain the norms of individual autonomy and run counter to established practices of working within the disciplinary silos entrenched in many universities (Parker et al. 1995).

The complexity of continual improvement also poses difficulties for adopting this innovation in higher education. While the tools and methods do not appear complex by themselves, it is often unclear how these tools and methods are related in a problem-solving process, and what team and organizational strategies are required for their use. Many of the early attempts by universities and colleges to implement continual improvement occurred in management and engineering schools and benefited from partnerships with organizations in other industries that had learned how to analyze and improve processes, identify customer requirements, and measure and react appropriately to variation. Yet only a few health professions education programs have established such partnerships. In higher education most faculty members view improvements in the process of teaching as individual activities, not cross-functional projects. While student feedback is a standard part of teaching, such feedback is often too late, too general, or too limited to offer much assistance in redesigning learning experiences.

The complexity of continual improvement and the absence of a clear vision about applying these ideas in the classroom or laboratory have also limited trialability and observability. Individual faculty have created excellent courses, but these courses may be rarely seen by other faculty. Moreover, individual courses are insufficient to infuse continual improvement into a curriculum of study. Thus, small-scale experiments have had limited impact on broader curriculum reform.

Beyond the nature of continual improvement as an innovation in health professions education, there have been several organizational obstacles to integrating this knowledge in health professions curriculum. These obstacles stem from the characteristics of universities as highly "organic structures" (Burns and Stalker 1961) with loose rules and regulations, decentralized decision making, and a disjointed hierarchy of authority. Such structures create excellent contexts for creative work, but they prove highly immune to change themselves (Duncan 1976). Those attempting change in such organizations often face difficulties in formulating goals, recruiting those whose actions are necessary to achieve those goals, and developing a clear understanding of how to change the teaching and learning processes.

Models for Change

The most common method for implementing broad-scale organizational change is to begin at the top with the knowledge and enthusiasm of senior leaders and then deploy change throughout the organization. This model is often recommended because it helps to ensure a strategic emphasis on the change and an operational deployment of the means of achieving the change: Goals are established; resources committed; and training, information, and other supports are provided to assist those in the organization in making change (Kotter 1996). Most large organizations undertaking major transformations, such as continual improvement or reengineering, have adopted a top-down model for making that change.

Institutions of higher education face considerable difficulty in making top-down change. If the change involves transformation of the curriculum, teaching methods, or other aspects of the teaching process, then faculty must be convinced that such changes are in their best interest. Faculty are notoriously suspicious of changes advocated by university administrations, and they are vigilant about defending academic freedom over matters of course structure and content as well as the subject and methods of research. Traditional ways of launching continual improvement initiatives in industry, including broad-scale training and chartering improvement teams are unlikely to be successful in an environment where professionals control the key work processes—teaching and research.

A second model for change relies on grass-roots initiatives. Individual faculty members can make changes to their courses or launch new research that incorporates ideas from continual improvement. Small faculty groups can also change course sequences, course content, and curriculum goals. These changes, however, depend on goodwill from other faculty and benign neglect, if not direct support, from administrative leaders. Moreover, such changes are naturally volatile. The next person to teach the course may use different readings or focus on different content. The next curriculum coordinator may stress different goals. Grass-roots efforts are easy to initiate, but difficult to institutionalize.

Bringing about Successful Change

Successful changes in higher education, therefore, usually require a combination of the top-down and bottom-up approaches. Senior administrative leaders need to support the changes, but faculty and students must lead the change locally: learning, adapting new methods and ideas, and experimenting with new approaches. Harry Roberts of the University of Chicago argues that grass-roots efforts are more likely to succeed in the context of senior support (Roberts 1995). He notes that senior leaders' efforts to make change outside of the administrative processes that they command directly are unlikely to be successful unless they can create local champions.

Similarly, Susan West Engelkemeyer argues that aspects of both a top-down and bottom-up approach were needed to implement continual improvement initiatives at Babson College (Engelkemeyer 1995). In this case, several factors were crucial in engaging faculty and overcoming resistance: establishing a compelling need for change, based on an understanding of current performance and competitive challenges; creating opportunities for faculty involvement; concentrating on the educational goals rather than the application of tools and techniques; allowing latitude regarding the pace and structure of changes; allowing faculty to participate in identifying priority areas for change; and being flexible about the timing of specific changes.

One method for encouraging faculty to integrate concepts and tools of continual improvement lies in initiating partnerships with organizations that have already seen the benefits of using such tools. By reaching out to such partners outside of the university, academic organizations can draw on skills in other agencies and facilitate their own learning about improvement (Evans 1992; Gelmon 1997).

A second strategy for stimulating involvement lies in creating collaboratives that bring together a number of organizations to share data and experiences. This strategy expands the social support and resources available to local sites, while motivating participants to maintain their commitment. Such collaborations have played an important role in the development of continual improvement learning in health care, beginning with the National Demonstration Project in 1987, which bought together 21 health care organizations with experts from other industries (Berwick et al. 1990). Other collaborative efforts have focused on improving clinical care. The Northern New England Cardiovascular Disease Study Group, a collaboration of 23 cardiothoracic surgery teams in five medical centers in Northern New England (Kasper et al. 1992; O'Connor et al. 1993; O'Connor et al. 1996) and the Breakthrough Series sponsored by the Institute for Healthcare

Improvement (Carver et al. 1997; Baker 1997) have demonstrated how collaborative efforts facilitate improvement.

CREATING AN INTERDISCIPLINARY PROFESSIONAL EDUCATION COLLABORATIVE

Most early experimentation in continual improvement in health professions education was disciplinary, not interdisciplinary. Yet, as has been frequently recognized, many of the problems in service delivery stem from failures in handoffs between disciplines, or from poor communication between different providers. Recognizing the need to initiate interdisciplinary improvement efforts in health professions education, the Institute for Healthcare Improvement, with assistance from the Bureau of Health Professions and the Pew Health Professions Commission, initiated a working group in 1992 to plan a demonstration project to develop models for teaching and learning about interdisciplinary continual improvement in health care. This initiative, known as the Interdisciplinary Professional Education Collaborative (IPEC), sought to identify health administration, medicine, and nursing programs that were willing to work together to apply skills and knowledge in continual improvement. The planning committee, which included representatives from the three disciplines, sought local practice sites where groups of faculty and students could create learning laboratories, developing knowledge and skills to improve the health of individuals and communities. The criteria for selection in the collaborative included:

- evidence of commitment to and prior experience with doing and teaching continuous improvement
- evidence of commitment to participation across the three disciplines (medicine, nursing, and health administration)
- evidence of local resources to support the project
- commitment of resources to provide core support for the collaborative
- willingness to commit to a three-year effort

In 1994, four groups were selected to participate in the collaborative: (1) the Medical University of South Carolina; (2) a Pennsylvania group that included the Medical College of Pennsylvania and Hahnemann University (now the Allegheny University of the Health Sciences) along with La Salle College, Duquesne University, and Carnegie-Mellon University under the sponsorship of the Allegheny Health Education and Research Foundation; (3) Case Western Reserve University and Cleveland State University; and (4) George Washington University and George Mason University. In several sites, the requirement that each local site include participation from medicine, nursing, and health administration necessitated inter-university as well as interdisciplinary collaboration. The goals for the collaborative are listed in Exhibit 10–1.

A LESSON FROM THE LOCAL IMPROVEMENT
TEAM CASE STUDIES

All four university-based teams of educators faced multiple challenges in trying to create projects that incorporated continual improvement knowledge, worked across educational program and disciplinary boundaries, and, in three cases, spanned more than one university. Project work by students was often community-based efforts rather than institutionally focused. This focus raises a further challenge because continual improvement methods have been more thoroughly tested in institutional settings and greater resources exist in these settings (Knapp and Hotopp 1995).

Work began in April 1994 with a three-day meeting to clarify the aim of the collaborative, identify jointly shared needs, and create effective working relationships to support efforts, both at a local level and across the collaborative (Headrick et al. 1996).

At this meeting, participants recognized the disparity in knowledge and skills about continual improvement within the collaborative. To remedy this deficit, a workshop was held with broad participation from the four local site teams and the collaborative's advisors. This meeting helped improve understanding of the methods and tools of continual improvement and their application in health care. Moreover, it provided collective learning about models for change and forged understandings within local teams and across the collaborative of how such methods could be used to guide improvement. Two lessons emerged from this experience: (1) building shared knowledge and using common tools improved communication and helped to stimulate learning across the collaborative, and (2) develop-

Exhibit 10–1 Interdisciplinary Professional Education Collaborative Goals

---

Interdisciplinary Professional Education Collaborative:
First-Generation Collaborative Goals

Aim: To improve health care by equipping new health professionals with the ability to improve continually the health of the individuals and communities they serve. The collaborative seeks to prepare health care professionals with:

- an understanding of the knowledge that will drive continuous improvement in the daily work of health service delivery
- skills in the application of that knowledge
- a professional ethic that supports integrated work, and competency for integrated health professional work aimed at meeting individual and community health needs and making health services more cost-effective

---

ing a shared aim, both within the local sites as well as between them, accelerated learning and maintained focus.

Interdisciplinary collaboration has been difficult in health professions education because of strong commitments to discipline-specific models of education. Few medical schools, for example, have used interdisciplinary models in educating physicians (McPherson and Sachs 1982). Not surprisingly, creating effective interdisciplinary learning experiences was not easy for participants in the collaborative. The initial efforts of the South Carolina team illustrate some of the barriers in creating an effective interdisciplinary team.

For example, the various groups learned important lessons about the effectiveness of working on real problems and sharing work and common models as a means of establishing this collaboration. Faculty read articles and books together, discussed new ideas, and designed and taught workshops. Sometimes "interdisciplinary work" is only an invitation for others to join in a specific discipline's efforts and adopt the mental models that guide its work. The work of the South Carolina group illustrates the value of using new models that are not attached to a specific discipline (e.g., the clinical value compass) (Nelson et al. 1996a-d) or the Langley model for improvements (Langley et al. 1994)) and then jointly exploring their use. The South Carolina local interdisciplinary team (LIT) also recognized the need to explore the underlying issues defining their differences. Their exploration of the meaning of "health" frustrated some team members, but enriched the ability of individuals to work more effectively based on a more fundamental understanding of the mental models guiding their work.

While most new courses begin as didactic experiences, all the four local teams felt the need to incorporate practical experiences as part of the learning experiences and to recruit local expertise. The George Washington-George Mason team placed one of their initial student improvement teams at La Clinica del Pueblo, a Latino community health clinic. Students in Pittsburgh organized a community health fair, and, in Philadelphia, the initial team project was based at a community nursing center. These efforts to branch into the community reflected a sense that improving health required more than interventions to improve the processes of institutional care. A byproduct of this emphasis on incorporating practical work in the educational efforts was the acceleration of faculty knowledge. Experiencing and collaborating in the efforts of improvement teams working on real projects stimulated reflection and deepened appreciation for the ideas and tools of improvement.

The course innovations at the IPEC local sites were led by multiple faculties from different schools who brought different assumptions and varying experiences to bear on developing a new course. These initiatives were thus unlike most innovative courses where change has traditionally been the purview of individual instructors. Not surprisingly, therefore, one of the first tasks all the local faculty teams faced was understanding the differences among them, so that they could develop a common vocabulary and create learning experiences that met the needs and backgrounds of an equally diverse student group. Faculty and students on the Cleveland team consciously spent time focusing on understanding differences in the history, philosophy, analytical perspectives, and areas of practice of medicine, nursing, and health administration. These explorations have been incorporated into the ongoing learning experiences related to interdisciplinary teaching.

Even apparently simple logistics posed problems. Discovering a convenient time and place for meetings created enormous difficulties for many groups. The Pennsylvania group worked in Pittsburgh and Philadelphia. The Cleveland and Washington groups were based on different campuses, and the South Carolina faculty were spread among widely dispersed schools on a large urban campus. By necessity, groups often met early or late in the day. The need for coordination spawned innovation. The Cleveland group took advantage of the development of a "virtual campus," a telephone system that linked students and faculty electronically. The Pennsylvania group organized cross-site monthly video conferences in addition to periodic face-to-face meetings. All sites made extensive use of electronic mail to keep in touch with the work of faculty and students.

Logistical problems sometimes mask underlying differences in approach or philosophy. One challenge that several of the local teams faced was the range in prior knowledge, experiences, and expectations that different faculty and different institutions brought to the collaborative. In some cases, these differences led to the defection of team members. In Pennsylvania, each of the two sites used a different model to guide improvement efforts, which complicated learning. Despite these hurdles, the groups struggled to create a common approach that served their disparate needs and to overcome the barriers and frustrations that arise when organizations and individuals are at different stages of learning about continual improvement.

Faculty at the four pilot sites also had access to an impressive range of advisors and mentors with considerable experience in learning and implementing improvement in education and health care. A rich and supportive atmosphere of shared learning pervaded the collaborative's work, reinforcing individual initiatives and spurring continued efforts.

KEY ISSUES IN INSTITUTIONALIZING THE INITIATIVE

Several issues continue to present challenges to the local teams. What differences are there in improvement work in the community, and how do these differences influence the educational models developed in the collaborative? The George Washington-George Mason team expanded their focus through their funding as one of the Health Professions Schools in Service to the Nation (HPSISN) demonstration projects. These projects are funded by the Pew Foundation to support community-oriented primary care training for residents and nurse practitioners. The George Washington faculty viewed this new funding as an opportunity to expand the initial efforts to practice continual improvement in community settings. The models of continual improvement and community-oriented primary care, while seemingly compatible, emphasize different ideas and pose different demands on learners, however. The team has wrestled with understanding these differences and developing a model that incorporates the methods for improving care with the development of community-based practice.

One approach for accelerating the diffusion of these education initiatives lies in developing a broader model of professional learning that elucidates the similarities and differences between continual improvement, community-oriented primary care, and service learning. Batalden suggests that such a model needs to be based on an understanding of how learners progress in their appreciation of the problems and their grasp of the skills and knowledge needed to address these problems (Batalden 1996b). Moreover, he states that such a model needs to address how health professions education can be structured to encourage development and contributions across disciplines.

More broadly, given the resistance to change that seems to pervade academic organizations, what are the levers that are most likely to produce change? The IPEC was based on the implicit theory that working on specific improvement topics with organizational support will result in change. But will these efforts be stable enough to survive transitions in membership and the addition of the new responsibilities and new constraints that are emerging in health professions education?

The local teams have all recognized the importance of learning by working locally with existing improvement efforts on specific problems and continuing to inform and attract the sponsorship of the senior leaders of their organization. The South Carolina group, for example, undertook projects using faculty and student teams, taught different groups of students, and worked on improving their own knowledge of continual improvement. At the same time, the team was conscious of the need to keep university, and to a lesser extent hospital and other health agency, leadership aware of their efforts. These efforts to engage leadership have already reaped benefits. Despite the departure of their initial team leader and champion in 1996, there was a relatively smooth transition to new leadership, a change facilitated by the support of senior academic leaders at the university who wanted to ensure that the initiative continued. In Pennsylvania, the senior leaders of Allegheny University of the Health Sciences used the experiences from this project to seed broader efforts within their programs and established a grant program to encourage similar initiatives.

FUTURE CHALLENGES

The four local IPEC teams have initiated significant local efforts to create viable, interdisciplinary professional education in continual improvement. These results stimulated the Bureau of Health Professions to support a second generation of the collaborative. Membership now includes 10 groups. While the first- and second-generation teams face a number of new challenges, the work of the first three years has yielded important results.

Returning to the earlier description of the characteristics of an innovation that are associated with the likelihood of its adoption, the four original teams demonstrated some of the ways in which health professions education can reframe continual improvement as an innovation, making it easier to adopt in other settings. Starting with small pilot courses reduced the learning barriers, improving the trialability and complexity of continual improvement in health professions education. Rather than searching for the "perfect approach" or trying to resolve all possible problems before launching a new course, the faculty groups embarked on experimental courses with small groups of students.

This pattern of small-scale change is different from the broad-scale curriculum redesign seen in some initiatives (Boyatzis et al. 1995). Moving from these small-scale improvements and pilot projects to institutionalization of continual improvement as a core competency in health professions education remains a challenge. Nevertheless, the local teams have recognized the importance of making their efforts more observable, informing local leaders and maintaining their support. Senior leadership and local faculty teams need structured opportunities to continue to share their understanding of how continual improvement can contribute to the improvement of educational experiences.

With increasing experience in offering interdisciplinary courses in continual improvement, the local teams are also able to demonstrate the compatibility of their work with the broader strategic goals of their universities. Integrating continual improvement is not the only demand on university administrators for curricular reform. Other stakeholders are clamoring for increasing the relevance of education for working in managed care environments, refocusing on the skills and knowledge needed for primary care, and developing community-oriented models for learning. At the same time, academic organizations face severe cost pressures as students, families, and employers resist further increases in educational costs and cross-subsidies from service delivery revenues are disappearing. Continual improvement efforts in health professions education will be more successful if academic groups are able to focus these efforts to develop solutions that also meet the other growing demands on leaders in health professions education. Shared learning across health professions education initiatives, such as those being facilitated by Campus Community Partnerships for Health, will also help to accelerate these changes by building on the experiences of a variety of projects across the disciplines. Last, there is an increasing pressure to link change in health professions education to real improvements in health and health care. The goal of improvement should be positive changes from the point of view of the customer (Joiner 1994). While students are the immediate customers of education focused on improvement, only those changes that ultimately improve the health of individuals and communities may be supported by those who fund such education. Thus it appears that the relative advantage of continual improvement as an innovation in health professions education may rest on demonstrating that better education can lead to more effective health care and thus better health for individuals and communities. This evidence is difficult to establish, but critical to success. Thus the second-generation teams have begun by focusing efforts on the health of specific populations in their communities, rather than on the design of better education. These lessons, and those mentioned earlier, are summarized in Table 10–1.

Everett Rogers, in his studies of innovation, remarks on the differences between the characteristics of those who are innovators and early adopters of an innovation and the great majority who follow (Rogers 1995). The challenge for the continuing work of the collaborative will be to design the change strategies and educational tools necessary to diffuse this work to the wider range of health professions education programs in the United States and Canada. The second generation of teams, which launched efforts in June 1997, will focus on specific community-based projects using a common improvement model and link their improvement efforts with education for students in a variety of health professions disciplines.

Table 10–1 Barriers to Change in Health Professions Education and Lessons from the Interdisciplinary Professional Education Collaborative

General Barriers	How Barriers Impede Learning	Lessons Learned
Characteristics of innovation*		
Relative advantage	Most faculty do not see how improvement knowledge assists them in teaching and research.	Focus on the linkages between changing education, improving health care services, and ameliorating the health of the population.
Compatibility	Faculty may view an emphasis on continual improvement as violating their autonomy in teaching and research.	Make participation in continual improvements a voluntary activity.
	The contribution of continual improvement to other curriculum goals (e.g., interdisciplinary education, community-based education) is unclear.	Take advantage of opportunities to link continual improvement ideas and methods to other initiatives such as service learning or community-based partnership.
Complexity	While no tools are difficult to learn, it is unclear when and how to use different improvement methods and tools.	Develop a workshop that helps faculty to develop shared understanding of core principles and tools. Treat initial courses as "pilots." Enlist students as collaborators; disclaim expertise.
Trialability	Courses are generally 10- to 15-weeks long and repeated yearly; individual course experiments may not be known by other faculty.	Start with small groups of students in pilot courses. Identify changes that will improve learning. Teach in faculty "teams."

continues

Table 10–1 continued

General Barriers	How Barriers Impede Learning	Lessons Learned
Observability	Faculty rarely see their peers teach; unless they are collaborations they often do not know the details of other faculty members' research.	Work in faculty teams to share learning. Collaborate with other facility on effective methods for teaching these new ideas. Identify key leaders who will support these efforts and keep them apprised of progress. Invite visitors to view and discuss these initiatives. Present learning at national meetings. Create a strategy for disseminating results.
Characteristics of academic settings		
Diffuse and decentralized authority	There is a loose hierarchy of academic environments. Administrators have limited influence on teaching and research.	Focus work on the front line with faculty and students, but secure senior-level interest and support where possible. Build alliances between faculty in different departments or schools. Identify common interests between faculty and develop shared aims.
Resource	Few resources are available for teaching innovations.	Work on faculty and student teams.
Functional structures	Discipline-based schools, each controlling teaching content and schedules, make disciplinary work difficult.	Be innovative in overcoming logistical barriers: Try alternative times and *continues*

Table 10–1 continued

General Barriers	How Barriers Impede Learning	Lessons Learned
		places to meet.
		Use technology such as "virtual campus."
		Use improvement ideas and methods to satisfy complementary curricular objectives such as "Interdisciplinary courses," "generalist training," or "service learning."
		Use interdisciplinary course listings and readings or project course numbers to secure course credits for faculty and students.
		Work on real problems to create greater interest among faculty and students.
		Collaborate with community partners.
		Use common methods.
		Have faculty learn together.
		Identify a shared mentor and work with that person.

*These characteristics were identified by Rogers (1995).

CHAPTER 11

Why Focus on Health Professional Development?

Paul B. Batalden

Most patients get health care from health professionals who work in very complex organizations (Greenlick 1996). Little prepares these professionals for work this way (Shugars et al. 1991). Caregivers are frustrated with their own ability to respond to the social pressures to remove cost while maintaining or improving the quality of care. They recognize that something is missing and are flocking to seminars and learning opportunities that offer a new way. Others are resigned to invest their energies outside medicine or "get out early" and take retirement at the first feasible time.

This frustration is compounded by pressures for social accountability that focus at the level of the organization or the individual caregiver, neither of which is the "functional front-line level" of caregiving where real change and improvement is possible. Increasing pressures for the publication of organization-level data on outcomes of care are creating new roles for accrediting organizations that now are preparing for public data releases about the care delivered in the organizations they accredit. For example, the Joint Commission on Accreditation of Healthcare Organizations announced its intention to use performance and outcomes measurement in its revised accreditation processes. Its pilot program for this integration is named Oryx. These issues were reviewed in the Joint Commission education program about the project in Boston, Massachu-

Source: Reprinted with permission from P.B. Batalden, Why Focus on Health Professional Development? *Quality Management in Health Care* Vol. 6, No. 2, pp. 52–61, ©1998, Aspen Publishers, Inc.

setts, on June 18, 1997. Comparative data on charges and other outcomes permit purchasers to ask new questions of accountability. The requirements by the Joint Commission and NCQA [National Committee on Quality Assurance] to use outcome measures and demonstrate continuous improvement to present new challenges and individual provider scorecards present a key to knowing from whom one should get one's care (U.S. General Accounting Office 1994).

The reality is that at the organization level there is very little that can be done to improve quality and value of care, and most of the individual health care providers working in complex organizations do not provide care as individuals; they work together with a small group of people and information support (Batalden et al. 1997). Together they make the decisions about the methods and daily care routines for the populations for whom they care.

This mismatch between the unit of analysis/accountability and the way care is actually given would be of little consequence if real changes in the value and quality of care were not desired. However, real changes are sought by recipients of care and by those paying for care. They perceive that provider "unresponsiveness" is a matter of will and seek political, regulatory, or "contractual" relief.

At the same time, we have witnessed a major change in the way manufacturing and service enterprises are being led. Built into the assumption structure are expectations about customer-driven design, process and system analysis, and improvement. While the leaders in other sectors were able to make these changes, it has been difficult for many of us in health care to consider these as relevant. Though we have learned the names and terms, we have had difficulty learning and incorporating these basic insights offered by W. Edwards Deming and others (Deming 1993; Batalden and Stoltz 1993). Some in health care have begun to see this requirement for new knowledge and its application (McLaughlin and Kaluzny 1994). Market pressures and regulatory pressures have helped increase the recognition of the terms and the pace of some change.

As health care leaders have worked to apply this knowledge and these skills, we have witnessed two large deployment strategies for the continual improvement of quality and value of health care: organization-centered and issue-centered, each of which has some strengths and important vulnerabilities. This chapter aims to explore these strategies and, in their context, consider the relevance of health professional development strategies for the improvement of health care today and tomorrow.

ORGANIZATION-CENTERED STRATEGY

Organization-centered improvement in health care has been alive in the United States for several decades, since the American College of Surgeons began accrediting hospitals (Brennan and Berwick 1996). A new chapter began when health care organizations, particularly hospitals, began to explore the lessons of continual improvement that were being learned concurrently in other sectors.

In 1980, new visibility for organization-wide efforts to improve quality came from the public television documentary, "If Japan Can, Why Can't We?" (Dobyns and Mason 1991). Early visibility in the U.S. for "Company-Wide Quality" (Mizuno 1988) or "Total Quality" came in manufacturing settings, most prominently in the automotive sector.

By the middle of the 1980s, efforts were underway in health care in the Alliant Hospital System in Kentucky and the Hospital Corporation of America in Nashville, Tennessee (McEachern and Neuhauser 1989). Many more in health care became interested as the Joint Commission on Accreditation of Healthcare Organizations and subsequently the National Committee on Quality Assurance incorporated this thinking into the accreditation processes. Several features, described below, characterized these efforts.

Focus on the context for work. Efforts were made to clarify what it meant to engage "quality" as a business or organizational strategy. Work on statements of mission, values, and vision was undertaken to create visibility for the centrality of the aim of continual improvement of services and products. These efforts were undertaken in part to foster a work environment that recognized and celebrated the value of learning at work. Deming wrote a set of guidelines for Western management, widely known as "Deming's Fourteen Points," that were extensively studied as descriptive of a workplace that was to be encouraged (Deming 1986). Health care versions of these points were made, and they facilitated study by health professionals and their organizations.

Knowledge of work as system, process. Building on and complementing the work of many general systems thinkers (Bertalanffy 1968; Ackoff 1981; Brockman 1977; Churchman 1971; Checkland 1981; Forrester 1990; Mitroff and Linstone 1993), Deming offered a view of the work of organizations as a system (Deming 1986). Adaptations of this model were made and used in health care (Batalden and Stoltz 1993; Batalden and Mohr 1997). With a description of health care as a system and process came adaptations of process and system change strategies as described below in *"Projects."*

Attention to patients, payers, communities as "beneficiaries" or "customers." By many wonderful leaders and learning experiences, health professionals have been prepared and socialized historically to understand the oft-quoted aphorism attributed to the Harvard Medical School professor Francis Peabody that "The secret of the care *of* the patient is in caring *for* the patient." Moving beyond the "patient-ness" of the patient in even more aggressive ways to understand the personal preferences, values, and aims *of* the person as we design and deliver our care and service *for* the person became the focus. Many methods for creating the new knowledge and understanding we needed were offshoots from the "customer" focus in sectors other than health care (Batalden and Nelson 1990; Nelson and Batalden 1993; Joint Commission 1992). It was no longer a matter of "patient relations" or "patient satisfying"; it became clear that we needed more insight into our efforts to *design* care. Coping with the reality of multiple—and sometimes apparently conflicting—customers' requirements of our work placed us alongside the many other sectors with similar struggles.

Projects. Using many different approaches to problem solving, process improvement, and innovation, we documented the possibility of local change for the design and redesign of service and care (Gustafson 1997). In many cases, the people leading the change had not been active before in those roles, and this newfound opportunity gave them additional pride in their work.

"Tribes" grew up around improvement methods and approaches. Sometimes the language of one was difficult for another to understand—so it was easier to classify the label than to understand the relation of the label to the underlying phenomenon. Sometimes the proprietary interests of the authoring individuals and organizations got in the way of easy dissemination and critical methods analysis. Despite these limits, methods and skills for changing health care in usual practice settings gained new visibility.

Leader's role in promoting learning. To bring these changes about, leaders had to move beyond "command and control" understandings of their own work (Taylor and Taylor 1994). Work done by Argyris and Schon (Argyris 1991; Argyris and Schon 1996) expanded our understanding of what it meant to learn in the work setting. This contribution became connected to the idea of testing change and learning from that testing in the workplace, which had been advocated by Walter Shewhart some years earlier (Shewhart 1986). Reginald Revans's observations on the helpfulness to patients and to the longevity of student and graduated nurses in the London hospitals promoted ease in asking "upward questions" and added to a new appreciation of the leader's job in promoting learning at work (Revans 1964). The work of Peter Senge and his colleagues at the Massachusetts Institute of Technology provided great visibility to the idea of a "learning organization" for work, identifying five disciplines as fundamental to the creation of such organizations (Senge 1990; Senge et al. 1996).

Organizational networks. The desire to create opportunities to share work underway in similar organizations led to the creation of multiple networks of organizations. [IHI's Quality Management Network (QMN), Group Practice Improvement Network (GPIN), The Healthcare Forum's Quality Improvement Networks (QINs), and HCA's Healthcare Quality Technology Network (HQTN) all had active, regular meetings and cross-network learning.] Of interest, these networks were settings for organizations and their leaders to come together to learn and accelerate their own efforts at organization-wide improvement.

At the same time these efforts were underway, massive changes in the nature of health care organization life were beginning to occur.

Organization definition changes weekly. The flurry of new partnerships, mergers, acquisitions, divestitures, joint ventures, etc., confused the "front-line" professionals. Agreements to provide contracted services seemed to rapidly move from one opportunistic source to another. These changes added confusion and complexity at the level of the caregiving personnel, as new procedures for connecting their services emerged continuously. Less concrete, but perhaps more consequential over the long term, caregivers began to wonder who they worked for.

Layoffs, cutbacks, hiring freezes, and highly targeted human resource programs. New mergers made it possible to consolidate some previously underutilized capacity. Oversupplies of certain medical specialty services became more visible as the relationships between populations and caregivers became contractual (Wennberg et al. 1996). The old patterns of working wherever you wanted as a graduated medical specialist gave way to considerations of where there was work.

Huge variations in caregiving as well as health resource capacity. The Dartmouth Health Atlas documents huge variations in caregiving and health resource capacity: beds, physicians, nurses, caregiving practices per thousand population. These variations prompted many to ask why they should bear the additional costs and morbidity experienced in their region. Often the caregivers were unaware of the population-based differences, adding to the sense of loss of control they were feeling (Wennberg et al. 1996).

Costs of care, the watchword. As similar clinical outcomes were being documented for lower costs, purchasers accelerated their pressures for cost reductions. With minimal agreement about measures of quality, assumptions that "all care is about the same, only the costs are different" led purchasers to engage in demand or target pricing strategies: The purchaser tells the health plan how much less they will pay for their health care premiums the next year. These pressures were often hard to fully communicate to the front-line caregivers who were being asked to work harder in the established methods of caregiving.

Outside of the health care sector and about the general "workplace" in society, larger trends were being noted.

Workplaces of the future will be less stable places of employment. Workers will move in and out of employment relationships. Charles Handy (1989) and others (Bridges 1994) described a workplace of the future that seemed to be a more accurate depiction of the workplace of the present for many. The forms of employment—a job—were migrating to term agreements to perform specific tasks (Bridges).

There will be less loyalty between worker and employer. Downsizing efforts that often accompanied work reengineering efforts led the still-employed to become less secure in their assumptions about the dependability of their workplace as a future source of employment. Without good measures of the full intellectual contribution individual workers were making, undocumented losses seemed to be occurring (Edvinsson and Malone 1997).

In summary, organization-centered strategies for the improvement of health care gave new emphasis and new energies to many features of organization life that were helpful to improving quality. However, the fundamental realities that organizations of all kinds were becoming less stable, organization-wide efforts of all kinds were becoming less dependable, and "quality" was becoming only another theme for the harried top leaders left the unmistakable impression that dependency on organization-centered strategies for the improvement of health care quality made the improvement effort vulnerable. As witness to this potential vulnerability, when the staff leaders (senior corporate quality executives) gathered from across sectors, they were worried about their futures (U.S. Conference Board 1996).

ISSUE-CENTERED PROGRAMMING

Improving health care by finding topics or conditions that could be improved, conducting tests of change, and disseminating those efforts is as old as the application of empiricism to health care. What seemed new was the public identification of gaps between what was known and what was usually done coupled with strategies to accelerate closing those gaps (Berwick 1994).

In his keynote address to the annual National Forum of the Institute for Healthcare Improvement, Donald Berwick challenged the group by naming specific conditions and clinical situations where the scientific evidence suggested one path for practice and the increasingly available data about our common practices suggested another path in use, indicating a real performance gap. Later, these observations were prominently featured in a widely circulated medical journal (Berwick 1994).

These observations were made possible by increasingly available comparative practice data made public by purchasers, private data companies, and public sources, including states. These data invited comparisons across provider settings and revealed wildly varying care processes. Variation in care across small areas had been known for years (Wennberg and Gittlesohn 1973). What was new was the extent of the variation and its significance for both clinical outcomes and costs (Wennberg et al. 1996).

Under the auspices of the Institute for Healthcare Improvement, a series of issue-specific efforts began in May 1995. The model brought together a panel of knowledgeable subject matter experts and a panel of people who had been able to make change in their practices. Together they developed a set of "change concepts" worth trying. Other teams of subject matter practitioners were invited to join a cooperative effort to rapidly test these concepts in their home settings and to compare experience meetings. Their collective experiences were made public in publications and a national "congress" for the larger interested public. The gains were impressive. Stretch goals of change: more than a 40 percent change in practice was achieved in more than 25 percent of participants, and more than a 20 percent change in practice in 78 percent of the first 147 organizational participants (Kilo 1997).

Concurrently there were several other issue-specific efforts underway:

- The Agency for Health Care Policy and Research (AHCPR) Patient Outcome Research and Treatment (PORT) teams gathered the scientific evidence supporting best practices for the conditions that PORT teams had been established to study (Salive et al. 1990).
- Guidelines for best practice in the management of specific conditions began to emerge from many sources: professional societies, proprietary companies, and publicly supported research studies, including the PORT teams. So many have emerged that guides to the guidelines were developed.
- Benchmarking efforts popularized by Xerox Corporation came alive in health care. Local benchmarking efforts coupled with public and private initiatives began searching for best practices. Attractively illustrated publications geared to rapid reading raised the consciousness of many leaders (Health Care Advisory Board 1993).
- Rapid cycle change methods proliferated (Langley et al. 1996; Nelson et al. 1996a-d). These methods encouraged participants to design and test change in dramatically reduced cycle times.
- Issue-based collaboratives and networks emerged. People working on common topics came together to share their efforts, such as the work of the Institute for Health Care Improvement (IHCI) and its ongoing Breakthrough Series Collaboratives.

The rush of issue-centered activity sharpened the focus for improvement, many changes were made, and networking increased among commonly motivated clinicians and other health care leaders. At the same time, it became clear that all this highly visible activity masked some real unevenness in execution—sometimes within the same systems. The idea that improvement could occur without explicit attention to the context for work grew. The popularity of "naming the issues" caught on and the impatience to "name" the next issue seemed to take precedence over deployment of systematic change. The longevity for an "issue" seemed to be getting shorter. Improving patient care, issue by issue, became the same as creating a "quick-fix skunkworks": delegating the responsibility for improvement to that group and assuming that they would accomplish all that was needed. Privately, some wondered about the sustainability of the larger numbers, faster issues, and activity vortex, that seemed to obscure unresolved deployment challenges and which seemed to exhaust dedicated (but finite) health professional resources. Some also wondered about the cost of this "late education" and wondered why the acquisition of this knowledge and these skills could not become a part of the regular preparation of health professionals.

PROFESSIONAL DEVELOPMENT-BASED STRATEGY

With this vulnerability of organization-centered strategies and the questions about the sustainability of issue-centered programming, the future for the improvement of health care seems less than certain. Fortunately, we have another option.

Health professionals have long been proud of their personal commitment to lifelong learning and to their role as leaders in the design and delivery of health care. What might be involved if we were to attempt to use that professional development process as a means of advancing the improvement of the quality and value of health care?

What Is the Process of Professional Preparation and Development?

The exact process varies for each professional discipline, but at a high level the processes resemble one another and can be illustrated with the case of medicine, though similar paths may be constructed for the other professions. The process can be described by the categories of formal educational preparation:

- basic health professional preparation leading to an MD degree
- graduate health professional preparation leading to specialty certification
- postgraduate health professional preparation for continuing medical education and certification

Each step of the process has a currently defined content of learning. That definition of content has been based on some expert assessment of what is now known, what is appropriate for the learner at this stage of his or her preparation, and what the profession in general has established as knowledge needed for competency as a professional at that developmental stage. State, national, and professional exams have been developed to assess the candidate's knowledge and skills.

How Might One Connect This New Knowledge to Existing Learning?

The growth of knowledge and expanding scope of practice has been titrated against the finite amount of time in the curriculum for professional education. As a result of these enormous curriculum content/time pressures, efforts to "add" new courses are not greeted with much joy. The challenge, instead, is to identify "insertion opportunities" into the existing learning opportunities: *Teach and learn about the familiar subject, but teach and learn about it in a way that enables you simultaneously to learn improvement knowledge and skills.*

This approach involves the following:

- identification of the "new information and new skills" (Batalden and Stoltz 1993; Berwick et al. 1992a and b; Berwick 1993)
- juxtaposition of that information and those skills with the existing curriculum
- creative learning methods development at the points of potential "junction" between the new knowledge and skills and the existing subject matter learning
- careful assessment to ascertain that the previously taught subject matter is mastered as well as the new improvement knowledge and skills

The following will be helpful for the acceleration of this change.

Cross-profession development models. Several experiments in community-based improvement that cross disciplinary boundaries have been undertaken. For examples, see Chapter 10 of this book and the special 1996 issue of the *Joint Commission Journal on Continuous Improvement* (Bellack 1996). Most patients get health care today from health professionals who are actively working collaboratively at the front line of patient care with other professionals. Each has been prepared within her or his own disciplinary, professional "silo." Everyday, they work together in processes that require them to reach common understandings about the design of change and improvement of care. Moreover, models of professional development that offer a theory of knowledge and skill acquisition that cross disciplines have the added attraction of offering opportunities for faculty collaboration in the creative development of these "insertion junctions" (Benner et al. 1995; Dreyfus and Dreyfus 1996). (See Exhibit 11–1, "Exploring the Stages of the Modified Dreyfus Model of Skill Acquisition.")

Faculty who understand the new information and skills and who can integrate them into their own way of teaching the current subject matter. Currently, a small but growing number of traditional academic faculty are prepared to teach this way about this material. (The IHI Health Professional Educators Registry Web site is under development pursuant to BHP Grant.) A small, but growing literature is developing that highlights efforts that faculty are making (Chessman et al. 1996; Elliott et al. 1996; Gelmon and Baker 1994; Gelmon et al. 1997; Gordon et al. 1996; Headrick et al. 1992; Headrick et al. 1995; Norman and Lutenbacher 1996; Parenti et al. 1994; Weingart 1996).

Clear guidance from accrediting and certifying bodies. Health professional education and development programs have extensive accreditation processes that offer explicit guidance to program directors regarding the content of the learning experiences. If these were clearer about their

---

Exhibit 11–1 Modified Dreyfus Model of Skill Acquisition

**Exploring the Stages of the Modified
Dreyfus Model of Skill Acquisition**

Explorer: What is the role all about?
Novice: What are the rules that can help me?
Advanced beginner: What do I need to remember about the setting/context for care?
Competent: What goes into a good plan for the care of the patient?
Proficient: How can I get some of the waste out of my life?
Expert: What complex cases do you have for me?
Master: What can I learn from the surprise that just happened to me?

expectations of graduates' abilities to improve health care, it might help interested programs.

Hiring policies that reinforce the value of acquiring these competencies. With the increased formalization of health care delivery settings, it is becoming the rule that health professionals are employed. If these employers can make their preferences clearly known, preparatory programs can do a better job of preparing their graduates for work in these ways (Batalden et al. 1989).

Are There Limits to the Use of the Professional Development Process for Improving Health Care?

"It is easier to relocate a graveyard than to change the academic curriculum" (Source unknown). Though commissions (Shugars et al. 1991) and study panels (Lohr et al. 1996) have recommended changes in the health work force preparation process, these pathways change slowly. Sometimes current health professional educational content reflects state laws and cannot simply be changed. More often, the momentum of the present situation prevails over new ideas. In addition, large invitations to change such "stable" curricular and learning processes invite reaction formations that can easily reject good ideas in the company of not-so-good ideas.

Integrating the Models to Offer More Robust Programming for Improving Health Care Quality and Value

Health care improvement that is undertaken with any one of the strategies as the major driver can expect experiences of the strengths and weaknesses we have already seen with them. Improvement that is able to harness the synergy of an integrated approach has the possibility of creating a potentially more robust strategy.

Such an effort offers the health care sector a potentially transforming and more durable model for the continual improvement of health care. Individual caregiving settings, such as the Dartmouth Hitchcock Medical Center and the Henry Ford Health System, are already demonstrating their integration of parts of the model. To illustrate:

A health system's leaders have been hard at work focusing the energies of the organization on the improvement of care. Through their organization-led efforts, they learn they must improve their care for women of childbearing age. They select the issues of childbirth care, including Caesarean births, and make the networking around those issues accessible to the local leaders. The professional development efforts for all levels of all related health professionals focuses learning in that setting on the knowledge and skills needed for the improvement of that health care. New possibilities emerge as the contributions of each of the efforts come to a common focus.

Working across, between, and within all the approaches offers creative health care leaders many new opportunities and access to many additional energies for learning and fostering the improvement of health care.

PART IV

Application

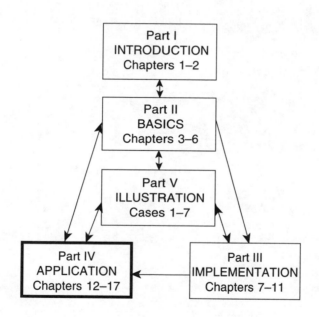

CHAPTER 12

CQI in Primary Care

Linda S. Kinsinger, Russell P. Harris, Arnold D. Kaluzny

Most Americans receive health care within a primary care setting. Quality and efficiency of services are issues for primary care just as for other areas of health care. Yet the never-ending demands of daily work are such that providers rarely have time to step back and gain perspective on the problem. Continuous quality improvement (CQI) is a potentially powerful tool for primary care providers to meet the challenges of quality and efficiency. This chapter places CQI in the context of other approaches to change in primary care practice and outlines one CQI initiative to produce change toward improved quality and efficiency of preventive care in this setting.

THE CHALLENGE OF CHANGE IN PRIMARY CARE

Medical practice must change constantly. Although there are age-old techniques that good physicians have always used, new scientific research daily adds to the evidence for or against various diagnostic and treatment approaches. The weight of evidence builds, and, at some point, it becomes clear that a new approach is best, that medical practice must shift to a new way of doing things. There is, for example, recent and convincing evidence that screening sigmoidoscopy decreases mortality from colorectal cancer, yet most physicians have not been routinely performing this procedure.

There is another reason why medical practice must constantly change: The problems of patients change over time. Although this change is slower than the pace of medical research, the problems that patients present to physicians in the 1990s are different in important ways from patients' problems in, say, the 1960s. AIDS and the resurgence of tuberculosis, for example, necessitate new approaches to patients with cough and weight loss. A higher percentage of patients is old, and has degenerative, incurable conditions, requiring very different management skills from an earlier practice with predominantly younger patients and acute medical problems. Domestic violence, while present in an earlier day, has now reached epidemic proportions in some areas.

Medical practice, however, and particularly primary care practice, is not well designed for change. Although primary care is in a transition from primarily solo and small group practices to larger groups and networks of practices, they are mostly run by people without organizational experience or expertise (i.e., physicians). In general, primary care providers are so overwhelmed with the daily workload that it is impossible for them to step back and determine programmatic needs, and develop and evaluate new programs. Primary care is much less well reimbursed than other, "procedural" specialties in medicine, and thus has fewer resources (e.g., personnel, computers, consultants) than other branches of medicine. Primary care has also evolved a very individualistic style of operating that makes its practitioners very suspicious of external influences, and of change itself.

There have been a number of attempts to change medical practice, with varying degrees of success. No approach, however, has found change simple or easy to accomplish. A recent review of 50 randomized controlled trials of continuing medical education (CME) found "a direct relationship between the intensity of the intervention and the number of studies with positive outcomes" (Davis et al. 1992). Traditional CME with lectures by experts, printed materials alone (Evans et al. 1986), journal articles (Haynes 1990), and consensus statements (Kosecoff et al. 1987) generally did not have a large impact on medical practice. Several approaches, such as "academic detailing" (Soumerai and Avorn 1990) and the influence of "opinion leaders" (Lomas et al. 1991), have been used successfully to change simple behaviors such as prescribing a specific drug or allowing a trial of vaginal birth as opposed to performing Caesarean section. These approaches need more study in other areas of medical practice to define more clearly their uses and limitations.

Continuous quality improvement (CQI) is a new approach to change in medical practice. By CQI, we mean an approach to change in organizations that begins with collecting data about an important issue to determine to what extent there are "performance gaps," opportunities for improvement. The organization then sets a goal to improve the outcome measured by the

data, and breaks down the task of achieving the goal into small, manage-
able steps. A plan for implementing the steps is developed and tried, and
the outcome of concern is monitored to determine if improvement indeed
takes place. Data from monitoring are given back to the organization
regularly to allow fine-tuning of the new approach and to reward those who
have made changes to improve the outcome. The entire process includes all
relevant members of the organization, working together to identify opportunities for improvement and new approaches to try.

To date most experience with the CQI technique in the medical field has
been within large medical institutions such as hospitals and HMOs rather
than private primary care practice. While some have been impressed with
its success in large institutions, the inherent problems of change in private
primary care practice noted above make it necessary to consider how to
adapt this potentially powerful technique to primary care. Its promise to
alter complex behavior, such as counseling for cessation of cigarette
smoking, should make research in this area a high priority.

PRACTICE CHARACTERISTICS AFFECTING CQI

There are several issues to consider in the adaptation of CQI to the
primary care setting. The fact that private medical practice is dominated by
physician-led practices with little management expertise and overwhelmed
with daily work, means that it is questionable whether practices by
themselves will be able to develop the data needed to define "performance
gaps" (i.e., areas where performance is not up to agreed-upon standards)
and detect improvement over time. As we suggest below, developing such
data may become the province of a respected second party, such as the
continuing medical education department of a university or a professional
association.

Although the CQI approach emphasizes change coming from within an
organization, this modification of CQI envisions the practice being initially motivated to seek change by a respected "outside" group pointing out
that performance is suboptimal. Clearly, the issue chosen by the "outside"
group must be one, such as preventive care, understood by all to be
important.

It is also doubtful that practices alone will have the time and expertise to
organize practice planning groups to develop new, detailed plans that can
be discussed with the rest of the staff, tried, evaluated, and fine-tuned to

perform the specific function in a different way. Again, a respected second party may be needed to assist the practice in working through this process. Such second parties must be chosen carefully, as the culture of many practicing physicians is to resist outside direction.

Another issue in adapting CQI to primary care practice is the lack of incentives to carry out the CQI process at all. While hospitals and other large health care organizations are often required to complete the CQI process to remain accredited, there are no such requirements for primary care practices. Again, outside, "external" groups may be needed to reward successful change.

Finally, the medical mindset that all tests and treatments must be exactly tailored to each patient, implying that no guideline can lump people into groups of patients needing the same procedure, greatly complicates developing automatic systems of any kind. The more one can identify groups of patients who need the same procedure(s), the higher the probability that processes such as CQI can develop systems that get the job done most efficiently. Another related but complicating idea is that physicians should not advocate specific procedures, but should only provide the patient with information and options, and leave the decision to him or her. This idea again limits what office systems can accomplish.

ONE MODEL OF CQI IN PRIMARY CARE: THE NORTH CAROLINA PRESCRIBE FOR HEALTH PROJECT

The North Carolina Prescribe for Health Project (NC-PFH), funded by the National Cancer Institute from 1991–1995, was an initiative designed to help community-based, primary care practices change how they provide preventive care, especially breast cancer screening, for their patients (Kinsinger et al. 1998). Many studies have documented that clinical preventive services are often not provided as recommended by national expert and advisory groups (Lewis 1988). For a variety of reasons, most preventive care seems to be delivered haphazardly—some patients receive it; many don't.

One of the reasons for the difficulty in reaching higher levels of performance relates to recent changes in the paradigm of preventive care itself. Guidelines for preventive care are undergoing change. As new research shows evidence of benefit of certain procedures, these are being recommended more strongly (an example is sigmoidoscopy for colorectal cancer screening). Some tests previously considered useful are no longer recommended when they are found not to have value for screening (routine chest radiographs, for example).

The list of preventive care procedures that has been shown to reduce mortality (the ultimate goal for preventive care) is actually rather short and does not include the long battery of routine tests that has often been done in the past. The idea of an annual head-to-toe physical examination has been replaced by the concept of a periodic visit, tailored to a patient's specific risk factors. Skills, such as counseling about personal behaviors, not often learned in medical school in the past, are now required. The new prevention paradigm calls for a changed type of physician-patient relationship, in which patients are encouraged to take a more active role in their own health, and patients and physicians become more like partners on a team, rather than following a hierarchical model. NC-PFH was an approach, using the principles of CQI, to help practices face and deal with these changes.

NC-PFH sought to improve performance of preventive care services by assisting primary care practices to develop a more organized system for preventive care. In using a CQI approach to accomplish this goal, the project encouraged change based on (1) data collected at base-line to document a "performance gap"; (2) plans by the practice for systematically accomplishing five "steps" in getting prevention done; and (3) feedback to the practice on how it was doing in meeting its goals for preventive care (Kaluzny et al. 1991). All members of the practice, staff as well as physicians, were involved in this process.

Primary care practices in two mostly rural areas of North Carolina, whose physicians were members of three sponsoring medical professional societies, the American College of Physicians, the American Academy of Family Physicians, and the National Medical Association, were randomly chosen to participate. The project was co-sponsored as well by the North Carolina Area Health Education Center (AHEC) Program. These professional organizations are known for their interest in the quality and content of medical practice and have been active in formulating guidelines for preventive care. One of the important reasons for working together with professional associations in NC-PFH was that such groups might well be involved in CQI-type interventions for their member physicians in the future.

Because the CQI approach included working with members of the group as a team, the NC-PFH project worked with whole practices, rather than individual physicians. Making changes in practice routines is a process that involves more than the physician alone. Deciding on changes to be made and implementing these changes requires the input and efforts of all members of the practice.

Base-Line

The first phase of the project involved collecting base-line data on preventive care procedures recommended or performed from each of the participating practices. The data consisted of (1) reviews of randomly selected medical records of patients; (2) brief anonymous questionnaires from consecutive patients in the waiting rooms, asking about preventive care procedures done in the last year or more; and (3) questionnaires of physicians and office staff members, determining their approach to delivering preventive care. Members of the project staff collected the data (except for completion of physician and staff questionnaires), so as not to impose a burden on already harried office staff members. They compiled information from medical record reviews and patient questionnaires on performance data and sent it back to physicians in an easy-to-read format. Figures 12–1 and 12–2 are examples of charts showing high and low rates of performance, respectively, of several preventive care procedures in two study practices.

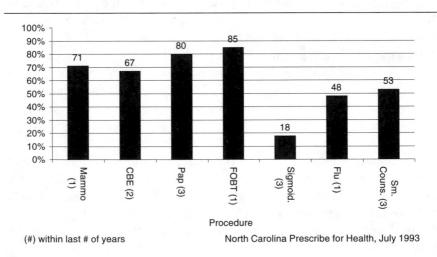

(#) within last # of years   North Carolina Prescribe for Health, July 1993

Figure 12–1 Preventive Care Performance (Chart Reviews, Patients 50 and Older)

Half of the 62 study practices that participated in NC-PFH were then chosen at random to receive a yearlong period of consultation and support from NC-PFH to try new strategies for increasing preventive care in their offices. The other half of the practices received support later in the project. The intervention phase involved a series of meetings with each practice, beginning with an initial meeting with physicians and staff to review their performance results and to set goals for increasing their rates of preventive care in areas in which the practice was interested. The purpose of the meeting was to identify preventive care procedures in which there may have been a "performance gap," that is, a difference between the rate at which the practice currently provided that service for eligible patients and the rate at which it would like to provide the service. The project encouraged practices to focus on a short list of preventive care procedures for older adults, especially breast, cervical, and colorectal cancer screening, smoking cessation counseling, and influenza immunizations. These procedures have been shown to be effective in reducing disease-specific mortality.

Action Steps

To deliver preventive care routinely to patients eligible for these services, the primary care practices must carry out five steps:

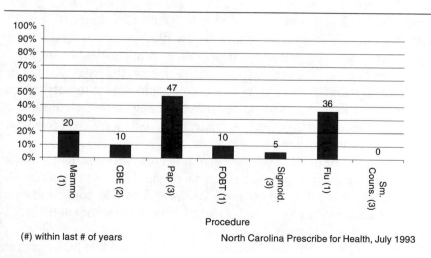

(#) within last # of years   North Carolina Prescribe for Health, July 1993

Figure 12–2 Preventive Care Performance (Chart Reviews, Patients 50 and Older)

1. identify patients' needs for preventive care services and prompt providers about these needs
2. recommend these services to patients
3. perform or order the services
4. follow-up the results of the services
5. recall patients at the next appropriate interval.

These five steps provide the framework of the office system (Leininger et al. 1996). Many practices already had methods in place for one or two of the steps, but few were routinely addressing all five steps in a systematic way.

Subsequent meetings with the practices centered on understanding the then-current method for carrying out the steps for preventive care and making revisions to get each step done more systematically for all eligible patients. Project team members worked with practice staff to document any systems already in place that accomplish one or more of these steps. Project members then assisted physicians and office staff together to consider various options for new ways to perform these functions, thus developing a revised system for preventive care. Practices were offered an assortment of "tools" to assist them in carrying out the functions. "Tools" included items such as flowsheets, sticky notes for charts that prompted providers about procedures that are due, patient brochures detailing which preventive services the practice recommended by age and gender group, stamps and crack-and-peel labels used as flowsheets for charts, stickers to indicate smoking status on the charts, tickler files with cards for tracking patient needs and self-addressed postcards to recall patients, and brief patient questionnaires to identify procedures done in the past (whether in the office or elsewhere), used as a prompt for physicians to perform or order the procedures. Practices selected from among these tools those that best fit their needs. To the extent possible, these tools were customized to the practice's specifications.

For example, one practice decided to routinely identify a patient's needs for preventive care by having the nurse check the chart and confirm with the patient as she is doing her in-take assessment. Then she communicated this information to the physician by using a removable sticky note on the encounter page. This note (Figure 12–3) listed several procedures for which the patient may be eligible. The nurse simply checked the boxes for those for which the patient is due. The physician then indicated performance or ordering of the prompted procedures by checking another box on

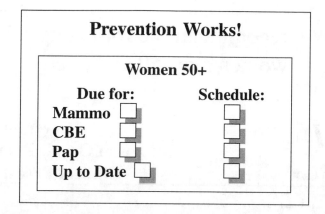

Figure 12–3 Eligible Procedure Note

---

the note and returning the note to the nurse or receptionist. The nurse gave all women patients over the age of 50 a brochure that told them which preventive care services the practices encouraged for them (Figure 12–4); this step was briefly documented in the chart. Patients were notified by phone of their test results. After the appropriate interval, the practice sent a reminder postcard, asking patients to call the office to set up an appointment for another preventive care visit.

Practices were encouraged to set a "start date," the date on which they put their revised plan into action. Project staff kept in close touch with the practices during this time. A month or so after the start date, project staff members made an observation visit to each practice to see how the system was working and to get feedback from practice staff. Project staff members made their observations in the waiting room/reception area and in the clinical area. They focused on a number of items, including use of the project's office system tools, availability and use of patient education materials on preventive care, patient waiting times, and interactions among staff, physicians, and patients. These visits were scheduled for one-half day and were conducted with the consent of the practice. The observations were presented back to the practice at a later follow-up meeting between practice physicians and staff, and project team members. These discussions often resulted in modifications of the preventive care office system.

In all, the NC-PFH team provided support and consultation to the practices in the intervention group for a period of 12 to 18 months. At the conclusion of the intervention phase, the NC-PFH team conducted a repeat practice survey in all study practices. This repeat survey included another

We recommend the following for women ages 50 and over:

✔ *1*

every year

Prevention Visit
Fecal Occult Blood Test
Clinical Breast Exam

✔ *1-2*

every one-two years

Mammogram

✔ *3*

every three years

Pap Smear

✔ *5*

every five years

Sigmoidoscopy
Cholesterol Screening

✔ *10*

every ten years

Tetanus Booster

Figure 12–4 Preventive Care Services Brochure

medical record review of randomly selected patients' charts and question-naires of physicians. The repeat study focused on preventive care performance during the study period and allowed comparisons between practices that had already received assistance to develop office systems for preventive care and those that had not. The NC-PFH team then offered the practices in the latter group brief assistance, through three-hour workshops, to develop and implement such systems.

Results

Preventive care procedures were recorded from the medical record reviews in one of two ways (for most procedures). A test was counted as "mentioned" if there was either any notation about the test in the visit notes or if a report was in the record. The test was counted as "reported" if there was only a report found in the record. That was done to give "credit" to the physician for recommending the procedure to the patient, even if the patient did not follow through with the recommendation. Physician questionnaires included items on their preventive care policy and their interest in preventive care for their patients. At follow-up, physicians in practices that had received assistance were also asked about the completeness of their office's system for preventive care.

The medical record reviews and physician questionnaires showed overall improvement in several practice-level indicators of office systems (Table 12–1). More practices had a written preventive care policy and were using flowsheets to track preventive care for their patients at follow-up compared to base-line. A larger number of practices were also involving staff in recommending preventive care, such as mammograms, to patients who were eligible for the procedure. Practices that received the assistance were more likely to have these indicators in place than were the practices not receiving the help. Although the intervention practices were also more likely to note an increased role for staff in identifying patients' needs for mammograms and an increased use of prompts and flowsheets by physicians, these differences were not statistically significant.

The proportion of women with mammogram and clinical breast examination (CBE) discussion and/or results in their charts was similar at baseline between intervention and control practices (Table 12–2). Over the course of the study period, the proportion of women's records with

Table 12–1 Practice-Level Measures of Office Systems (from Physician Questionnaires)

	Intervention Practices (%)			Control Practices (%)			Differ-ence** in Change	p	OR	CI
	Base-line	Follow up	Change*	Base-line	Follow Up	Change*				
Written policy	16	57	41	13	7	–6	47%	.01	14.2	(2.0 - 98.8)
Flowsheet entry	10	29	19	19	7	–12	31%	.02	9.9	(1.4 - 68.4)
Staff identify patients due	37	65	28	39	44	5	23%	.18	2.3	(0.7 - 8.0)
Physician use of prompt/flowsheet	35	65	30	29	44	15	15%	.51	1.5	(0.5 - 4.9)
Staff recommend mammograms	41	58	17	48	33	–15	32%	.04	3.6	(1.0 - 12.4)

* Change from baseline to follow-up
** Difference in change in intervention practices compared to control practices

Table 12–2 Performance of Breast Cancer Screening in Last Year for Women Age 50 or Older by Chart Review

	Intervention Practices (%)			Control Practices (%)			Difference** in Change	p	OR	95% CI
	Base-line	Follow up	Change*	Base-line	Follow Up	Change*				
Mammogram mention	38.7	51.4	12.7	40.5	44.0	3.5	9.2	.01	1.5	(1.1, 2.0)
Mammogram report	28.0	32.7	4.7	30.6	34.0	3.4	1.3	.56	1.1	(0.8, 1.4)
Clinical breast exam (CBE)	41.1	46.4	5.3	44.6	43.9	-0.7	6.0	.06	1.3	(1.0, 1.6)
Mammogram mention and CBE	28.2	38.7	10.5	30.3	32.6	2.3	8.2	.01	1.4	(1.1, 1.9)

* Change from baseline to follow-up
** Difference in change in intervention practices compared to control practices

mention of a mammogram in the last year increased significantly more in the intervention, compared with control, practices (12.7 percent vs. 3.5 percent, respectively; p=.014, 95 percent confidence interval [CI] 1.1, 2.0). The proportion of women's records with a mention of CBE in the last year showed a trend toward an increase in intervention practices (5.3 percent increase), compared with control practices (0.7 percent decrease; p=.058). There was, however, no difference between intervention and control practices in the change in the proportion of women's records with a mammogram report in the last year (4.7 percent increase compared with a 3/4 percent increase respectively; p=.56). There was also no difference in the change in the proportion of women's records with a Pap smear report (for women who had not had a hysterectomy), or of men's and women's records with a sigmoidoscopy or fecal occult blood test for colorectal cancer screening.

We saw no difference in base-line performance or change in performance between physicians of different specialties (family physicians vs. general internists), different practice size (solo vs. group) or age (younger vs. older physicians). Physicians' change in performance over time was not associated with their beliefs in the effectiveness of cancer screening procedures, their stated readiness to change their cancer screening activities, or their perceptions of community standards of practice for cancer screening procedures.

SUMMARY

The NC-PFH project applied the principles of CQI to the challenge of improving preventive care in primary care practice. Each practice's own data, collected for them from chart reviews and patient questionnaires, were used to identify potential target areas for attention. The task of delivering preventive care was broken down into five separate steps and each step was addressed individually. The process involved the practice as a whole, including physicians and staff working together to solve a problem. Strategies were developed to monitor the process and to feed back to the practice the results of their efforts. The problem of lack of management expertise within practices and the reluctance to allow "outsiders" to work closely with them was overcome by the structure of the project, which was offered as a consultation, and by the sponsorship of the project by the medical professional organizations to which the physicians belonged.

The lack of strongly favorable results was disappointing. Despite a moderately intensive intervention, practices were not able to implement complete office systems for screening patients for cancer. Some increase was seen in the development of written policies, use of flowsheets, and involvement of office staff in recommending mammograms, but no indicator was present in more than two-thirds of intervention practices. The mean number of the five indicators in intervention practices was only 2.8. Given the lack of success in helping practices to develop office systems, it is not surprising that there was little impact on actual performance of cancer screening activities. Although there was an increase in the proportion of eligible women whose records indicated some mention or discussion of mammography, the proportion of women with reports of completed mammograms did not change significantly.

Why didn't this intervention work better? There are several possible explanations. First, nearly all physicians and office staff members endorsed mammograms and clinical breast examinations as important screening procedures for breast cancer, but many had difficulty understanding the need for a systems approach to accomplish screening goals. Many physicians were either skeptical that it is possible for a busy practice to screen a high percentage of eligible patients, or were inclined to solve the problem by simply "trying harder" themselves. Second, because this was a randomized, controlled trial, the project worked with practices individually, that is, in isolation from other, nearby practices. We made no attempt to use social influences in the local medical community to change the community standard for breast cancer screening or to influence physician behavior through key local leaders.

Third, few medical practices in the study had computer capabilities beyond billing and appointment functions. Only one practice had a fully electronic medical record. Therefore, we were not able to take advantage of this potentially useful tool which could help practices organize their patient records to establish a tracking system for breast cancer screening or a "denominator" of eligible patients who were "due" for screening during a specified period of time.

In the practices that experienced large changes, the office staff, especially the nurses, played a critical role. These nurses embraced their role as patient educators and became more active in discussing breast cancer screening with women patients. Some were able to act on "standing orders" from their physicians to order mammograms for women who were due for them; others encouraged patients to talk with the physician about getting a breast examination and a mammogram.

Overall, we focused the intervention primarily on "enabling" factors, as defined by Green and Kreuter in the PRECEDE health promotion planning framework (Green and Kreuter 1991). These are factors that facilitate the performance of actions by individuals and organizations through changes in the work environment, skills training, and provision of resources to support new work patterns. We did not, however, emphasize "predisposing" factors, those pertaining to attitudes, beliefs, values, and perceived needs, or "reinforcing" factors, including social support and feedback. Although the physicians in the study practices intellectually understood the reasons for change (the value of improved screening for breast cancer), they didn't feel any strong internal or external pressure to commit to the effort needed to effect those changes in their day-to-day activities. Thus they were able to modify their behavior somewhat but not enough to lead to substantially increased breast cancer screening.

Few other trials of CQI interventions in primary care practices have been published in the literature. Goldberg et al. reported on a randomized controlled trial of academic detailing techniques and CQI teams in Seattle, which focused on implementing guidelines for the treatment of hypertension and recognition and treatment of depression (Goldberg et al. 1998). The study was conducted in four clinics of different organizations, providers, and patient populations. Despite a considerable effort by providers and staff, little change occurred in increasing compliance with the guidelines. Goldberg states that, "although CQI teams could sometimes work in chronic disease care, they were no 'magic bullet.'"

THE FUTURE OF CQI IN PRIMARY CARE

Primary care medical practice will continue to face change, as research continues to discover new information, as the health care system undergoes a reconfiguration, and as society demands an increasing level of quality and accountability from medical care. The application of CQI to this process of change in primary care practice holds potential for helping physicians and their staff adapt to different ways of doing things. CQI techniques may be more effective in primary care practices when physicians and staff sense pressure to change their ways of providing care. Managed care organizations, health insurance companies, and professional liability carriers could offer incentives to providers for assessing the quality of care in primary care practices through the process of CQI. Additionally, area health education centers and academic health centers could take a leading role in helping practices adjust to change by developing a new type of continuing medical education that is based on self-directed learning and set in the physician's own practice. Such a CME program could enable physicians not only to keep abreast of the ever-changing field of medicine but also to change their practice to better serve their patients.

CHAPTER 13

CQI in Managed Care

Leif I. Solberg, Thomas E. Kottke, and Milo L. Brekke

Managed care and CQI as an oxymoron? Magnified by patient concerns about restrictions on choice of physician or coverage for specific services, editorials in most of the leading medical journals express concern that the managed care threat to quality requires serious attention (Bodenheimer 1996; Kassirer 1995; Clancy and Brody 1995; Ellwood and Lundberg 1996; Dalen 1996; Silver 1997). For example, the editors of *The New England Journal of Medicine*, in their introduction to a series of articles on quality, say that the rapidly heightening visibility and worry over quality is primarily because "the quality of health care is now seriously threatened by our rapid shift to managed care" (Angell and Kassirer 1996, 883).

This reaction and the legislative actions based on it can be seen as examples of conclusion by hunch and anecdote rather than by following the continuous quality improvement (CQI) precept of reliance on data-based thinking. Recent thorough reviews of the published evidence on the relationship between managed care and quality have noted that there is no clear answer to whether managed care is better or worse than other care arrangements (Miller and Luft 1994; Miller and Luft 1997; Hellinger 1998). With the possible exception of a few studies of chronic illness in the elderly, however, these reviews conclude that there is no evidence that managed care members receive inferior care or have outcomes inferior to those covered by indemnity insurance. In fact, a panel of the Institute of Medicine recently concluded that "quality of care is the problem, not managed care"(Chassin et al. 1998, 1000).

(Supported in part by grant #ROI HS08091 from the Agency for Health Care Policy and Research.)

298

Nevertheless, this chapter describes the growing need for managed care plans to address quality improvement as well as cost control, both to compete successfully and to garner the necessary support of the public and the medical care/public health establishment. It uses the example of a preventive services clinical trial to illustrate the challenges and needs of such an effort. If managed care plans can successfully help care delivery organizations transform themselves to better meet the health care needs of our times, they will deserve a continuing prominent place in the nation's care system and will overcome the skepticism and hostility that they currently face.

FROM COST TO QUALITY: A MANAGED CARE EVOLUTION

Ironically, the founders of the movement to make HMOs the dominant form of health care believed that it would produce higher quality than the then-existing cottage industry of medical care (Ellwood et al. 1971). Although this was long before CQI appeared on the American scene, they argued that HMOs would have "a vested interest in regulating output, performance, and costs in the public interest" (298) through better organization, integration, and coordination of care. It seemed obvious that the features Enthoven described as essential to managed care would naturally lead health plans to make use of whatever techniques worked to improve costs, care quality, and health outcomes (Enthoven 1988):

1. restricted choice of provider
2. extensive peer review system
3. negotiated prices with physicians
4. risk-sharing arrangement with physicians
5. responsibility for a defined population
6. integration of insurance and direct provision of services under a fixed prospective budget

It appears, however, that these theoretical pressures lead to different emphases on quality, depending on the extent of managed care penetration and competition in the marketplace. Goldsmith et al. (1995) have developed a useful conceptual framework for thinking about this evolution from cost to quality and value through three stages (see Table 13–1). Nelson et al. (1998) and others suggest a very similar notion. Although imperfect,

Goldsmith's framework helps explain why so many marketplaces thus far have focused primarily on cost competition. During Stage I, all of a managed care plan's focus is on the management of costs, primarily through the reduction of inpatient care. Managed care plans could thrive economically during this stage of "*event-driven cost avoidance*" without having to pay much attention to quality. Newly formed plans could achieve these cost-focused goals through various administrative and regulatory mechanisms without much need to work with hospitals and physicians to restructure the way that they provide care. McEachern et al. (1995) describe the strategies typically used during Stage I as making superficial changes in care delivery compared to the fundamental changes required in later Stages II and III. As all types of health insurance organizations achieve similar levels of hospital use and costs and as managed care becomes the dominant form of coverage, however, this strategy no longer

Table 13–1 Evolutionary Stages of Managed Care

	Stage I	*Stage II*	*Stage III*
Focus	Event-driven cost avoidance	Value improvement	Health improvement
Main Objective	Reduce hospital use	Control resource intensity and improve care delivery process	Population-based health status improvement
Secondary Objective	Reduce use of subspecialists	Increase consumer satisfaction	Reduced health services cost
	Utilization review	Capitation of specialists	Pooled risk capitation
Methods	Provider discounting	Clinical guidelines and pathways	Risk appraisal
		Outcome monitoring	Targeted intervention:
		Controlling services:	• at-risk individuals/ families
		• drugs	• community/ environment factors
		• procedures	Case management
		• tests	Multidisciplinary teams
		TQM/CQI	TQM/CQI

works to differentiate among health plans. They must find new ways to compete or engage in destructive price wars.

In Stage II, competition is forced to focus on value, combining more sophisticated approaches to cost containment with efforts to change the actual delivery of care. These care delivery changes require clinicians not only to cooperate with their implementation but also to provide the major change leadership (McEachern et al. 1995). Berwick (1994) has made a valuable contribution by pointing this out and by identifying "eleven worthy aims" for the clinical leadership of this reform of our health system. Interestingly, many of those aims address the resource management issues identified in Table 13–1. Others are related to the increasingly important need to devise and implement clinical guidelines and pathways. Since these care delivery changes are really process improvements, CQI is a potentially valuable tool to facilitate such changes.

Few health plans have successfully made much headway on these challenges in Stage II and Goldsmith et al. (1995) suggest that "it may take as much as a decade to actually achieve control over the value of their product through value improvement." (22) Once they have, the new strategies identified in Stage III will become necessary, focusing then on moving to population-based health status improvement. Although Goldsmith didn't include CQI as a method in this stage, we believe that it is equally important here.

BARRIERS TO MANAGED CARE USE OF CQI TO IMPROVE VALUE/HEALTH

In addition to the need for a managed care plan to develop an effective understanding and application of CQI principles in its own internal operations, at least four major barriers stand in the way of making effective use of CQI for the changes needed in Stages II and III. These barriers arise from the fact that clinicians must be actively involved in formulating and facilitating the changes:

1. Lack of financial incentives and tension to change at the medical group and clinician level
2. Low readiness of care delivery organizations to change long-standing care patterns and to use CQI concepts and techniques, especially in ambulatory care

3. Low readiness of managed care organizations to use CQI techniques themselves as well as low understanding of how to facilitate CQI and change management in their contracted care systems
4. Mutual misunderstanding and mistrust between managed care and clinicians, heightened by the techniques used during Stage I

Incentive to Change

Until a significant proportion of the patients of a medical group are covered by a risk or capitation payment system, it is very hard to interest the group in changing care patterns, since such changes will actually cost them money. Furthermore, even when that threshold is reached for the group as a whole, most groups have productivity incentives for individual clinicians that may defeat the group's overall interest in reducing unnecessary care. When these problems coexist with an absence of public measurements of accountability and with local purchasers who are only interested in cost management, only farsighted and brave (foolish?) clinicians will want to change.

Clinic Readiness

There are many factors involved in the primitive state of readiness of most care delivery organizations to undertake planned organizational change to improve care processes. Some of these factors, like the tradition-bound attitudes and expectations of both physicians and patients, are hard to modify regardless of an organization's desires and abilities. Most medical groups, however, also lack organizational infrastructure for change as well as leaders with the vision, understanding, skills, and experience needed to undertake the difficult task of planned change in processes. In fact, most medical groups still consist of clinicians who have banded together for efficiency and for the power to negotiate with various purchasers and regulators. Although they share space, they do not think of themselves as groups with a need to operate care processes in a common way. Other barriers include absence of top management commitment, incomplete quality infrastructure, limited resources, physicians' professional autonomy, incentive systems, turf issues, limited availability of data, and conflicts with the cost and efficiency of service (Jackson et al. 1994; Reeves and Bednar 1993; Lowery 1996).

Moreover, although the data-based thinking of CQI would seem to be a good fit for physicians, involving them is widely recognized as a major challenge. In addition, their concept that measurement needs to be of research quality interferes with their use of measurement for improvement (Solberg et al. 1997e). Although there are some published examples of use of CQI by medical groups (as compared to hospitals), we have evaluated this experience in smaller groups in a region that is relatively far advanced in improvement interest and CQI pervasiveness and found it lacking (Solberg et al. 1998a). Zairi and Matthew (1995) suggested the same deficiency in their study of TQM in English general practices, especially in the areas of measurement and standards. In a recently published review of CQI in clinical practice for the Institute of Medicine, Shortell et al. (1998) concluded that it required both an organization with a considerable degree of readiness and a supportive external environment.

Managed Care Readiness

Kaluzny (1992) has described how the interaction model developed by Hakansson to explain supplier-customer relationships in industrial markets can be applied to the interaction between clinician organizations and the managed care plans with which they contract. He noted that the relationships, exchange of information and funds, and dependencies created by their interactions provide an opportunity for the managed care plan to encourage and facilitate clinician activities (such as CQI).

Even where there is both incentive and potential for managed care plans to help medical groups learn to use CQI to improve care delivery processes, there are also readiness barriers to such actions within the plans. Not least of these is their lack of CQI culture, experience, and use internally. It is interesting that the literature on CQI in health care is virtually devoid of any reference to use of CQI concepts and techniques within managed care plans. In a literature with abundant descriptions and even a few evaluations of CQI in hospitals, we have been able to find only one article for HMO CQI. That study of six HMOs with "exemplary quality improvement programs" was striking in several ways (Hillman and Goldfarb 1995):

1. Five of the six plans were nonprofit, at a time when that was a disappearing life form.

2. It focused almost entirely on HMO actions to affect the quality of care provided to members by contracting clinician groups, suggesting by omission that CQI was not a part of internal operational improvement efforts.
3. It emphasized activities more commonly associated with quality assurance than quality improvement or CQI—data collection for accountability, establishment of standards, measuring outcomes, recruitment/credentialing, and preparing for external accreditation by the National Committee on Quality Assurance (NCQA).

The point is that it will be difficult for managed care plans to facilitate CQI activities by their care-providing affiliates if they are not committed to it internally, both for credibility and as a way to build skill and experience. In addition, managed care plans have mostly used arms-length and micromanaging ways to reduce costs during Stage I and have little experience with how to develop and sustain the collaborative relationships with providers that are necessary for CQI. Finally, most managed care personnel have limited experience (or credibility) with the realities of providing care.

Managed Care and Clinician Suspicion

Numerous surveys have documented the widespread unease or hostility that clinicians feel about the changes being forced on them, which they largely attribute to managed care. Less well-documented is a similar feeling among many managed care leaders that clinicians are the major barrier to cost and quality improvements. Much of this suspicion has been created on both sides by the approaches used in Stage I, but it can easily continue into a new focus on quality, since clinician behavior is more important to success here.

**IMPROVE: A TEST OF MANAGED CARE CQI FOR
IMPROVING THE QUALITY OF PRIMARY CARE
PREVENTIVE SERVICES**

Over the past five years, we have been involved in a randomized controlled trial of a CQI-based intervention in primary care clinics which has been sponsored by two large managed care plans in the Midwest with funding by the Agency for Health Care Policy and Research (AHCPR) (Solberg et al. 1995; Solberg et al. 1996). Since there is only one other published trial of CQI in any industry (Goldberg et al. 1998), this trial has provided us with an extraordinary opportunity to increase our understanding of the potential of this Stage II/III strategy. Although the focus for this trial was on the delivery of clinical preventive services, the concepts, methods, and lessons should apply to any effort to facilitate CQI use by medical groups.

Background

The primary stimulus to planning this trial grew out of the need to find a way to improve preventive services in primary care. Although there has been some reduction in the gap between population rates for important preventive services and the modest goals of "Healthy People 2000," no clear answer exists for how to speed this up (McGinnis and Lee 1995). There is now a fairly extensive literature on the need for a systems approach to this problem; a need to build office systems that change the care environment to make it more likely that needed preventive services will be provided. We have summarized this literature as well as provided a specification and literature support for the various processes involved in such an office prevention system (see Exhibit 13–1) (Solberg et al. 1997d). CQI concepts are the basis for this system, recognizing that the identification of individual patient needs for services and the provision of services found to be needed are basically organizational processes, similar to an appointment or billing system. Unfortunately, these processes have heretofore been largely missing or disorganized and, like much of medical care, dependent on the memory and actions of individual clinicians who are too busy addressing the immediate needs and wants of their patients (Solberg et al. 1998c; Kottke et al. 1993).

The remaining unsolved problem is to discover how to stimulate the development, implementation, and maintenance of these prevention processes in medical practice. Except for one trial (Dietrich et al. 1992), various approaches to this problem have had only modest or no effect (Ruffin 1998). Because managed care plans have the potential for interaction effects as noted by Kaluzny above (1992) as well as the ability to provide external help for clinics, we proposed and were funded for a

Exhibit 13–1 The Prevention System

---

1. Guidelines
The process by which a clinical organization develops, obtains broad buy-in, and updates a specific uniform set of preventive services for defined age/gender/risk groups. Without organizational agreement on the recommended services, effective and efficient prevention systems cannot be developed.

2. Screen
The process of obtaining health risk and previous preventive service information in a standard way about all patients of a clinic in order to identify their specific prevention needs.

3. Summarize
The process of organizing and updating the information obtained in the screening process so that it is all in one place and easily accessible for review by those needing to know the current prevention status of a particular patient. Without a continuously current summarization of each patient's preventive service status, it is not possible to keep members up-to-date on the recommended services.

4. Cue/Remind
The process of reminding clinic staff and clinicians about their need to undertake necessary prevention system tasks.

5. Follow-Up
The process of communicating to patients the results of preventive services along with appropriate explanations and recommendations.

6. Resources
The process of selecting, gathering, organizing, and maintaining patient education and referral information needed by both patients and clinic personnel.

7. Counsel
The process of assisting patients and their families to make needed changes in their behavior.

8. Track and Recall
The process of reminding patients about their needs for specific preventive services, especially those without acute care visits.

9. Patient Activation
The process of encouraging patients to take greater responsibility for their own preventive services and behavior changes.

10. Prevention Visits
The process of providing all of the preventive services needed by a patient during a single visit designed and organized for that purpose. This special visit may not be necessary in the future for many patients who have their preventive service needs met during their visits for other reasons.

---

scientific trial of an HMO-sponsored effort to facilitate CQI methods in clinics to institute prevention systems (Solberg et al. 1996). The trial focused on the improvement of rates of providing eight preventive services that had strong evidentiary and clinician support and represented a diverse set of delivery needs (see Exhibit 13–2).

Trial Design

This trial was called IMPROVE (Improving Prevention through Organization, Vision, and Empowerment). It was all the more unusual because it was actually sponsored by a collaboration of two HMOs who otherwise compete in the same regional market (Solberg et al. 1995). Forty-four primary care clinics contracting with one or both of these HMOs agreed to participate in response to a joint recruitment letter from the medical directors of the two plans, and were randomized into 22 intervention and 22 control clinics. These were fairly typical clinics for the area, representing 33 of the 71 medical groups contracting with these plans. They averaged seven to eight adult primary care physicians and 45 percent prepaid patients (although only half of that number was from the two sponsoring plans).

The intervention involved training two people from each intervention clinic in how to lead and facilitate an internal multidisciplinary team through a seven-step CQI process that was fairly typical for the early 1990s (see Exhibit 13–3). The training and improvement process addressed each of the 10 philosophical elements and most of the 8 structural elements described in Chapter 1 of this book. The training was not theoretical,

---

Exhibit 13–2 Preventive Services Addressed by IMPROVE

I. **Cancer Screening:**
    Clinical breast exam and mammography every 2 years from age 50
    Pap smears every 2 years from age 20
II. **Heart Disease Risk Factor Screening:**
    Tobacco use at each visit from age 20
    Blood pressure at least yearly from age 20
    Blood cholesterol every 5 years from age 20
III. **Immunizations:**
    Influenza yearly from age 65
    Pneumococcus once from age 65

Exhibit 13–3 The Process Improvement Model

1. Identify the problem.
2. Collect data to understand your current process and customer needs and expectations.
3. Analyze the data to understand root causes.
4. Develop alternative solutions that address the root causes.
5. Generate recommendations to implement the best alternatives and test them in a pilot study.
6. Implement the tested new process using systematic preparation steps, including orientation and training.
7. Use an iterative cycle through these steps to evaluate the new process and continue to improve it until it is good enough.

however, but very task-oriented around preventive services and the systems that have been demonstrated to be effective. It was spread out in seven sessions over a six-month period to be just-in-time, followed by bimonthly opportunities for the trainees to meet for networking about their techniques, tools, progress, and problems. In addition, consultants from the project visited or called them periodically over the 22 months of the intervention to reinforce their efforts and to problem solve with them.

In order to evaluate the trial, all clinic personnel, the clinic CQI team members, and patients visiting the clinics completed surveys, both before the intervention began and near its end. The charts of the surveyed patients were also audited to provide another way of assessing clinic behavior. Both quantitative and qualitative data were gathered to document the intervention experience. These data provided us with many lessons about both preventive services and CQI in this setting.

Preventive Services Findings

During the original recruitment for the trial, we learned that many of the medical groups in our area had substantial interest in improving preventive services. When asked what were their principal reasons for participating in this trial, 87 percent of the recruited clinics said that it was to improve their prevention rates and 82 percent said it was to improve their efficiency in delivering these services (Solberg et al. 1996). Most of those that declined did so regretfully (because of temporary turmoil) while expressing interest in the issue.

Measurement of the rates of these services before the intervention began was especially valuable in understanding the problems of low rates. Actually, the rates at which visiting patients reported being up-to-date for these services before the clinician encounter were fairly good by national standards (Kottke et al. 1997a). If they needed a service, however, they only had a 6 percent to 29 percent chance of receiving a recommendation for the service during their visit (except for blood pressure, which was performed about 90 percent of the time, whether it was needed or not). Thus, after the visit the up-to-date rate for these services had only increased an average of 6 percent. Interestingly, the 20 percent of patients who were there specifically for a complete physical were only a little more likely to be offered needed services. Since patients reported making an average of four visits to the clinic a year, and since patient reports tend to overestimate both the recency of services and recommendations by clinicians, it is unlikely that the current overall rates will improve without a major change in approach.

In order to better understand the reason for these low rates, we measured the presence of functioning prevention systems in these clinics (Solberg et al. 1998c). This was evaluated by asking the clinicians and nurses who had to use them, including questions about each of the 10 processes described in Exhibit 13–1 for each of the 7 services in Exhibit 13–2. Not surprisingly, they reported that most of these processes were not present in any organized way. Where present, they were only in effect as individual processes for individual services, with *follow-up*, *guidelines*, and *resources* accounting for 60 percent of the total existing processes. Since none of these three is directly related to the delivery rates of the services being measured, it is not surprising that the rates were as low as they were. We also demonstrated that there was great variation between clinics and, more important, within clinics in the relative rates at which various services were provided (Solberg et al. 1997c). In other words, a clinic that had the highest rate of the 44 for providing mammography was just as likely to be among the lowest as the highest for other services. This tended to confirm the lack of systems.

Our surveys also shed light on relevant customer attitudes, both those of clinicians and patients. Clinicians were nearly unanimous in regarding these services as very important, and were nearly as strongly agreed that patients wanted these services (Solberg et al. 1997b). Although they supported systems changes as important to improved rates, they had very mixed feelings about whether their clinic should improve the way they provided these services. That may explain why we found very little correlation between these attitudes and the actual rate at which individual clinics provided each service. Unfortunately, we also found very little correlation between these rates and patient satisfaction with either preventive services or overall satisfaction with care (Kottke et al. 1997b). Thus, neither clinician nor patient attitudes appear to be a particularly important driver for improvement.

We especially studied the rates at which these clinics provided these services to their patients with low incomes, no insurance, or medical assistance (Solberg et al. 1997a). Since it is widely recognized that such people are less likely to be up-to-date on preventive services (and we confirmed that), it has been assumed by many that clinicians are less likely to recommend needed services to them. Not only did we find that low socioeconomic status (SES) patients received such recommendations at the same rate as higher SES patients with insurance, they were just as likely to have the recommended services actually performed.

Unfortunately, the post-intervention measurements revealed that only a few services increased in intervention clinics more than they did in control clinics (Solberg et al. 1999). This was confirmed by both patient report and chart audit. Even worse, when we looked at the rate changes in various subsets of intervention clinics that had appeared to do the best job of process improvement, they had not done much better than their counterparts.

Our measurement of the presence of functioning processes in these clinics sheds some light on the cause of this discouraging finding (Solberg et al. 1998b). Although the intervention clinics did significantly increase their use of prevention processes, it was far from ideal or complete. At base-line, both intervention and control clinics reported having 11 to 12 process/service combinations in place out of a theoretically complete 73 (7 aren't needed, e.g., follow-up for immunizations). Thus, the doubling in the intervention clinics (to 26) was still only one-third of what was needed for complete systems. The key finding is that the reminder process was still largely absent, despite the fact that the teams had all chosen to continue to rely on the physician to order needed services rather than delegating this task to nursing staff. Reminder systems are the process that has by far the strongest evidence base for affecting preventive service rates (Solberg et al. 1997d).

CQI Findings

This trial provided the first opportunity to study the extent of CQI penetration in primary care clinics. Although this region may be relatively advanced in its stage of managed care, its exposure to CQI, and its transition from solo to group practice, it offers a glimpse of what may happen in other regions in the future and provides a context for the CQI lessons of this trial.

From the beginning of recruitment we had evidence of interest in CQI. More than two-thirds (71 percent) of the participating clinics said that they were doing so in order to obtain training and experience with CQI (Solberg et al. 1996). Twenty of the 44 reported having had at least one process improvement team, and they identified at least 89 previous teams (Solberg et al. 1998a). Unlike the experience in hospitals where most teams have addressed problems in administrative processes, half of these clinic teams had worked on improving clinical processes. One-third of these had chosen preventive care, although they were much more restrictive than our proposal, focusing on specific services like flu shots. We surveyed the members of what each clinic identified as its most successful previous team (pre-IMPROVE) and found them to be surprisingly multidisciplinary. Only 40 percent of these teams reported recycling through evaluating their changes, however, perhaps explaining why only 60 percent reported making successful improvements.

At base-line, we also surveyed all clinicians and nurses and found that large majorities reported understanding and supporting CQI (Solberg et al. 1998a). When it came to questions that required more detailed knowledge about CQI (e.g., variation reduction or not blaming problems on individuals), however, there was much less agreement and more neutral responses. Only 53 percent reported that their clinic leadership was firmly committed to using CQI.

We also conducted a survey of all clinic personnel as a way to obtain a self-assessment of the existing culture for quality in these organizations, using the criteria from the Malcolm Baldrige National Quality Award (Solberg et al. 1998a). The mean clinic scores overall and for the seven Baldrige categories were similar to scores from hospitals or businesses of various types and lower than scores from two companies that had won the Baldrige award. Thus, the clinics' support for quality as assessed by all their personnel was not in keeping with the belief among many health care professionals that their field is more quality-minded than other lines of work.

All of the 22 intervention clinics established multidisciplinary teams to work on IMPROVE and all had identified sponsors from clinic management. All but one clinic's team leader/facilitator attended the training sessions. Both surveys and anecdotes reassured us that the trainees found the process both valuable and enjoyable. Nearly all worked diligently on the improvement process, although only about 60 percent reported implementing their new systems at the time of the post-intervention data collection. Surveys of the clinic teams at that time confirmed that nearly all of the teams had completed at least 12 of the 17 activities we had suggested as important (Solberg et al. 1998b). The primary area of incompletion was in evaluating the changes made and using that information to repeatedly cycle through the process.

In retrospect, it was surprising that these teams and clinics stuck with their task as well as they did. Not only was the CQI process used a slow and time-consuming one, but it had been carried out through a period of enormous turmoil in these clinics and the region. We measured that turmoil and found that during the first year of the intervention, 64 percent of the clinics had undergone a change in ownership or affiliation, 77 percent had lived through change in at least one major internal system (e.g., billing, lab, records), and 45 percent had changed clinic manager, medical director, or both at least once (Magnan et al. 1997). Moreover, six teams changed leaders, seven changed facilitators, and eight experienced a change in sponsor during this time.

In order to better understand the efforts and barriers that these process improvement teams faced, we undertook two qualitative evaluation efforts. One involved the two clinics that served as pilots during development of the intervention and the other studied a randomly selected subsample of intervention clinics at one point in their improvement work. These studies have been published (Fischer et al. 1997; Fischer et al. 1998) and are summarized by Fischer in Chapter 8 of this book.

Postlude

At the end of the intervention, we asked the control clinics whether they wanted to receive a comparable but improved version of the intervention (Magnan et al. 1998). Everything they had heard from the intervention clinics was so positive that 17 of them said they wanted to and were able to undertake it at that time. In addition, the project team used this opportunity to train and involve regular staff members from both HMOs in the new intervention, and they identified another 18 medical groups that they would like to have participate. Eleven of these groups chose to do so and these 29 clinics/groups went through the experience with even more enthusiasm than the first group. Unfortunately, we do not have similar measurements of this experience, but both the training and the team efforts seemed to go much more smoothly and quickly than they had the first time.

The same gratifying response from the original participants led to modifying this approach to use it for chronic disease management for diabetes before we had the final results from IMPROVE. This new project, called IDEAL (Improving Diabetes through Empowerment, Active collaboration, and Leadership), is being conducted in collaboration with the Minnesota Department of Health and has been similarly well received by the eight clinics that have participated in it (Solberg 1997). Although we do not have results yet from this second randomized controlled trial, repeat data collections by several of the participating clinics have shown promising improvements in the rates of key diabetes services.

Another spinoff of the IMPROVE project has been a brief uncontrolled test of a modified way to provide assistance with process improvement. This project continued the collaboration between the two health plans (HealthPartners and Blue Cross and Blue Shield of Minnesota) in a contract with another part of the Minnesota Department of Health. This five-month project with three community clinics provided an opportunity to test the use of externally provided experienced facilitators for clinic teams that were working on building prevention systems. These teams worked much faster than did those in any of the other efforts, but they tended to founder when the facilitators were withdrawn at the end of the contract.

LESSONS FROM IMPROVE

In addition to the findings that have been described above, IMPROVE and its offspring have many lessons for those interested in CQI and in managed care. Some of these come from what went right, but as usual there is more to learn from what did not.

CQI Lessons

We believe that the immediate reason that the rates we measured did not increase significantly is because the systems put in place to accomplish that were incomplete and perhaps misdirected. The situation is much more complicated than that, however, with many factors contributing to the lack of rate change. In fact, it seems to us that a whole chain of factors must be satisfied to obtain the desired improvements. Some of these factors are the same as those noted briefly at the beginning of this chapter as barriers to managed care facilitation of clinical CQI. The lesson is that each of these factors needs to be satisfied in order to obtain quality improvement in clinical settings, regardless of whether the means chosen are called CQI.

High Priority Organizational Commitment to Change

In order to achieve the type of fundamental system change that we were aiming for, both clinic leadership and the clinicians must see the change as a very important priority and be deeply committed to it. Usually that means that there must be either a financial or a deeply personal benefit in the new way of behaving as well as a belief that the change is possible. Most of this tension for change may need to come from the external world in the form of incentives, comparative performance feedback, professional peer pressure, or regulatory/purchaser requirements, but ultimately it must be seen internally as important for organizational survival. A strategy of generating tension for change from multiple sources may be more effective at generating change than focused efforts from a single source.

Our own data suggest that patients are unlikely to serve as a sufficient driver, at least at present (Kottke et al. 1997b). Only about one-third of patients indicated that they would like to receive more preventive services from their physician. The other two-thirds were either indifferent or wanted to receive fewer services.

In addition, our survey of clinicians demonstrated that, despite belief in the importance of these preventive services, they did not have a sense that improvement was necessary (Solberg et al. 1997b). With the possible exception of tobacco cessation advice, nearly as many respondents disagreed with the need to improve each service as agreed. Since they had no way to know exactly how well they were doing, this ambiguous response could mean that they thought that they were already doing quite well. It seems more likely, however, that improving prevention just didn't have sufficient organizational priority at a time when a great many issues seemed more likely to affect survival, especially since only two-thirds of the respondents reported that their leadership was committed to this task. Both of the sponsoring HMOs as well as the local business coalition on health have emphasized the need to improve preventive services, but until very recently there was no financial carrot attached to that. Thus, change motivation appeared to be borderline at best.

Organizational Ability to Manage Change

This is a complex factor that includes a variety of knowledge and skills at both top and middle leadership levels, along with a supportive organizational structure and culture and a successful experience with previous change efforts. The role of senior organizational leaders is particularly important in ensuring the presence of this ability as well as in supporting specific improvement efforts. Caldwell (1998), Weiner et al. (1997), Bender (1995), Masters (1996), and Jackson et al. (1994), among others, have described the many barriers in typical medical practices that interfere with their ability to undertake the changes increasingly being demanded of them. Although we have worked with hundreds of clinics and medical groups over the past 15 years, we have seen few examples where this organizational ability is in very good shape. Our quality culture survey measure suggests the same problem existed for these clinics. Crabtree et al. (1998) have provided a valuable documentation of this issue by their observational study of 84 practices in Ohio in relation to preventive services delivery. They note that these practices are complex, and conclude that those wanting to stimulate change "need to have a more comprehensive approach than is now commonly used to assess practices that encompass a broad spectrum of variables." (403)

Even so, there must also be what we have come to speak of as a "tolerable level of turmoil" both externally and internally, for a clinic to be ready for successful change. As noted above, that was clearly not the case for most of these clinics (Magnan et al. 1997). One clinic team had to stop functioning for six months after the clinic was bought by a hospital that eliminated most benefits and made everyone fearful. Other teams told us that they hung on to their IMPROVE team activities as the only thing going on that they could feel good about. In some ways it is remarkable that the prevention rates did not deteriorate during this time.

The type of CQI process being used may be key to this ability to manage change. We hoped that we were basically providing a vehicle and the training/support needed for change. The CQI model we used was probably not up to the task, requiring so much time and effort that most teams lacked the will to evaluate the success of their efforts and learn that more change was needed. It is certainly possible that some version of the approach recently used by the Institute for Healthcare Improvement (IHI) might have been more successful with its emphasis on rapid cycle tests of small changes (Nolan 1997; Berwick 1996; Berwick 1998).

Even with an effective change model, however, leadership of the change by our trainees probably wasn't optimal. Although they were mostly creative, dedicated, and industrious, this was a first experience with this kind of change leadership for many. Our experience with the later health department project that used experienced team leadership from the HMOs made clear how much faster a team can work with such leadership. That model still requires a way to transition to clinic ownership, however, and it is not clear that many HMOs are prepared to devote that many resources to this task. Finally, we learned that simply designating a clinic manager as team sponsor and encouraging active support wasn't enough. In the second round, we tried to correct for this by putting on a special training session for the sponsors and by making a much greater effort to visit them regularly and to identify specific actions for them to take in support of their teams.

Substantive Change Content

Clearly the best change management in the world will accomplish little if the changes made are not substantial, with good reason to believe that they can result in significant improvement. Skeptics of CQI have correctly noted that there is often so much emphasis on the process of identifying problems and on original thinking by team members unaware of existing knowledge, that they develop only superficial changes such as educational programs or new chart forms that will be as unused as previous ones have been. In the only other scientific trial of CQI, Goldberg et al. (1998) pointed out that this was one of the major problems with their team efforts. He has gone so far as to suggest limiting the scope of a CQI team's activities by having them concentrate on tailoring a change with demonstrated efficacy rather than picking one (Goldberg 1998).

In order to minimize this problem, we emphasized from the beginning that this was a test of the combination of a change process plus proven care process content knowledge. An emphasis on system changes and on the individual process components of an overall prevention system (Bigelow and Arndt 1995) was a dominant part of the training and consulting. Thus, we were providing the teams with the change concepts emphasized by Nolan (1997) and others (Batalden et al. 1996) as fundamental to real improvement. As Berwick has noted (1996, 620), "new systems do not bubble up from below," and we would add that they also will not appear *de novo* in an adequately sophisticated form just because a team of people is working on a problem requiring such systems. Although the clinic teams responded well to our training on prevention system processes in their plans for change, our measurements of what was actually changed suggest several problems that ultimately led to the lack of benefit.

One problem was the reported absence of implementation of a reminder process to stimulate the clinicians to make use of the information about prevention needs that was identified for individual patients by screening and using a summary sheet. Only a few clinics seem to have instituted reminders. A bigger problem may have been the reliance on reminders rather than building the new system around task delegation to nonphysicians. Although we included this approach in the training, the extensive research evidence for the effectiveness of reminder systems led us to emphasize ensuring that the clinician was aware of an individual patient's prevention needs (McCarthy et al. 1997). In retrospect, adding prevention topics to a clinician's agenda that was already too busy for a brief visit may not be a successful strategy in real life.

Effective Development and Implementation of Improvements

Even if there is high motivation, good readiness, and sound content, the teams and their clinic leadership must effectively carry out the development and implementation of system changes. This category overlaps with motivation and readiness, but the slow pace of the improvement process in most clinics, the fact that only 60 percent reported implementation after 18 months, and the lack of evaluation and a second cycle of improvement by that time suggest that whatever changes were made were less likely to have achieved their goals.

We do not blame the teams or clinics for this problem. In fact, their enthusiasm and dedication was a constant inspiration to the intervention group, as reflected by some of the individual clinic IMPROVE stories that have been published (Hogan et al. 1997; Heiniger et al. 1997; Moriarity

1996; Magnan et al. 1998). It may have had as much to do with our CQI model, their inexperience, and the motivation and readiness issues noted above as anything else. An equally important barrier may have been the major paradigm shift required by patients and clinicians to include a clinic agenda (identification and delivery of needed preventive services) in a brief visit already busy with the need to meet other patient and medical needs.

Time: Sufficient but Not Too Much

Even if everything else works well, any change of the magnitude required by this project needs sufficient time to take hold. Other experiences with a medical group collaborative working on the improvement of preventive services (Mosser 1996) suggest that at least two years and, some clinics have argued, three to five years are needed. They tell us that this task requires an organizational transformation before major change in systems can be obtained. If so, changing organization culture, systems, and other readiness issues noted above certainly will take time. In fact many of the team leaders and facilitators have told us that IMPROVE has been very helpful to them in this larger task and they continue to make use of the lessons learned for addressing all types of challenges facing them. Unfortunately, we do not have the quantitative information from which to provide a definitive assessment of this.

On the other hand, allowing too much time for specific innovations to evolve probably also impedes adoption. The IHI strategy of rapid cycles and ambitious stretch goals is based on this experience (Berwick 1996). Implementation of preventive services systems in the IMPROVE project might have been more successful if we had been more aggressive with the participating clinics to keep preventive services on the change agenda and with the teams to shorten their Plan-Do-Check-Act (PDCA) cycles. The trick is to push for change while understanding that real change takes a lot of time.

Managed Care Lessons

It is easier to summarize the lessons for managed care plans from this experiment, although the preceding section on CQI constitutes a major part of those lessons as it applies to working with clinics on improvement. Other lessons include collaboration between competitors and with clinics.

Collaboration between Competitors Is Both Feasible and Useful

As described more fully in other publications (Solberg et al. 1995; Magnan et al. 1998), competing managed care plans can jointly provide a clinic intervention designed to improve the quality of patient care. Our experience with this has gone very well. Success depends upon the partners sharing a common aim and recognizing that it requires a common effort. Since most medical groups and clinics in this region, like an increasing proportion of the country, provide care for most of the HMOs in the region, and since clinicians do not find it possible or desirable to treat various plan patients differently, it is impossible to improve the care for only one HMO's patients. By working together, several HMOs have much more influence with the providing medical groups. Those groups are particularly grateful for the opportunity to reduce the duplication that is often created by the different requirements of competing HMOs. Another reason to work together is that HMOs often have different strengths and can complement each other in supporting the clinic changes.

Collaboration with Clinics Is Also Feasible and Useful

The IMPROVE project changed the relationship between plans and clinicians, making it possible to address the issues of value and health improvement that require clinician leadership and cooperation in evolutionary Stages II and III. Just as the need to cooperate with the clinics they shared brought two HMOs together, the presence of those HMOs as neutral intermediaries facilitated networking and sharing between clinics and medical groups that normally do not do that. These networking sessions were clearly the most popular parts of the intervention, both for learning and motivation.

CONCLUSIONS AND RECOMMENDATIONS

Although the IMPROVE trial did not result in significantly increased rates of the targeted preventive services, it did lead to a great deal of information about clinics, the change process, and prevention. We believe it also helped the participating clinics to increase their readiness for any other organizational change they will surely confront in the near future. In most cases, it seems to have helped them to begin an important transformation of their managerial and operating styles. In the long run, CQI may turn out to be more valuable for assisting in this transformation than in facilitating specific process change.

What the trial says about the ability of CQI concepts and techniques to produce measurable changes in the quantity or quality of clinical services (much less patient outcomes) is much less clear. We have identified a number of barriers to change in this trial (above), any one of which might have prevented the rate changes desired. Not the least of these barriers is the type of CQI process being followed and the magnitude of change in thinking and action that is required for preventive services improvement. In addition, it can be argued that CQI may not be as good for designing and creating an entirely new system where none has previously existed as it is for making refinements and even major changes in a system that already exists.

Perhaps greater awareness of these barriers and challenges as well as the need for a more efficient and effective CQI process will make it more likely that others will be more successful in the future. After all, successful improvements in any other aspect of medicine or in other industries typically require a great many failures and disappointments before the correct approach is demonstrated. Unfortunately, there have been more anecdotes and "boosterism" in the CQI movement than dispassionate assessment of the value of specific approaches, preventing needed learning. This may have been shortsighted, contributing to what is becoming somewhat of a reaction to CQI among clinicians in much the same way as managed care has produced this reaction or overreaction.

We hope, therefore, that others will continue to explore the potential that seems evident in the concepts that underlie CQI. We also hope that, as they approach the challenges of addressing value and health improvement, managed care plans will also transform themselves, learning how to work collaboratively with their competitors and their clinicians. In order to increase the likelihood of such a collaborative effort's success, we make the following recommendations based on the lessons of IMPROVE:

1. Before beginning to facilitate a clinic change process, be sure that adequate incentives are in place, that disincentives for improvement are eliminated, and that the targeted clinics have indeed committed themselves to the desired changes.
2. In order to learn whether the groups and clinics are adequately ready to engage in the change, use some type of assessment process.

Unfortunately, there is no currently available validated tool for this assessment, so for the time being it may require a subjective guess as to this readiness in both desire and ability. We and others (Crabtree et al. 1998) are working on this task, however. Crabtree's group, for example is developing a "practice genogram" (McIlvain et al. 1998). They believe that this technique holds promise for enhancing data gathering, increasing understanding of the complexity of practices as adaptive systems, and increasing understanding of current and potential approaches to changing practices. In addition to knowing whether a particular group is ready to undertake the effort, an effective assessment can identify needed changes in the organization and can tailor assistance in the change process.

3. Be sure that the content changes are substantial enough to lead to real improvements. Ideally, the selected change concepts should be based on both research and real-life demonstration of feasibility and value. Then ensure that the change agents in each clinic thoroughly understand these concepts and have access to both detailed examples and expert consultation in the application of those concepts.

4. Be equally sure that the improvement process chosen fits with the size and nature of the task and that it is on an ambitious but feasible time line. Although the concepts and techniques currently used in the IHI Breakthrough series sound promising, they have not yet been adequately evaluated and we probably have much to learn about the improvement process, especially as it applies to the front lines of care delivery.

5. Start slow and small with both collaborations and with quality improvement projects. Your first efforts will never be as good as later ones.

6. Make extensive use of measurement in repetitive cycles, both in the improvement process and in assessing the value of that process. Be sure to understand the differences between measurement for improvement and measurement for research or accountability, however, so that the measurements do not get in the way of the goal (Solberg et al. 1997e).

Finally, managed care plans will perform a great service for the nation as well as themselves if they apply themselves to the improvement of health care quality, using CQI as well as other approaches. The stages of managed care evolution concepts of Goldsmith et al. suggest that a steadily increasing proportion of managed care plans will find themselves in the stage of needing to do this for their own competitive survival (Goldsmith et al. 1995). The National Roundtable on Health Care Quality, convened by the Institute of Medicine, however, has suggested that the national interest requires "a major, systematic effort to overhaul how we deliver health care services . . . [because] serious and widespread quality problems exist throughout American medicine" (Chassin et al. 1998, 1000). The Roundtable classified the problems as *underuse, overuse*, and *misuse* and said that they occur everywhere and equally frequently in managed care and fee-for-service (FFS) care systems, harming large numbers of people as a result. "Quality of care is the problem, not managed care."

CHAPTER 14

CQI in Contract Research Organizations

William A. Sollecito

Clinical contract research organizations (CROs) are unique organizations that combine a range of services from consulting to labor-intensive tasks such as data processing. In organizational terms they range somewhere between academia and industry, and the successful CROs have drawn the best techniques from both. One common characteristic of most successful CROs is the application of continuous quality improvement (CQI) techniques. The distinguishing characteristics of CQI include four major areas described below.

1. customer focus
2. training and empowerment
3. leadership
4. statistical process control/statistical thinking

Before discussing the CQI characteristics demonstrated by CROs, it may be useful to review briefly the development of CROs, since this will help in explaining the bases for application of CQI in the CRO industry.

GROWTH OF CROs

During the past 20 years the clinical contract research industry has grown at a remarkable rate. The growth has occurred for two reasons. First, the pharmaceutical industry in the United States and throughout the world

Source: Portions of this chapter have been adapted from W.A. Sollecito and A.D. Kaluzny, Continuous Quality Improvement in Contract Research Organizations—The Customer Focus, *Quality Management in Health Care*, Vol. 7, No. 3, pp. 7–21, © 1999, Aspen Publishers, Inc.

has undergone a transition that has included strategic use of outsourcing in drug development. Second, CROs have responded to this demand through entrepreneurial leadership rooted in the application of both scientific and sound business practices. The scientific procedures developed by CROs have focused strongly on techniques to provide customer satisfaction and reinforce the strategic value of their role in pharmaceutical development.

This discussion will be limited to the use of CROs by the pharmaceutical and biotechnology industries, which has accounted for the majority of CRO use in recent years. In this context a *contract research organization* can be defined as an organization contracted by a sponsor (client) to perform one or more of the functions and duties related to carrying out clinical trials designed to obtain regulatory approval to market a new pharmaceutical or biotechnology product. The services that CROs perform for their clients range from consulting and advice about the design of drug development programs to labor-intensive services that are part of the drug development process. These services include clinical monitoring of investigatorial sites, data management and statistical analysis, and presentations of regulatory submissions for review by regulatory agencies, such as the U.S. Food and Drug Administration (FDA). Exhibit 14–1 lists the most common clinical services provided by CROs.

Pharmaceutical Industry Trends

The process of developing a new pharmaceutical product is time consuming and very expensive. On average it takes 10 years from the time a molecule is discovered until a product is marketed, at a cost of $259 million

---

Exhibit 14–1 Typical Clinical* Services Performed by a CRO

- Site identification and coordination
- Project planning/management
- Clinical monitoring/auditing
- Data management and biostatistics
- Clinical trials laboratory services
- Regulatory affairs
- Medical support
- Safety monitoring
- Health economics/outcomes research
- Management of clinical trial materials

*Performed during clinical stages of a drug development program (Phase II–IV) (in 1990) dollars (DiMasi et al. 1991). The expense of this process is offset by the profits to be gained through marketing of successful products; however, only about one in 60,000 compounds discovered results in a highly successful marketed product (U.S. Congress, OTA 1993). The reasons for this include the complexity and number of stages (phases) a product must pass through (Pocock 1983) in the drug development process. One of the most important limitations on profitability is the limited patent protection given to pharmaceutical products. For many products developed in recent decades, patents had a lifetime of 17 years, although in 1995 this was extended to 20 years. There have been other extensions based on recent legislation in the U.S. and other major health markets (Schweitzer 1997); however, the length of patent protection relative to drug development is quite short.

An important factor is that during the 1980s there was significant variation among pharmaceutical companies in drug development time. Figure 14–1 illustrates this by presenting the average time (prior to regulatory submission) of the clinical phase (human testing) of new pharmaceutical products approved during the period 1981 to 1989. For the 10 companies listed each bar represents development time in years for all products developed by the company during that time frame. The average clinical development time ranged from a maximum of almost 10 years for two companies to less than 3 years for one company. This wide range in clinical development time gave CROs an indication that there was significant variability in the efficiency of drug development. Some companies were clearly more efficient than others were and there was room for improvement in the process (Sollecito 1993).

As a direct consequence of the lengthy drug development time relative to short patent protection, there is intense interest in accelerating the process in order to improve profitability in the pharmaceutical and biotechnology industry. This is also a concern from the medical care and public health perspective, since a shorter development time for important therapies will bring greater benefits to patients and communities. Thus, it becomes critical for all concerned to define efficient processes for drug development and regulatory review, and to continuously improve these processes over time.

Regulatory Issues

In reviewing drug development, it is important to emphasize the role of worldwide regulatory agencies in guiding the process. Regulatory agen-

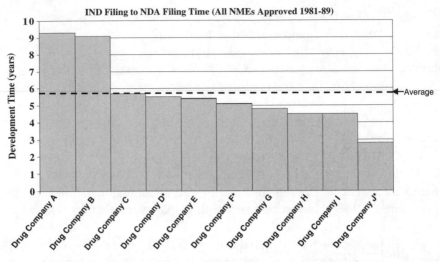

*Development times for foreign companies may be understated where substantial pre-IND work was carried out overseas.

Figure 14–1 New Molecular Entities Approved (1981–1989); Selection of Major Pharmaceutical Companies

---

cies, such as the FDA in the United States, have a clear mandate to protect the public's health through laws, regulations, and guidelines that provide oversight of the drug development process. The history and stages that define this process are well documented (Miller and Millstein 1996) and are carefully adhered to by all pharmaceutical and biotechnology companies, as well as by CROs. One of the key development rules, which is directly related to the underlying philosophy of CQI, is that process errors should be prevented or detected at their earliest stage; in no case is it acceptable for errors to be first detected during review by the regulatory agency. This is an important basis for CQI in the pharmaceutical and CRO industry and will be expounded upon further, later in this chapter.

In summary, drug development is a long and complex process involving clinical trials that may involve several thousand patients and requires adherence to guidelines and laws that are enforced by regulatory agencies. In this setting, efficiency and CQI are essential for achieving success.

Cost Containment

The introduction of cost containment in medical care by managed care organizations and government agencies has had a significant impact on the pharmaceutical sector. From 1982 to 1996, the percentage of private sector employees receiving health benefits through a managed care plan grew from 8 percent to 77 percent with HMOs having an estimated 59 million members in 1996 (Pharmaceutical Researchers and Manufacturers of America 1998).

Virtually every health care organization that reimburses for drugs, whether public or private, utilizes some form of cost containment strategy with regard to pharmaceuticals. These include manufacturer discounts, formularies, generic and therapeutic substitution, and drug utilization review (Schweitzer 1997). Once again, the impact on the pharmaceutical sector has led to a focus on improving efficiency in drug development.

The Biotechnology Challenge

Another important challenge has come from within the pharmaceutical sector itself as biotechnology companies emerged in the 1980s to develop products that would directly compete with pharmaceutical products. Many of the biotech companies made a strategic decision not to become the same as "big pharmaceutical" companies; many decided that in order to be truly competitive, they had to develop new procedures and processes with an emphasis on lean organizational structures and efficient research and development (R & D) processes. This led to alliances with pharmaceutical and financial partners and a development strategy that emphasized outsourcing to CROs rather than building infrastructure. The biotech industry quickly embraced the "Virtual Model" (Byrne 1993) as a way of improving the process of drug development.

The biotechnology industry represents a very high-risk R & D process, which is given intense scrutiny by financial partners and other investors. As a result biotech companies have focused on the use of high-tech innovations and CQI procedures to ensure maximum efficiency for themselves and their (virtual) partners, including CROs.

Outsourcing Trends

The primary impact on the CRO industry of the trends described above was that during the 1980s and 1990s there was a significant increase in outsourcing by the pharmaceutical and biotechnology industry, which led to the foundation and then substantial growth of CROs worldwide.

What started out as piecemeal consulting prior to 1980 evolved into full-scale clinical services in the early 1990s and has now evolved further to include diverse services such as contract sales and disease management services. In 1992, the top 10 CROs in the world had approximately 4,000 employees and revenues of $350,000,000 (excluding investigator grants) (Tassignon 1992). Meteoric growth has occurred since 1992; in 1996 the top 10 CROs had doubled in size compared to 1992, and worldwide the total number of CROs was approximately 600. Several large companies have now grown to the stage where they have gone public to raise capital to support further growth. For example, Quintiles Transnational Corp., the largest CRO in the world today, averaged 50 percent growth per year from 1994 to 1997 and had revenues of $800 million dollars in 1997; revenues for the top four CROs were about $1.8 billion dollars (Quintiles Annual Report 1997).

Outsourcing in the pharmaceutical industry has also led to the growth of other contract services, including contract clinical laboratories, to provide specialized blood and other tests required during clinical trials. A recent phenomenon is the growth of site management organizations (SMOs). During the clinical trial stage, clinical investigators who cover the entire range from investigators in academic medical centers to private practitioners carry out actual patient testing. These represent independent contractors who work directly for pharmaceutical companies or as subcontractors to CROs. As a direct consequence of the independence of these highly valued practitioners, there is little control over processes. This has resulted in a need to monitor quality because of the importance of the data collected during patient testing. The development of SMOs represents an attempt to form organizations of investigators with the goal of improving efficiency through standardized training and improved administrative procedures. The use of SMOs in the pharmaceutical industry is still in the development stage but it represents another example of how CQI procedures can be applied and may lead to further growth in the contract research sector.

HOW CROs WORK

Initially, when CROs worked with clients the scope of work was fairly narrow and working relationships were fairly informal. As the use of CROs increased, a number of different organizations emerged and CROs began to compete in order to sustain critical mass and grow. From the earliest days, CROs developed a reputation for excellence, which in turn led to greater acceptance and increased utilization of CROs. This process was explained by Tassignon (1992) in describing the emerging relationship between CROs and the pharmaceutical industry: "The unwritten deal between the pharmaceutical industry and clinical CROs can be defined as follows: 'You, the sponsors, delegate the conduction of the clinical studies to us, CROs, and we guarantee you quality, timeliness, adequate manpower and predictable costs'" (38).

Early on it became clear that CROs would have to compete on two levels, among themselves and against the internal clinical development teams at sponsor companies, many of whom initially felt that no CROs could offer the same level of services they could provide. Senior management in pharmaceutical and biotech companies, however, soon began to advocate outsourcing as a way to replace the fixed costs that were historically associated with drug development infrastructure by variable costs that the use of CROs represented. In addition, with CROs the expectation was that time lines would be met and the highest goal of quality would be guaranteed. CROs had to rise to these challenges; CQI procedures provided the way not only to win clients but to manage operations efficiently and meet all three objectives: highest quality, on time, at the lowest cost. Tassignon (1992) provides a historical perspective that helps to explain why CROs emphasized quality above all else:

> Quality first. The history of drug development is unfortunately tainted with stories of fraud and negligence. . . . The CRO industry is, of course, not immune to fraud, but such temptations would mean the death of a CRO. The higher the reputation of the CRO for quality data, the greater the "exportability" of clinical reports to regulatory bodies worldwide . . . procedural sloppiness would cost them the client. Timeliness has traditionally been the nightmare of drug developers . . . CROs can offer an improve-

ment, for several reasons. First of all, they are accountable for the agreed upon milestones in the contract that binds them to their clients. Secondly, CROs work on very innovative drugs. . . . Thirdly, the CRO is organized exclusively for the purpose of conducting clinical studies. Speed of execution as well as cost effectiveness are decisive competitive advantages. Whereas the industry tends to promote strategic thinkers to the top, CROs tend to reward "doers," people who get the job done within time and budget constraints (38–39).

As the CRO industry matured, pharmaceutical sponsors began to develop standardized ways to manage CROs. These included the formation of contract research management teams and the implementation of formalized proposal, bidding, and contract processes. Once again this fostered the use of CQI because CROs often had to bid against each other in order to win the contract. Unlike government contracting, the pharmaceutical industry often awarded contracts not based on the lowest bid, but rather on the CRO's ability to implement innovative solutions to development problems. Many of these innovations represented process improvement initiatives by the CROs. This was particularly true in data management, an area where the pharmaceutical industry had been plagued for many years by inefficiency, high costs, and long delays. During the 1980s and 1990s, when the CRO industry was maturing, many new breakthroughs occurred in information technology that were directly applicable to improving large-scale data management in pharmaceutical clinical trials. These included the introduction of microcomputers and improvements in telecommunications such as fax and touch-tone technology for transmitting data. Because of their competitive positions CROs were able to embrace and further develop these tools to benefit both themselves and their clients.

Once awarded, the contract between a sponsor and a CRO is very specific in defining procedures for interacting and includes CQI tools such as production flow diagrams, Gantt charts, patient enrollment graphs, and performance metrics which allow both the CRO and sponsor to monitor and improve performance.

Another important aspect of the drug development process that contributes to implementation of CQI is the project management systems employed by CROs to carry out studies. Many of the large CROs, such as Quintiles Transnational, have structured themselves as matrix organizations with a mission-oriented project management system (Sollecito 1993).

From the perspective of implementing CQI, a matrix is the ideal organizational structure. The Quintiles' project management system uses a value-added approach that emphasizes "the why and how of serving the client" and eliminates waste (i.e., anything that does not add value). The essential components of this approach are a clear understanding that every project has a customer and a sense of serving the customer by the project team (Dotson and Wallman 1994). Another critical component of CQI that is illustrated by the Quintiles' project management system is careful focus on the importance of communication and development of systems that facilitate clear communication between the CRO and sponsor as well as within the CRO project team (Sollecito and Dotson 1995). Effective application of project management techniques is a major reason for the growth and success of CROs in their earliest stages of development. These techniques have allowed CQI processes to be implemented on a large scale, involving networks of sponsor affiliates, clinical investigation sites, and even other CROs. Many CROs have introduced improvements in project management techniques in the pharmaceutical industry, which led to the evolution of Virtual Drug Development Models, sometimes involving multiple sponsors and multiple CROs (Sollecito 1994). This trend is expected to continue in the future as CROs become more market driven, research driven, and customer driven. The use of virtual drug development models is expected to lead to the creation of cooperative virtual organizations responsible for using the resources of all partners (CROs and sponsors) to get the job done (Rudy 1996, 42). At each stage in the evolution of the CRO industry, innovation and continuous improvement have been the key to success and further growth.

CQI CUSTOMER FOCUS

By its very nature the CRO industry is customer driven. The customer defines the projects that CROs work on and every project has a specific life cycle; further the decision as to whether or not additional work is performed for a specific client is determined in large part by performance on the most recently completed project for that customer. Two unique aspects of CRO projects are that first, the work performed by CROs is scientific in nature, requiring a high level of expertise, and second, sponsors make a conscious choice to assign work to CROs that in an earlier time they might have done themselves. Thus, the CRO is asked to meet and exceed standards that are defined not only relative to other CROs' performance, but also relative to the expected performance of the sponsor.

The pharmaceutical sponsor, however, represents only one of the components of the customer matrix that CROs deal with. As depicted in Table 14–1, this matrix of customers can be divided into two dimensions along the lines of classical definitions of external and internal customers. The primary distinction is that all internal customers supplement, support, or are part of the virtual team that provides services along with the CRO to meet the needs of external customers.

The complexity of implementing CQI procedures in drug development is directly related to the interrelationships of the various customers and suppliers depicted in Table 14–1. This is especially true for CROs, which are frequently at the center of this complex matrix in terms of coordinating the needs of both internal and external customers.

Table 14–1 CRO/Drug Development Customer Matrix

Internal Customers/ Suppliers	External Customers			
	Sponsors	Regulatory agency(ies)	Physician-practitioners	Patients
Other CROs				
Other divisions (within CROs)				
Clinical trials laboratories*				
Drug supply and distribution facilities				
Physician-investigators				

*Includes clinical laboratories that provide blood and urine analysis as well as specialized laboratories that provide other specialized evaluations.

External Customers

Physician-Practitioners and Patients

Because of their important role in funding all drug development activities, typical sponsors (pharmaceutical or biotechnology companies) may perceive themselves as the ultimate customer for work performed by CROs. Both sponsors and CROs, however, are actually working to meet the needs of patients and their representative, the physician-practitioner who treats them.

The needs of patients must be kept in mind throughout the drug development process; they provide a direct source of motivation to ensure the highest quality of clinical development activities. The ultimate goal in drug development, as in all medical care, is to prevent and treat illness; thus the patient is the ultimate customer. Feedback on patients' needs and patient satisfaction does not usually come directly from patients themselves, but rather from their caregivers. Thus, the pharmaceutical industry pays a great deal of attention to working with physicians to keep them aware of new therapies that are available and to seek their feedback on the effectiveness of new therapies in treating patients (i.e., in meeting the ultimate customers' need). Other measures of patient satisfaction come from patient surveys.

CROs are most directly involved in this process through provision of contract sales services or post-marketing safety monitoring services. The ultimate responsibility for patient satisfaction rests with the sponsor, but in a true CQI environment, this is shared by the CRO. One direct measure of quality, which is a direct reflection on the drug development process, is the number of safety problems that occur in a treated population after a drug is approved and distributed. When these problems occur, the most serious concern is the negative impact on the health of the population. Other negative impacts include criticism of the sponsors and their agents, such as CROs, and criticism of the regulatory agency. By its very nature, the drug development process does not allow for all potential safety problems to be identified in advance, due to sample size and other clinical design considerations. Sponsors, regulators, and CROs, however, share a responsibility for using the information derived from safety problems that occur in the patient population to respond quickly and to improve processes to prevent future reoccurrence of problems. The most dramatic form of response is the recall of a newly approved product; most often the response is less dramatic and, in the spirit of ongoing improvement, involves the issuance of revised guidelines about use of the drug with possible warnings to be observed. This is a joint responsibility of the regulatory agency and the sponsor—to first provide a patient safety monitoring process, and once that is in place, to act quickly when problems are detected. Hospitals and "health advocacy organizations," such as Public Citizen, that monitor and publish guidelines about the use of drugs, are other agents of patient care. Another important component of this patient representative hierarchy are the managed care organizations and the federal agencies responsible for health care (e.g., Medicare). These organizations and agencies have an impact on the assessment of and feedback on newly approved pharmaceutical products. Their impact is almost entirely on the sponsor and the regulatory agency, but is a source of information to be used in continuous improvement by all components of the drug development customer matrix, including CROs.

Regulatory Agencies

One of the most important external customers for CROs and sponsors alike is the regulatory agency. In this discussion, comments will be limited to the FDA, although they are applicable to other agencies as well.

The FDA defines customer expectations in a pyramid that includes laws, regulations, and guidelines (Miller and Millstein 1996). The purpose of these hierarchical prescriptions is to share information and ensure compliance in the development of new pharmaceutical and biotechnology products. The goal is to make the approval process as simple as possible, while still focusing on the most critical mandate—to protect the health and safety of the U.S. population.

In the context of CQI, the FDA laws, regulations, and guidelines provide a roadmap of customer expectations from a customer who has complete authority over the approval process. Failure to meet these expectations may lead to costly delays in the approval of new drugs and may also lead to punitive actions (e.g., blacklisting of investigators who are found guilty of fraud); in extreme cases, the FDA has authority to pursue legal remedies.

CROs and others in the drug development process have an obligation to understand and comply with FDA regulations and guidelines. Although in most cases legal responsibility remains with the sponsor, the CRO must be aware of FDA requirements in meeting its obligations to the sponsor.

Because of these obligations, CROs have added regulatory personnel to their organizations; more important, they have adopted procedures that promote a view of the FDA as a customer rather than as a bureaucratic impediment in the drug development process.

An important aspect of interacting with the FDA is compliance with quality assurance (QA) regulations. FDA inspectors have the legal right to audit sponsors and have done so on many occasions as part of their ongoing QA process; they also carry out "for-cause" audits when they encounter a problem during a regulatory review. These same procedures apply to CROs and other participants in the drug development process. Thus, the concept of "conformance quality" is an important part of the drug development process. As a result, drug developers, including CROs, have instituted elaborate mechanisms for demonstrating compliance, such as standard operating procedures (SOPs), which include detailed training records for all employees.

Training processes and records are in fact a critical part of complying with FDA regulations and they also represent CQI components within most large CROs; smaller CROs subcontract with professional training organizations to accomplish the same task. Most training focuses on good clinical practice guidelines that have been established by regulatory agencies throughout the world to ensure consistency and high quality within the drug development process.

Drug developers, CROs, and regulatory agencies make use of benchmarking to develop consistent worldwide standards. Formal initiatives, such as the International Conference on Harmonization (ICH), help to ensure consistency in standards. Informal benchmarking is carried out continually by reviewing public documents that record policies and summarize outcomes of drug reviews within and between regulatory agencies. An example of this was once illustrated by a Japanese sponsor, who said: "When the FDA gets a cold, the Japanese regulatory authorities sneeze."

Sponsors and CROs continually conduct benchmarking activities, not only to be in compliance with FDA and other regulators, but also as part of continuous improvement initiatives. Most CROs and sponsors pay close attention to presentations, publications, and other documentation of FDA opinions or revisions to guidelines. For CROs it is a source of pride and also good business practice to demonstrate knowledge of and conformance with the latest FDA guidelines.

An example of how the FDA functions as a customer is the fact that the FDA has undergone CQI processes to improve its performance with "suppliers" (e.g., pharmaceutical sponsors and CROs). Part of this process has included charging *user fees* to sponsors as they submit "new drug applications" (NDAs). The FDA has used these fees to hire staff and provide for other FDA needs to facilitate speedier and more efficient review of NDAs (Miller and Millstein 1996). The user fee initiative has also enabled the FDA to review processes internally and, most recently, there has been a movement by the FDA to develop "Good Review Practices"—clearly a CQI initiative within the agency.

An important way in which CROs and sponsors interact with the FDA as a customer is through the interactive review process. Following predefined rules and guidelines, CROs and sponsors meet with FDA reviewers during the drug development process. These interactions lead to review and improvement in study design, study protocols, and overall strategy prior to submission of NDAs. During and after NDA submission there is a dialogue on the review of findings that sometimes speeds up or clarifies the review process. CROs and sponsors use these interactions to continuously review and improve processes for future submissions, as well as to make changes in current applications. One clear advantage to this process is that it helps to clarify the "unwritten rules" that some FDA reviewers have; knowledge of these rules facilitates improvement in design of future studies.

One example of FDA customer behavior and its impact on CROs and sponsors is the cooperative development of technological improvements, such as "computer assisted new drug applications" (CANDAs). As new technology became available to transfer data electronically, the FDA, sponsors, and CROs began to work cooperatively to use this technology to improve the NDA submission and review process. Through formal and informal discussions, meetings and presentations, CROs and sponsors worked diligently to develop CANDAs that would meet and exceed the FDA's expectations. This benefited the FDA, whose review task was simplified, and it benefited sponsors, whose products were approved in a more efficient and timely manner. Of course, the most important beneficiary of the process was the ultimate customer, the patient, who obtained earlier access to improved treatments.

Pharmaceutical Sponsors

A CRO's primary customers are the pharmaceutical and biotechnology companies, or sponsors, who make the decision to develop new drugs and who hire the CRO to carry out all or part of drug development programs. Because of the competitive nature of the CRO industry, it is critical that CROs understand and meet sponsor needs and demands; further, it is critical that CROs practice continuous improvement. In most contracting businesses (construction, etc.) and especially in scientific endeavors such as drug development, "You are only as good as your last project."

CROs keep in close touch with customer demands in several ways. First, CRO/sponsor relationships are defined by carefully crafted contracts that spell out expectations and often include performance metrics that are used to trigger payments and evaluate conformance to expectations. CROs also obtain customer feedback through formal client satisfaction surveys that are usually conducted after project completion.

Another important mechanism, which falls more within the quality assurance than the quality improvement area, is the audit process. In the same way that regulatory agencies audit both sponsors and CROs, sponsors conduct their own periodic audits of CROs and other subcontractors and suppliers, including investigator sites. These audits take the form of site visits at various times during a project. Sponsors almost always conduct such audits prior to awarding a contract. CROs are required to present their overall procedures and experience, including training processes and SOPs, as well as project-specific plans. This process is an important reason for CQI procedures to be in place; it is part of the "survival plan" of most CROs since it is a critical means of guaranteeing contract awards. Sponsors also conduct audits and site visits periodically during the course of a program's execution. Specialized contract research management groups along with clinical (scientific) staff and members of corporate QA teams conduct the site visits made prior to the award of a contract. Independent corporate QA personnel usually conduct post-award audits. The CRO usually receives feedback from audits via a formal mechanism and uses it to make improvements or changes where needed.

The Role of Project Management in Ensuring External Customer Satisfaction

The most important mechanism for ensuring customer satisfaction and continuous improvement during the execution of a project is the CRO project management system. Although project teams vary in structure in different CROs, the common denominator is that each project team has the responsibility for maintaining close communication with and meeting the needs of the client. Project managers are the primary contact with the client, and part of their responsibility is to maintain ongoing communication with sponsors as well as with team members, other affiliates of the CRO (e.g., on worldwide projects, teams in other parts of the world), suppliers, and other internal customers. The project team is directly responsible for adhering to contract metrics and project time lines, and most important, is responsible for the overall quality of the project.

In a typical matrix organization (Grove 1983), the project (mission-oriented) team is responsible for interacting with corporate (function-oriented) departments to ensure that customer requirements are met (or exceeded) and that improvements are implemented as necessary. Thus, the CRO's project management team is critical for guaranteeing not only that improvements are made where necessary on specific projects, but also that the corporate side of the matrix organization maintains the strict CQI focus required to succeed on all projects.

The underlying philosophy of project management in the CRO industry is that every project has multiple customers whose needs have to be identified and the CRO project team becomes an extension of the sponsor's team (the extended team approach). This requires open communication with a sponsor, including sharing of problems and solutions (i.e., trust). The goal of a project team is to add value to the process regardless of whether the CRO is one component of a larger drug development program or is managing an entire program. The CQI tools and procedures that CRO project management teams use include the following: formal communication mechanisms such as defined team structures (see Figure 14–2 as an example), clearly identified communication lines, and regular meetings with internal customers (e.g., project team), suppliers, and external customers (sponsors and FDA) to provide status reports and seek feedback for continuous improvement. They also make use of traditional management tools such as Gantt charts that are now available in project management software.

Internal Customers/Suppliers

Clinical research is by its very nature an interdisciplinary process and CROs are often at the center of the process. In addition to working with a range of external customers, CROs are involved with a variety of internal customers and suppliers. Depending on the nature of the contractual

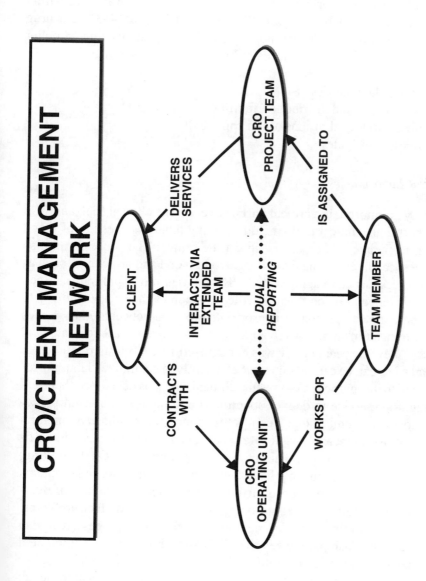

Figure 14–2 CRO/Client Management Network

relationship with the sponsor, a CRO can be a small part of the supplier chain or play a central coordinating role. Often, in recent years, the CROs, especially the larger worldwide CROs, have been in a central coordination role, such as that depicted by the network in Figure 14–3. In a drug development program, the components of the internal customer/supplier network include four major pieces, which the CRO has to manage:

1. clinical laboratories
2. drug supply and distribution facilities
3. other CROs or divisions of the same CRO
4. investigative sites

Clinical Laboratories

Safety monitoring is a critical part of every large clinical trial, and with few exceptions clinical trials include routine laboratory testing of blood and urine samples, often at multiple time points. The process can also involve specialized testing that goes beyond blood and urine tests, such as magnetic resonance imaging tests (MRIs) in neurology programs. When CROs play a central coordinating role, it becomes their responsibility to coordinate the completion of appropriate lab tests between clinical sites and the transfer of "machine readable" data into the database for statistical analysis. Several years ago it was recognized that lab tests required for clinical trials can be carried out most efficiently in centralized laboratories dedicated to this purpose. As a result, clinical trial labs developed that used overnight air service to deliver specimens and highly automated procedures to avoid cumbersome reentry of laboratory results. Automation facilitated overnight analysis of safety data and allowed for quick identification of safety problems. This is another example of CQI in the drug development process; not only have data transcription errors and problems related to spoiled samples been virtually eliminated, but the use of overnight processing allows for rapid flagging of outliers and other problems.

From the customer/supplier perspective, this new process has also simplified relationships between the CRO and laboratory. The automated centralized clinical trial laboratory represents a state-of-the-art supplier that greatly improves the outcomes for all. As an internal supplier the lab requires that CROs develop specialized procedures to deal with the direct receipt of computerized files and that CROs become familiar with the process of how lab samples are collected and shipped via overnight

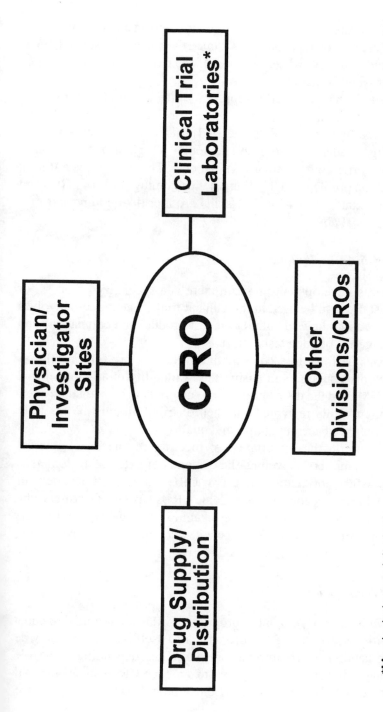

*May include specialty tests.

Figure 14–3 Contract Research Internal Customer/Supplier Network carriers. As a further example of continuous improvement, some CROs (e.g., Quintiles and Covance) have developed their own automated laboratories and made this critical service part of the overall package that they offer to external customers.

Specialized testing laboratories represent a special problem for CROs. Although CROs are ultimately responsible for delivery of all data, the specialized labs often required specialized tests which can only be performed in large academic centers and do not have high priority compared to tests being carried out for their own patients. This represents a timing and coordination problem that challenges the planning skills of CROs and is yet another example of why CQI skills are a critical component of a CRO's operational abilities.

Drug Supply and Distribution

In every drug development program there is a specialized process for supplying test drugs to be used in the clinical trials. The process involves considerations about how to "blind" the test product and comparator and how to package the blinded test materials.

When CROs perform in a coordinating role, they are responsible for working with drug suppliers to ensure the availability of all clinical trial materials (CTM) and the distribution of all materials to investigative sites. CTMs are often highly regulated and their distribution must be carefully managed in regard to accountability and quality.

A clear focus on the importance of meeting the needs of internal customers and suppliers as well as the demands of external customers is key to successful coordination of CTM. CROs have used a variety of methods to achieve this coordination. Some CROs have used partners who were responsible for new modes of packaging. At the other end of the spectrum, some of the larger CROs have developed their own packaging facilities to participate in the process directly.

Other CROs or Divisions

In worldwide drug development programs, CROs are required to coordinate activities with other CROs or, if the CRO itself is a large worldwide CRO, with other divisions of its own company. Thus, depending on the role the CRO plays, it may be a supplier (to another CRO) or an internal customer (receiving data and services from another CRO). In either case it is critical to establish procedures that are highly compatible with internal customers and suppliers and transparent to the external customer; it is not the external customer's job to make such arrangements work, it is the job of the internal customer and supplier. Coordinating centers such as the CRO depicted in Figure 14–3 have this primary responsibility. This is another situation where efficient project management systems are critical; as teams interact, it is important to treat each other as internal customers rather than competitors and work together for the benefit of all. CQI plays a role in this process since each interaction contributes to a databank of experience that all can benefit from over time. A customer focus by all parties is the key to success. Some components of a project are absolutely critical and cannot easily be shared; in such a case one partner assumes the responsibility to develop the process for all. A simple example of this is the responsibility for coordinating data management in a worldwide program. Small variations in data collection or coding on variables can lead to substantial inefficiencies and quality problems. This is easily avoided by giving one party the responsibility for defining data management procedures for all and then monitoring the process over time through a series of interim database transfers or reports to verify that all parties are adhering to the process. The process can be extended not only to multiple CROs but also to multiple laboratories and drug suppliers, perhaps in different parts of the world. Simple procedures such as standardization of reporting units and attention to time zone differences become very important and remain simple only if they are addressed with a CQI focus on "customer delight."

Investigative Sites

Perhaps the most difficult and most important part of the internal customer/supplier network in clinical trials is the physician investigator site. All data and decisions in drug development, especially in the later stages, emanate from physicians treating patients with the new therapies that are being tested. Investigative sites represent "mini-organizations" that have strong scientific and patient care missions but that essentially function as businesses which have access to patients and can provide data on patients who receive the experimental treatments being tested. From a production perspective, investigators are suppliers in the initial stage of the drug development process. This relationship is complicated, however, by the fact that the physicians and their patients are also representatives of the patient-providers who are the ultimate (external) customers in drug development. In addition, investigators sometimes play the important business role of promoting new drugs after they are approved, through publications and presentations at professional meetings. Perhaps the most important complicating factor is that physician investigators are carrying out scientific missions in the drug development process and are subject to all of the uncertainties and complications of the scientific process. In short, it is very difficult for CROs or sponsors to manage the role of the physician investigator in a drug development program.

This is the one area in which CQI principles have been applied least effectively in drug development. The industry has seemed over the years to be content to accept that the benefits of investigators' involvement far outweigh the problems, and the system has been structured to compensate for these problems rather than eliminate them.

For example, one of the most cost-intensive aspects of clinical trials is clinical monitoring; this is essentially a QA process in which experienced clinical personnel, often nurses, review data generated by investigators and make site visits to check data quality (vs. source medical records) and correct case record forms. Processes have focused on correcting errors after the fact, rather than preventing errors before they occur. The CQI principle that error prevention is more cost-effective than error correction has clearly not been fully realized in this aspect of drug development. There is, on the other hand, a recognition that time and money are saved by detecting errors early in a process, since in most drug development programs clinical monitoring of individual cases occurs as soon as possible after a patient visit. One form of quality improvement that has facilitated this to a limited extent is the use of electronic means of data transmission (most commonly fax) to obtain the (paper) case report forms as soon as possible and allow for timely review by clinical monitors. Until very recently, however, technology such as remote data entry has not been fully utilized to facilitate this process.

To understand the cause of this situation and seek CQI solutions, parallels can be drawn to the role of physicians in medical care, in general. Discussing the role of physicians in a hospital environment, Labovitz and Lowenhaupt (1993) point out that to realize the full potential of CQI in a health care environment, the needs of internal customers must be met. This is best done through a customer-supplier dialogue in which suppliers take the initiative to understand their internal customer's needs and make their own requirements clear. These authors go on to say, "Unfortunately physicians—the most critical group of internal customers—are unaccustomed to collaborative efforts and are often unwilling to participate in CQI training. The solution is to use the customer-supplier dialogue to understand physicians' unique needs so that they can be trained effectively and drawn into the CQI process" (39).

Training opportunities for investigators do exist within the drug development process and CROs can play a stronger role. At the beginning of each clinical trial, one or more "investigator meetings" are scheduled to explain the study protocol, the unique features of the trial, and the new therapy to investigators and their study coordinators (nonphysician study staff who carry out trial-related activities at the site). Very often when CROs are involved in trials, they are responsible for conducting investigator meetings, where CQI dialogue and training similar to that described by Labovitz and Lowenhaupt could be carried out.

Attempts by CROs to implement CQI methods at investigator sites have included two recent initiatives: (1) training of study coordinators by CROs and provision of recruiting services to hire study coordinators, and (2) establishment of alliances between large CROs and academic medical centers. For example, Quintiles has announced such alliances with several academic medical centers including the Cleveland Clinic (Center Watch 1997b). The purpose of these alliances is to facilitate better interaction and sharing of resources and scientific knowledge between institutions, including training capabilities. Parexel, a large CRO which has a separate division devoted to training, recently announced an alliance with the School of Nursing of the University of North Carolina at Chapel Hill (Center Watch 1997a) for the purpose of training study coordinators. These relationships clearly present opportunities for dialogue as part of the CQI process.

One other major development in recent years which has the potential to promote CQI processes between investigator sites and the CROs and other participants in the drug development supplier-customer chain is the birth of site management organizations (SMOs). These organizations represent associations of clinical investigative sites in various forms, some more structured than others. They have multiple purposes, some business and some scientific, but most include improving the consistency of operations and training; all include speeding up (improving the efficiency) of the patient enrollment process. The potential for CQI in SMOs is clear, and the potential for CROs and SMOs to work together to improve the quality of the entire drug development process is there. Whether or not this occurs is primarily a business question that will only be answered over time.

In summary, in recent years, CROs have played a unique role in coordinating the various elements of the drug development customer matrix. Because CROs play a dual role—as a party without a vested interest in the success or failure of new pharmaceutical products and as a scientific member of a virtual team that facilitates the introduction of new beneficial therapies—they are in an important position to apply the customer-driven procedures of CQI. Successes in project management of large development programs have sustained the growth of the CRO industry and provide further opportunities for adding value to the drug development process through the application of CQI.

TRAINING AND EMPOWERMENT

According to Deming's classic work *Out of the Crisis* (1986), the transformation of an organization into a high-quality operation involves two major aspects of empowerment of employees—training and employee involvement. In achieving a CQI management style CROs have invested in both of these areas.

In a start-up industry such as the CRO industry of the 1980s, it was critical to train employees in the basics of drug development first, and then later in the more advanced skills necessary for success. The founders of the first CROs had experience; however, many of their early employees were drawn from academia or other areas and were formed into cohesive teams only through formal and informal (on-the-job) training.

Training, as prescribed by Deming and others, was carried out by the top management of the company and started out usually by describing a vision of how CROs could provide uniquely efficient services and in the long run transform the drug development process. As the CRO industry matured, formalized training, in many cases still provided by senior managers, became a standard part of the recruitment and development of new employees. This was especially important for clinical monitoring and data management skills. One critical skill area that emerged as CROs took more direct control of the drug development process was project management.

In contrast to pharmaceutical sponsors, whose project management process often required that physicians or other senior staff be in charge of project teams, CROs tended to assign project managers based on management potential, including an ability to understand and meet customer needs.

Like many small industries, the CRO industry required employees to "wear many hats"; the key skills for success were a willingness to accept challenges and a desire to excel and succeed. The project management process in CROs involved employees in all of the major aspects that Deming associated with quality management (1986). Project management team members participated in operating decisions, made suggestions, and assumed a high degree of responsibility for overall performance. Their role often included planning and monitoring performance along with clients, and always included direct interactions with clients.

Empowerment and Project Management Processes

The key to empowerment of project management teams is the close identification with the customer and the customers' product. Project teams in CROs often become extensions of the sponsor's project team, with a high degree of interaction within teams as well as among team members in the sponsor and CRO organizations. For example, statisticians on the sponsor team and CRO team interact directly to decide on analysis plans and carry out the data analysis, and they collaborate on the summary of findings. Project managers coordinate efforts between the two teams and facilitate communication, but they also have responsibility for guaranteeing that time lines are met and budgets adhered to. All members of both the sponsor and CRO teams share the responsibility for quality; all members of both teams are empowered to make the project a success.

An important source of empowerment, which develops over time once trust is earned on both sides, is the ability to share, rather than cover up, problems as they occur. Despite the fact that a CRO may be carrying out the day-to-day activities, the sponsor company's upper management expects its employees, along with the CRO's employees, to be responsible for delivering the expected products. Thus a sense of shared responsibility and trust becomes a critical way of working.

Another important source of empowerment of drug development teams is a sense of ownership of the sponsor's products. The CRO team is not merely providing services that are specified in a contract, rather they develop a sense of pride and desire to exceed customer expectations. This comes directly from the desire to add value, rather than just meet deadlines, and it is even further emphasized when the drug being developed has the potential to improve quality of life or save lives.

Why do sponsors empower project teams in CROs? The answer to this question has two components. The first is historical. In the early days of CRO involvement, the work was essentially piecemeal. Later, because CROs consistently delivered high-quality services on time, trust was built and the pharmaceutical industry began to expand the depth and breadth of CRO services; then control of the drug development process began to be shared. That is, pharmaceutical sponsors, and especially biotechnology companies, were willing to give up control of certain phases of drug development to other "partners," including CROs. This is very empowering, not only to the individual teams involved, but also to the CRO industry as a whole.

The second reason sponsors empower project teams at CROs relates to the growth of the CRO industry. As CROs became larger entities, clients no longer identified with founders or principal managers in CROs; instead, the linkage with a CRO came through the project manager and project team, who became an extension of the sponsor's internal team. The process by which CROs are chosen has tended to increase this identification. As the industry has expanded, the process for awarding contracts to CROs has become one that requires CROs to prove in great detail that they are qualified to carry out a project. This process includes establishing performance metrics and time lines to be adhered to, as well as establishing scientific credentials and process improvement initiatives. As a result, once a sponsor awards a large contract to a CRO there is great confidence in the choice made. As a safety net, contracts specify what additional data about the project status the CRO will provide to the sponsor to reassure the sponsor of the soundness of their decision. As CRO teams meet their deadlines and adhere to contract metrics, greater confidence is developed and this leads to further empowerment.

Thus the project management process has grown and expanded as CROs took on more responsibility for managing or co-managing drug development programs. The empowerment associated with this growth has provided a structure within which CQI became a standard mode of operation.

CRO Recognition and Experience

As noted by Melum and Sinioris (1992), recognition plays an important role in motivating successful team performance. In the CRO environment there are two forms of recognition: first, formal acknowledgment by a sponsor of the important role a CRO has played in a successful drug development program, and second (and most important), the awarding of new contracts to a CRO based on high-quality performance. One of the highest forms of recognition comes when the ultimate client, the regulatory agency, recommends a CRO to a sponsor.

Through awarding of new contracts based on high performance, CROs build experience and team training. Carrying out additional work for the same client builds further trust. The other major benefit that CROs derive from repeat work is that on-the-job training across a wide range of projects creates a high level of knowledge of the various kinds of drug protocols, clinical trials, and drug development programs that are being used. As CROs develop extensive knowledge of the "art" of drug development (i.e., "what works and what doesn't work"), their experience becomes invaluable for CQI. It also is an important source of empowerment as project teams become more confident of their ability to predict, prevent, and resolve problems efficiently and, once again, add value as members of a drug development team, not merely as service providers.

This kind of experience has also led pharmaceutical and biotechnology sponsors to adopt more of a "virtual development" model in recent years. Further, there have been formal initiatives to create drug development partnerships and alliances between sponsors and CROs. Such initiatives provide a high level of recognition and empowerment; they also foster a high level of education and training as partners become willing to share technology and training resources to benefit all members of the alliance.

LEADERSHIP

The importance of leadership as a component of CQI has been noted by many authors and is discussed elsewhere in this text. In Chapter 1, it is pointed out that one of the key structural elements of CQI implementation is "top management leadership to make the process effective and foster its integration into the institutional fabric of the organization." Melum and Sinioris (1992) speak to the importance of leadership, not only from the top levels of an organization but at all levels—"from the chief executive officer (CEO) and chief operating officer (COO) to vice-presidents, middle managers and front-line supervisors—and leadership throughout the organization" (9).

A definition of leadership that is applicable in CQI has been proposed by Crosby (1979): "Leading means stating objectives in a way that is precisely understood, ensuring the commitment of individuals to those objectives, defining the methods of measurement and then providing the impetus to get things done."

Leadership has been crucial for CROs. Taking a historical view once again may be useful. Many CROs were founded by pharmaceutical industry personnel who had insiders' experience in drug development and saw ways to "do it better." Others who founded CROs were academic consultants who could view the process objectively from outside the pharmaceutical industry and who had experience in solving many of the problems confronted by the industry. Both groups had a common vision of how to improve the drug development process. These founders of CROs also had an entrepreneurial approach which allowed them to go beyond the traditional limits that industry had imposed on itself.

One of the greatest barriers to effective leadership is a belief in the infallibility of the leader (Crosby 1979). CROs have avoided this pitfall over the years by the very nature of their business. Every contract has to be won on the basis of a competitive bidding process and, as stated earlier, CROs have had to compete both with other CROs and with the internal drug development teams of sponsor organizations. This has led CROs to reevaluate customer demand constantly and find new, more efficient ways to meet these demands. The need to maintain profitability and protect the welfare of their employees gives CROs a further impetus to focus on CQI. Finally, in order to win additional contracts, CROs have to prove that the methods they have developed do work; each new proposal is judged not only on the merits of what is proposed, but also on past successes or failures. Thus, CROs must demonstrate another critical leadership skill, the ability to lead by example. As the CRO industry matured, an expression that was often heard from sponsors during the proposal process was: "Don't just tell me what you can do, show me what you have done!" This justifiable attitude on the part of sponsors led to very detailed site visits and presentations by CROs to demonstrate that they truly could "walk the talk." This also empowered teams to be the best and to exceed customer expectations through the application of new technology and new approaches to maximizing efficiency in the drug development process.

Another aspect of leadership that CROs demonstrate is the ability to manage resistance. This is referred to by Melum and Sinioris (1992) in relation to total quality management (TQM) and is, of course, equally applicable to CQI. These authors note that resistance is a fact of life in TQM because it involves managing change. In the CRO environment, resistance can come from within and from outside the organization. Although sponsors have consciously chosen CROs to assist them in their drug development efforts, being middle managers and experienced scientists, they tend to be more comfortable with tried and true methods of drug development. CROs have to manage this resistance at the same time they are balancing the need to evoke customer satisfaction. It is through the skills of experienced project managers and senior scientists within the CRO that sponsors are convinced to "think outside the box" and try new approaches. The ability to train project managers in such skills is critical to CRO success. Sometimes it is the senior managers of the sponsor company who have more of a "big picture" view and encourage their own development staff to allow CROs to demonstrate the effectiveness of new approaches.

To a lesser degree, but also of concern, is the need to manage resistance to change within the CRO. This problem becomes more acute as a CRO grows and has to juggle many different project needs. It is sometimes possible under stress for CROs—especially the large CROs—to fall into the trap of doing it only their way. This problem has multiple dimensions. For example, the CRO may stop listening to customer needs because it is easier to do things in a standardized format that has worked for other sponsors, or the CRO may refuse to look for new ways to improve. This loss of momentum in the application of CQI requires attention and diligence at all levels.

The solution to both problems is leadership, from the top levels and throughout the ranks of CROs. Once again, the project management system provides a powerful vehicle for addressing the problem. The project manager must be a strong leader who promotes the goal of meeting and exceeding client expectations. One of the important ways to do this is to explain clearly and carefully why and how to accomplish these goals. Each team member, in turn, has a leadership role in motivating other team members. In a typical matrix structure, each team member will be drawn from a function-oriented department or section within the CRO. In addition to leading within the team, the team member also has the role of leading and motivating other staff members within his or her own department, including managing resistance to changes being proposed.

Value Added

One of the key objectives of visionary leadership in a CRO is to add value not only to the sponsor's drug development program, but also to the sponsor organization itself through interactions with the CRO team and the leadership and innovation demonstrated by the CRO. A further important goal is to add value to the CRO from the experience gained on each completed drug development program. This is accomplished by developing long-term relationships with sponsors and sharing knowledge and resources wherever possible. Value is also added within the CRO by identifying organizational leaders from among the ranks of successful project managers and project team members, and by using the knowledge and experience accumulated from each drug development project to build the overall expertise of the CRO. This, in turn, demonstrates a track record of successful projects and CQI to potential clients, and opens doors to new challenges and chances to improve further.

In summary, leadership yields a high level of excellence that is achieved by knowing and doing. This level of excellence raises the quality not only of CROs but of the entire industry as CROs and sponsors work together to develop new standards of excellence in drug development.

STATISTICAL PROCESS CONTROL/STATISTICAL THINKING

The need to apply statistical process control as part of an ongoing evaluation of system variability and improvement is an important aspect of CQI that has its roots in QA. Much has been written on this topic, especially by Deming, who describes the careful use of statistical analysis in CQI (1986). It is important to avoid the use of statistics to instill fear or to create artificial reward systems. Instead, statistical thinking should be emphasized. Earlier, in Chapter 1, statistical thinking is discussed as part of CQI implementation; it includes:

- how to look at variation as a generator of errors and costs
- how to speak with data and manage with facts
- how to take the guesswork out of decision making
- how to reduce variation and unnecessary complexity through the use of the seven standard tools of data analysis and display

Statistical thinking requires the understanding and effective use of statistical measurement and analysis. The CRO industry is a data-driven industry and it requires the collection and analysis of large amounts of data.

Various statistical process measures have been developed and used in a variety of ways in the CRO industry. Some are *performance metrics* that help sponsors gauge compliance with contract specifications; CROs also benefit from using these as measures of quality improvement (see Exhibit 14–2). A common example of this is the use of patient enrollment graphs that plot the number of patients expected to be enrolled in a study during a given time period against actual members enrolled (see Figure 14–4). Taken by itself this not a CQI tool but, rather, a measure of supplier (investigative site) performance. It can be very effective, however, as a CQI tool when combined with other quality metrics, such as the proportion of patients enrolled who are later identified as protocol violators or the proportion of dropouts or other patients who can no longer be evaluated. Rather than using such metrics as tools to penalize for poor performance, CROs have used these statistical tools to measure and improve their own internal performance while at the same time meeting the customer's need to have performance metrics written into contracts. A good example of statistical analysis of process measurement and improvement is data management.

Exhibit 14–2 Examples of CRO Performance Metrics

Quantitative
- Number of patients enrolled in study
  –Expected vs. actual (by time point)
- Number of pages of data processed
  –Received
  –Edited
  –Entered
- Number of patients completed
  –Completed trial
  –All data clarifications resolved
  –Locked in database

Qualitative
- Number of patients excluded due to protocol violations
- Number of dropouts/lost to follow-up
- Number of clinically evaluable patients
- Number of tags/DCFs generated
- Data management error rate

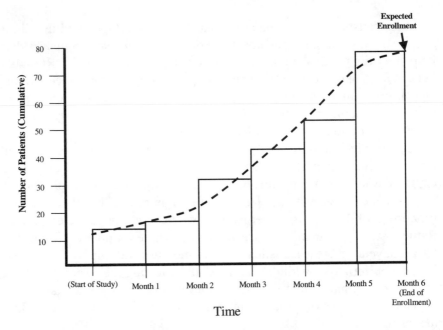

Note: Bars indicate cumulative total of actual patients enrolled.

Figure 14–4 Patient Enrollment Graph

Data Management: Process Measurement

Despite technological breakthroughs, data management in pharmaceutical clinical trials remains limited by manual activities. Although in recent years the process has become more automated, it still relies on labor-intensive procedures starting with paper data collection forms or case report forms completed by investigators and culminating in an electronic database which is compatible for statistical analysis procedures (Figure 14–5). Despite the large investments made in the clinical trial process, the data management step has traditionally been the weak link in the chain, and because new drug applications rely so heavily on manually processed data, it is a critical path to success.

In the early 1980s this was a particular problem in the drug development industry; data management operations in many large pharmaceutical organizations were "black boxes"; the process was not well understood and represented a bottleneck in the clinical trial execution. This presented an

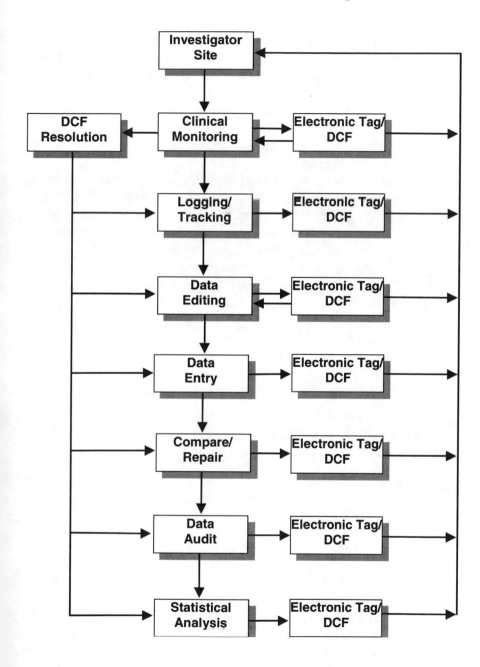

Figure 14–5 Flowchart of Data Management System

opportunity for newly developing CROs to improve the process, and in fact this was one of the key contributions of Quintiles, which started as a statistics and data management company. It was also a classic example of how to apply CQI processes.

The first step was to describe the process in a traditional production flowchart as in Figure 14–5. This figure represents the process as it was carried out prior to the use of electronic data collection steps. It is a process still used by many organizations.

Because of the number of manual procedures that had to be performed, various quality control and quality assurance steps had to be built in to ensure the quality of the database. Data management error rates are a good indicator of the quality of the entire system, including clinical monitoring effectiveness, data collection, data editing, and data entry, and these error rates are amenable to quantification and review.

Some of the process improvements that were introduced and which are now part of standard procedures in most clinical trial operations include the following:

- electronic range and consistency checks
- electronic tags
- automated data clarification forms (DCFs) to document queries
- double entry of all data
- 100 percent source verification of key safety information
- automated transfer of laboratory data files
- audits of final databases

Electronic Data Clarification

Two of these processes are worth further discussion because they are statistical processes that are applicable to other areas of health care. The first is the use of electronic tags and associated data clarification forms (DCFs). Initially, when paper case report forms were received from investigative sites, data management personnel, who were known as data editors, manually reviewed all forms using predefined edit checks and put "yellow sticky tags" on pages where errors were found. These errors were queried by having clinical monitors review the data and/or visit the investigative site and determine the correct value. As new technology became available, clinical monitors conducted the same review process on computer (after initial entry and basic range checks had been completed). Instead of manually checking the data, the checking process involved using electronic flags on variables that needed resolution; at the same time a "tag file" consisting of all data clarification forms to be resolved was automatically created listing all case report form (CRF) items that needed verification. The clinical staff and/or the original clinical investigator then reviewed each of these items for corrections. They removed the tags electronically as each DCF was resolved. A database could not be "closed" until all tags in the tag file and all DCFs had been resolved. Thus, the new system provided an automatic self-checking mechanism.

Much of this process improvement initiative is still in place today and, in fact, some developers of data management software include the electronic tag system as part of their basic package. Working together, CROs and sponsors developed these procedures as a way of improving the efficiency of the data checking system and the overall quality of the final database.

Data Processing Error Measurement

Another simple example of a CQI application is the use of data audits to verify the error rate in a database. This is a classic example of how industrial production methods for batch error checking have been applied in clinical trial data management. The overall objective of the process is to assure the sponsor that the error rate in a data processing operation is below some predetermined acceptable level. For example, an "acceptable" industry standard is 25 errors per 10,000 fields checked. Some CROs are so confident of their data management quality that they use error rates in marketing materials and write them into contracts. Error rate measurement represents a process improvement in that it uses scientific sampling approaches, which are now standard in industry, to avoid 100 percent verification of all data, an inefficient process that often leads to new (unmeasurable) errors.

Exhibit 14–3 describes the error rate measurement process. Briefly, the key to the system is that it is carried out after all data management steps, including all query resolutions, have been completed, and just prior to formally locking the database. A sampling methodology, either a ratio sample or a true random sample, is used to select patients' cases to be

Exhibit 14–3 Outline of Database Audit Procedure

Process
- Proofreading of original CRF vs. system printout
- Document findings by source of error
- Error correction

Sampling Approach
- Statistical sampling techniques
- Simple random sample/Ratio sample of patients/fields
  –Stratification by investigator
  –Audit 100% of data for sampled patients
  –Audit 100% of patients for key safety measures

Summary of Results
- Formal report/Control chart
- Primary goal: Systematic errors/System problems
- Secondary goal: Documentation of random errors
- Target: Error rate < 25 errors/10,000 fields

audited. In multicenter clinical trials, the sample is stratified to ensure representation of all investigators, because they are an important source of possible variation in quality. Once the sample is selected (usually representing no more than 10 percent of the cases), a 100 percent audit is carried out for all data items in the sampled CRFs. All errors found are documented, investigated and corrected. An important goal of this process is to identify systematic errors such as those that might be due to an electronic/programming problem in the system or to inadequate training. In addition to this sample, critical information such as listings of adverse reactions, a key safety indicator, may be audited on a 100 percent basis.

Audit findings are documented and summarized in a format similar to that used for standard control charts, to allow for ongoing internal process improvement and also to be made available to external customers, both sponsors and regulatory authorities, as needed. In cases where error rates are higher than expected, additional sampling or other investigation of the process is carried out.

As new technology becomes available and especially as more electronic methods are used to simplify "the black box" of clinical data management, it becomes critical to use process improvement technologies such as those described here and to develop new techniques to assess quality and further improve the process on a continual basis.

CONCLUSION

The CRO industry is relatively young. It just began in the 1980s, but it has achieved rapid growth and success. Much of the success of CROs in the pharmaceutical sector can be traced at least in part to the implementation of CQI processes.

CROs have exhibited each of the three CQI strategies described by Linder (1991). Because of the regulatory nature of pharmaceutical development, CROs have had to conform to requirements. They have used CQI to gain a competitive advantage, not only in competing with other CROs, but also in competing with internal drug development teams in sponsor organizations. They have also used CQI as a process improvement tool and, together with their sponsors, have developed many new tools and approaches to drug development. Wherever possible, CROs have used technology to seek solutions to bottlenecks and to accelerate the registration process for new products. Quality improvement has been critical in order to meet the requirements of the ultimate customers—regulatory agencies, which are responsible for approving new drugs; physician-practitioners, who must have confidence in the safety and efficacy of new drugs being dispensed; and finally and most important, patients, whose well-being depends on the quality of the new drugs they are taking.

In carrying out these processes, CROs have effectively used complex project management systems and have applied virtual approaches to emphasize cooperation and partnership with sponsors. Their approach can be described as co-configuration, a concept described in Chapter 1 as a futuristic approach to the application of CQI. This approach is one example of how the CRO industry has been ahead of many other components of health and medical care. It also explains why so much success has been achieved so quickly.

The future challenge for the CRO industry is whether it can maintain the customer focus, the level of empowerment, and the leadership it has built into its organizations. CQI processes are hard to develop and maintain. When CROs were small and growing, CQI was necessary for survival; now that many CROs have achieved financial and business success, the key question is whether they will be able to sustain the CQI philosophies and processes that got them where they are today.

CHAPTER 15

CQI in Public Health Organizations

Glen P. Mays, Theresa Hatzell,
Arnold D. Kaluzny, and Paul K. Halverson

Public health and continuous quality improvement (CQI) have an affinity that defies their lack of common ancestry. As a field of practice, public health focuses on the health of communities and populations. Like CQI, public health practice uses a systems perspective in identifying problems and developing interventions—recognizing the multiple inputs, outputs, and processes that affect health at the population level. Also like CQI, public health practice is firmly grounded in scientific methods that allow the measurement of problems and the tracking of system performance over time. Epidemiological investigation, population surveillance, and community health assessment are among public health's core methodologies for measuring and improving health at the population level. Additionally, both CQI and public health practice are based on the premise that meaningful improvements cannot be achieved without the involvement of key stakeholders within the system. In medical care organizations these stakeholders consist of senior administrators and core operational staff, but in the field of public health they often include public officials, community organizations, health care professionals, the media, and members of the public at large.

When successful, both CQI and public health practice reflect elements of *mass customization* in their strategies for performance improvement. CQI processes in medical care organizations focus on tailoring operations to individual patient needs and expectations, often with the aid of powerful information systems. At their best, public health organizations also tailor their interventions to specific community health needs and risks. Through the process of community diagnosis, these organizations identify clinically relevant subpopulations within their communities, evaluate health

360

needs and resources within each subpopulation, and design community interventions to address these needs using guidance and direction from the communities themselves. Community health information systems are being used to support these public health activities in a growing number of communities (Starr 1997).

Despite similarities in concept and method, the successful implementation of CQI within public health organizations is rarely automatic. This chapter examines both the opportunities and the challenges that public health organizations face in applying CQI methods to community health problems. First, this chapter identifies a set of critical dimensions that characterize CQI strategies within public health organizations. These dimensions must be considered—either explicitly or implicitly—when designing and implementing CQI efforts in public health organizations. Second, the chapter reviews the range of performance assessment and quality improvement tools and processes that have been developed over the past decade for public health organizations. These processes, which are grounded in core concepts of CQI, offer public health organizations valuable strategies for improving community health. Finally, this chapter identifies a set of barriers to CQI implementation that are commonly encountered within public health organizations. Potential strategies for addressing these barriers are considered. Throughout we examine examples of CQI efforts in both governmental and nongovernmental public health settings in order to illustrate the benefits and challenges of CQI in these diverse multiorganizational environments.

CRITICAL DIMENSIONS OF PUBLIC HEALTH QUALITY IMPROVEMENT INITIATIVES

As in other settings, quality improvement efforts in public health organizations must be linked to a core organizational mission. Although the specifics of this mission vary across organizations, a general and widely recognized statement of the public health mission is given by the Institute of Medicine (1988):

> The mission of public health is to fulfill society's interest in assuring conditions in which people can be healthy. Its aim is to generate organized community effort to address the public interest in health by applying scientific and technical knowledge to

prevent disease and promote health. The mission of public health
is addressed by private organizations and individuals, as well as
by public agencies (7).

From this statement, it becomes clear that public health performance
flows from the efforts of a wide array of organizations, and that public
health outcomes are defined and evaluated from a societal perspective
which reflects "the public interest in health." These concepts of *performance* and *outcomes*—which differ substantially from those used often in
the field of medical care—have important implications for how CQI
methods are implemented within public health organizations.

Several critical dimensions of CQI implementation are evident in the
process improvement efforts that many public health organizations undertake. These dimensions determine the focus of the improvement effort, the
organizations and individuals involved, and the specific measurement and
decision-making strategies that are used. Each of the dimensions examined
below must be considered either explicitly or implicitly by public health
organizations involved in CQI efforts.

Defining Public Health

In order to measure and improve performance, public health organizations require a clear definition of core public health activities. Such a
definition has historically been the topic of much debate and discussion,
and there continues to be substantial variation in how public health
organizations define the scope of public health practice. In 1988 the
Institute of Medicine (IOM) devised a simple conceptual framework for
describing core public health activities that has served as the basis for
many recent performance measurement efforts (Institute of Medicine
1988). The IOM framework identifies three core public health functions:

- *Assessment* is the regular and systematic collection, analysis, and
  dissemination of information on the health of the community, which
  enables community health needs to be identified.
- *Policy Development* is the exercise of the responsibility to serve the
  public interest in the development of comprehensive public health

plans and policies by promoting the use of scientific knowledge in decision making.

- *Assurance* is the guarantee to constituents that health services necessary to achieve public health goals are provided to the community by the composite actions of public and private organizations—a responsibility that may be carried out through regulation, contract, or direct service provision.

Subsequent work by the U.S. Centers for Disease Control and Prevention (CDC) led to the specification of 10 public health practices that link directly with the three IOM core functions (Dyall 1995). These practices, which were identified by a working group of public health experts convened by the CDC during 1991 and 1992, include the following:

1. *Assess* the health need of the community. (Assessment)
2. *Investigate* the occurrence of health effects and health hazards of the community. (Assessment)
3. *Analyze* the determinants of identified health needs. (Assessment)
4. *Advocate* for public health, build constituencies and identify resources in the community. (Policy Development)
5. *Set priorities* among health needs. (Policy Development)
6. *Develop plans* and policies to address priority health needs. (Policy Development)
7. *Manage* resources and develop organizational structure. (Assurance)
8. *Implement* public health programs and services. (Assurance)
9. *Evaluate* programs and provide quality assurance. (Assurance)
10. *Inform and educate* the public. (Assurance)

Under the CDC's sponsorship, several groups of researchers have used these definitions of public health practice to develop systems of surveillance for measuring the adequacy of public health practice in local geopolitical jurisdictions (Miller et al. 1994b; Turnock et al. 1994). Each of the 10 practices was linked to a set of measurable public health indicators for this purpose. The methods and results of these surveys are reviewed below.

Another federal effort to define the scope of public health practice occurred during the national policy debate over health care reform that took place throughout 1993 and 1994. An expert committee convened by the U.S. Department of Health and Human Services (HHS) identified a set of 10 essential public health services—ostensibly independent of the IOM and CDC formulations, but conceptually similar to these earlier efforts (Baker et al. 1994). The identified services include the following:

1. Monitor health status to identify and solve community health problems.
2. Diagnose and investigate health problems and health hazards in the community.
3. Inform, educate and empower people about health issues.
4. Mobilize community partnerships and action to solve health problems.
5. Develop policies and plans that support individual and community health efforts.
6. Enforce laws and regulations that protect health and ensure safety.
7. Link people to needed personal health services and ensure the provision of health care when otherwise unavailable.
8. Ensure a competent work force—public health and personal health care.
9. Evaluate effectiveness, accessibility, and quality of personal and population-based health services.
10. Conduct research for new insights and innovative solutions to health problems.

The federal government has tested this framework in evaluations of state public health agency expenditures and in assessments of state programs funded through the federal Maternal and Child Health Block Grant (Eilbert et al. 1997). The essential services framework has achieved broad support at the federal level, but appears to be used sparsely within state and local public health organizations at present (Mays et al. 1998a).

Another effort to define the scope of public health practice was initiated by the World Health Organization (WHO) in 1997, drawing on the knowledge and experiences of an international collection of public health experts (Bettcher et al. 1998). Using a Delphi process with 145 public health administrators, educators, researchers, and practitioners, the WHO study identified and prioritized a list of 37 essential public health functions that fell within nine general categories:

1. Prevention, surveillance, and control of communicable and noncommunicable diseases
2. Monitoring of the health situation (health status, determinants, risks, and interventions)
3. Health promotion
4. Occupational health
5. Protection of the environment
6. Public health legislation and regulations
7. Public health management
8. Specific public health services (school health, emergency services, and laboratory services)
9. Personal health care for vulnerable and high-risk populations

With straightforward modifications, the frameworks that the IOM, CDC, HHS, and WHO developed approximate each other, but it is unlikely that any one of them represents the last word for defining the complex role of public health in modern society. A recent survey of state public health organizations reveals that many of them are using the above frameworks in their efforts to measure and improve public health performance, but that few of them use any single approach in an unaltered form (Mays et al. 1998a). Many rely on locally developed definitions of public health practice. Although the means are still imperfect, the need to define the public health mission in measurable terms has become widely accepted; many constructive efforts are underway. Considering the great variability in structure and function of public health organizations, it is not surprising that a variety of approaches now exist for defining the scope of public health practice. To be successful, the approach that is used must provide a good fit with the public health needs, capacities, and priorities existing in that setting.

CQI Focus: Internal versus External Processes

A basic distinction must be made between performance improvement efforts that focus on an internal activity conducted directly by the public health organization, and those that involve an external process that depends on the actions of multiple organizations and individuals. For example, an internal CQI effort conducted by a local health department might focus on improving the immunization delivery practices of staff who work in clinics operated by the department. By contrast, an external CQI effort might focus on improving immunization practices among private physicians and clinics that operate within the local health department's jurisdiction. Both of these activities potentially relate to a local health department's mission of improving community immunization rates and reducing the incidence of vaccine-preventable diseases. Internal and external processes, however, may address markedly different facets of the public health problem under study, and they may require vastly different allocations of resources, skills, legal authority, and political clout.

In choosing the appropriate focus for a CQI effort, public health organizations need to consider a variety of factors, including:

- the nature of the public health problem being targeted
- the internal strengths and weaknesses of their organization
- the current and potential roles played by external organizations and individuals in the problem under study
- the public health organization's current and potential relationships with these external entities

In some cases, an external focus may be ruled out due to insufficient resources and skills, or due to a lack of political will in the external environment. In other cases, an internal focus may be inappropriate because of the limited effects that internal processes have on the public health problem under study. For example, improving immunization rates only among health department clients may be insufficient to achieve meaningful improvements in community immunization coverage. Therefore, an external CQI effort that targets the immunization practices of all community providers may be needed. In still other cases, an internal CQI effort may serve as an important initial demonstration to generate support for subsequent external efforts. This strategy follows an approach based on staged successes or "small wins," which has become an essential ingredient of many CQI efforts.

Role of Public Health Organizations in the CQI Process

A second critical dimension of CQI implementation involves the roles that public health organizations play in implementing CQI processes. The adoption of CQI often follows a staged process that includes awareness of a problem, identification of an intervention, implementation of the intervention, and finally institutionalization of the intervention (Hernandez et al. in press). Public health organizations may assume roles in any or all of these stages. For internally focused CQI efforts, these stages may all occur within the public health organization. For externally focused CQI efforts, however, other organizations may play critical roles in the adoption process. Public health organizations may play an *initiating* role for CQI efforts by raising awareness about a public health problem, only to let other organizations assume responsibility for implementing and institutionalizing a CQI process to address the problem. Public health organizations may play a *convening* role in CQI efforts by bringing organizations and individuals together for the purpose of identifying and implementing an intervention. During the process of CQI implementation, public health organizations may choose among several alternative levels of involvement, including:

- a *governing* role, wherein the public health organization assumes primary responsibility for directing and managing the CQI process
- a *participatory* role, which entails shared responsibility for managing the CQI process with other organizations
- a *contributing* role, which involves providing information, resources, and expertise to a CQI process that is actively managed by other organizations

The public health organization's role in CQI efforts will depend on its own mission, skills, and resources and those of other organizations having an interest in the public health problems being addressed. By encouraging other organizations to assume key responsibilities in public health CQI efforts, public health organizations sacrifice some measure of control over these efforts. In return, however, public health organizations benefit from the additional expertise and resources that other organizations contribute. These arrangements may also offer public health organizations opportunities to learn about CQI methods from other health organizations already skilled in these approaches, such as hospitals, managed care plans, medical practices, and laboratories. For example, in one community a private hospital assumes primary responsibility for a CQI process aimed at improving the delivery of prenatal care to low-income pregnant women. The local public health agency participates extensively in this process, but the hospital assumes primary responsibility for the core activities of convening and educating local providers, implementing a community-wide outreach and referral service for patients, and evaluating the community's performance in prenatal care delivery.

Source of Public Health Authority and Control

A third critical dimension of CQI implementation involves the source of public health decision-making authority and control. Governmental public health functions are carried out at federal, state, and local levels, with overlapping jurisdictions of authority existing for many public health issues. CQI efforts must be responsive to these different levels of authority. An important task for public health organizations, therefore, entails identifying the most appropriate level for operating a CQI effort and encouraging CQI implementation at that level. Some public health problems are most effectively addressed through interventions at state or national levels rather than at the local level. Enhanced legal authority or political will may exist at these higher levels; and superior resources may be available to address the problem. Many public health problems extend beyond the boundaries of a single local community, and therefore require broader governmental authority. Moreover, the problem may flow from a characteristic of a state or federal program, rather than from an element of local program implementation. For example, environmental health problems such as water quality and hazardous waste disposal often fall into this category because many state governments retain substantial regulatory authority over these issues. Rather than attempting to lead a CQI effort at the local level, local public health agencies may achieve better results by contributing to state-level or federal-level CQI implementation.

Conversely, other public health issues involve primarily local populations, resources, and health needs. Often, these issues can be addressed most effectively through community-level efforts rather than large-scale state or national interventions. For example, the task of improving the accessibility of family planning services within a community is likely to be most responsive to a local CQI effort. In this case, local community organizations primarily control the processes of service delivery, outreach, and education, which therefore makes them amenable to local improvement efforts. In other cases, local CQI efforts may be implemented because larger-scale state or national efforts are not feasible due to a lack of political will. For example, some local communities have initiated CQI efforts around the task of improving health insurance coverage for the uninsured, largely because state and federal initiatives to address this problem have failed to be implemented.

CQI activities may also involve public health organizations at multiple levels of authority. Local CQI efforts may be implemented as components of larger state or national CQI efforts, with linkages maintained through communication and information flows among the various levels of public health authority. These approaches are designed to address gaps in performance simultaneously at these multiple levels of authority, and are particularly relevant in cases where performance at one level has substantial influence on performance at another level. For example, the Florida Department of Health maintains a state-level CQI process for improving public health outcomes within the state regarding issues such as infant mortality, adolescent pregnancy, and the incidence of communicable diseases (Speake et al. 1995). As part of this effort, individual CQI processes are implemented at each local public health unit within the state. These local CQI efforts identify strategies for improving the delivery of public health services at the community level. These efforts also generate information about local resource needs and priorities that feed into the state-level CQI process, which uses this information to improve decision making regarding state budget allocations, policy making, and program development.

The administrative relationships that exist among local, state, and federal public health organizations play important roles in CQI implementation. In states such as Florida, local public health agencies are organized as centralized administrative units of the state public health agency. The state agency maintains direct authority for many public health activities within the state. In other states, local public health organizations are decentralized and operate under the direct authority of local governments and local boards of health. In still other states, local public health agencies operate under state authority for some public health functions (such as communicable disease control and environmental health protection), and under local authority for other functions (such as health promotion and disease prevention activities and community health assessment). Centralized public health jurisdictions may offer state agencies enhanced authority for organizing and coordinating CQI processes at the local level, while decentralized jurisdictions may offer greater opportunities for incorporating local needs, priorities, and values in the CQI process.

Federal public health agency relationships with state and local public health organizations also play important roles in CQI efforts. Federal agencies interact with state and local organizations primarily through the provision of public health funding, technical assistance, and regulatory oversight. Much federal public health funding is now disbursed through block grants and similar "pass-through" arrangements to state health agencies, rather than through categorical grants made directly to local public health organizations. Increasingly, federal agencies are using these funding vehicles to encourage quality improvement initiatives at the state level. For example, the Maternal and Child Health Block Grant administered by the U.S. Health Resources and Services Administration requires state grantees to conduct formal needs assessment processes, and to develop performance objectives and measures for their programs. Other federal agencies are developing similar performance measurement criteria for their public health funding programs, pursuant to requirements under the federal *Government Performance and Results Act of 1993*. These federal efforts, many of which are described in detail below, provide additional motivation for public health organizations to implement CQI processes.

Federal agencies may also encourage CQI implementation through their regulatory authority. Agencies such as the U.S. Environmental Protection Agency (EPA) use their regulatory authority to enforce compliance with federal public health standards such as those concerning air quality, water quality, and solid waste disposal. State and local public health organizations that do not meet these standards are required to adopt remediation processes, which offer opportunities for the application of CQI methods. Since 1995, the EPA's *Reinventing Environmental Protection* initiative has emphasized the use of CQI methods in helping communities achieve and exceed federal public health standards (U.S. Environmental Protection Agency 1998).

Finally, federal public health agencies encourage the implementation of CQI methods through their technical assistance role with state and local public health organizations. The CDC's Public Health Practice Program Office, for example, provides information and assistance to state and local public health agencies seeking to implement CQI methods. The CDC carries out its technical assistance role in partnership with professional associations such as the National Association of County and City Health Officials and the Association of State and Territorial Health Officials. Through these partnerships, the CDC has been instrumental in developing numerous resources for quality improvement processes, many of which are discussed below. Other federal agencies, such as the U.S. Health Resources and Services Administration, also provide CQI technical assistance to public health organizations.

Public Participation and Accountability

Another important dimension of CQI implementation in public health organizations is the extent of public participation and accountability. An essential component of the public health mission lies in responsiveness to community needs, values, and priorities. Some public health organizations ensure this responsiveness through the direct involvement of community representatives in public health decision making and governance. These organizations may operate under governing boards comprised of community representatives, or they may appoint community members to serve on public health task forces empowered to address specific community health issues. Other public health organizations rely on indirect approaches for ensuring responsiveness and accountability to the public. Many use formal processes for assessing community health needs and identifying public health priorities. Some organizations also rely on governing boards comprised of publicly elected officials to reflect public interests and priorities.

These same levels of public participation often extend to CQI initiatives within public health organizations. Some organizations directly involve community representatives in their quality improvement processes. Projects supported by the W.K. Kellogg Foundation's *Community-based Public Health Initiative* use this approach (Mays et al. 1999b). Each of the seven demonstration projects sponsored through this initiative bring together public health organizations, academic institutions, and community-based organizations to form collaborative processes for identifying community health needs, developing and implementing interventions, and evaluating outcomes. Representatives from community-based organizations—including churches, neighborhood associations, and other local groups—share responsibility for problem identification, intervention, and evaluation with the governmental public health organizations and academic institutions. Steering committees comprised of representatives from each participating organization use consensus-driven processes to decide how to improve public health services within the community. This approach is designed to ensure that improvement processes focus on issues of high importance for community members, and that they involve organizations and individuals having the greatest knowledge of and experience with community health problems. Although Kellogg support for these projects officially ended in 1996, most of them continue to operate successfully. A new demonstration effort launched jointly by Kellogg and the Robert Wood Johnson Foundation, entitled *Turning Point: Collaborating for a New Century in Public Health*, also emphasizes direct community participation in public health improvement processes (W.K. Kellogg Foundation 1997).

Other public health organizations use CQI processes that involve more indirect levels of community participation. These processes typically rely on community representatives to obtain information about community health needs and priorities; however, they often do not directly involve these representatives in the decision-making processes that govern the implementation and evaluation of quality improvement efforts. For example, many public health organizations invite community participation in their community health assessment processes. Through these processes, organizations collect information about community perceptions regarding the most pressing public health issues, and elicit opinions about the most promising strategies for addressing these issues. In many of these efforts, direct community participation is limited to the tasks of problem identification, planning, and priority setting. Decisions regarding what interventions to implement, how to implement them, and how to evaluate them remain the direct responsibility of public health organizations.

The degree of community participation may have important implications for the success of CQI efforts. Direct forms of community participation often ensure that the CQI process maintains a high degree of responsiveness to public health problems as experienced by community members. Direct participation may add substantial time to the CQI process, since community members must learn about CQI concepts and build trust and familiarity with other participants in the process. CQI processes involving direct community participation may also experience added difficulties in reaching consensus about key problems and potential interventions, given the diversity of opinion and perspective that is likely to exist among participants. Alternative levels of community participation may therefore entail trade-offs in administrative responsiveness, feasibility, and efficiency.

Performance Measurement and Evaluation

Performance measurement is an essential element of any CQI process. Public health CQI efforts vary widely in the approaches used to measure and evaluate public health performance. This variation results, in part, from the alternative ways that public health organizations define the scope of public health practice. This variation also stems from the alternative types of indicators that exist for a given public health activity, and the alternative methods for assessing the value of a given indicator. Like performance measures in medical care, public health indicators may reflect the *structural dimensions* of public health practice, the clinical and administrative *processes* used in practice, and the *outcomes* that result from these processes. Also like those in medical care, public health indicators may reflect elements of technical quality, effectiveness, appropriateness, comprehensiveness, accessibility, and efficiency.

Methods for assessing the value of a given indicator also vary substantially, but they uniformly entail comparisons (Gerzoff 1997). Some quality improvement initiatives rely on comparisons with *a priori* standards identified by experts, such as the national *Healthy People 2000: National Health Objectives for the Year 2000,* published by the U.S. Public Health Service. These comparisons have the advantage of being relatively simple to carry out once data are available, and of being widely recognizable and understandable. These comparisons, however, have the disadvantage of focusing only on a single level of performance, so that continued improvement is de-emphasized once the standard is met. Some quality improvement initiatives use comparisons over time—also called *trend analysis*—so that continuous improvement in performance can be detected and measured for a given indicator. This method addresses the problem with *a priori* standards noted above, but it has limited ability to value how much improvement is adequate and desirable over a given period of time. Finally, some improvement initiatives rely on benchmark comparisons with other public health organizations, so that performance can be evaluated in relation to similar organizations and/or leading organizations in the field. Combining methods based on *a priori* standards, trend analysis, and benchmarking can be particularly powerful for measuring and motivating continuous improvement in public health performance.

IMPLEMENTATION OF QUALITY IMPROVEMENT INITIATIVES IN PUBLIC HEALTH

Over the past decade, a wide array of performance assessment and quality improvement activities have been implemented within the field of public health at local, state, and national levels. These efforts reflect the concepts and methods of CQI in varying ways and with varying degrees of success. More important, these activities create opportunities for public health organizations to access models, tools, and insight for their own CQI efforts. Six general types of activities are most prominent in the current landscape of public health improvement efforts:

- community health assessment and planning tools
- public health practice guidelines
- community health report cards
- public health information networks
- performance contracting systems
- public health performance measurement systems

These activities are examined and compared below.

Community Health Assessment and Planning Tools

A number of tools have been developed to assist public health organizations in identifying and assessing community health problems within their jurisdictions, and in planning strategies to address these problems. These tools serve as important foundations and frameworks for implementing CQI efforts within public health organizations.

National Health Objectives

Perhaps the most prominent public health planning tools of the past two decades have been those developed by the U.S. Public Health Service to identify measurable national health objectives. These efforts identified a set of high-priority health issues, formulated national improvement goals for each issue, and specified measurement criteria and data sources to be used in assessing improvement. Objectives were identified for the years 1980 to 1990 in the document entitled *1990 Health Objectives*, and from 1990 to 2000 in the document *Healthy People 2000: National Health Objectives for the Year 2000*. Draft objectives are currently under development for the *Healthy People 2010* document, which will cover the period from 2000 to 2010. The *Healthy People 2000* document includes objectives in 22 general areas of health as outlined in Exhibit 15–1. In each area, three types of health objectives are identified: those that target *health status outcomes* for the health issue; those that target *health services and interventions*; and those that target *health risk factors*. For example, a health outcome objective in the area of child health states: "Reduce the infant mortality rate to no more than 7 per 1,000 live births" (American Public Health Association 1992, 14). Similarly, a health services objective in this area is to increase the proportion of primary care providers who provide age-appropriate preconception care and counseling to at least 60 percent (15). A health risk factor objective in this area is to increase the proportion of mothers who achieve the minimum recommended weight gain during their pregnancies to at least 85 percent (15).

Exhibit 15–1 Priority Areas for the *Healthy People 2000* National Health Objectives

1. Physical activity and fitness
2. Nutrition
3. Tobacco
4. Alcohol and other drugs
5. Family planning
6. Mental health and mental disorders
7. Violent and abusive behavior
8. Educational and community-based programs
9. Unintentional injuries
10. Occupational safety and health
11. Environmental health
12. Food and drug safety
13. Oral health
14. Maternal and infant health
15. Heart disease and stroke
16. Cancer
17. Diabetes
18. HIV Infection
19. Sexually transmitted diseases
20. Immunization and infectious diseases
21. Clinical preventive services
22. Surveillance and data systems

These national objectives have assisted many public health organizations in their improvement processes by identifying a set of priority health issues in need of attention, and by offering measurable goals against which performance may be judged. As a CQI tool, however, these objectives are limited in that they are not sensitive to public health problems of local and regional interest that may not be reflected in broad national trends and priorities. Additionally, these national objectives identify specific performance levels to be achieved rather than establishing a process for continual improvement. To complement the national objectives and address some of their limitations, several additional community health planning tools have been developed in conjunction with the U.S. Public Health Service's efforts.

Health Planning Tools

One of the most prominent of these tools, the *Planned Approach to Community Health* (PATCH), was developed by the U.S. Centers for Disease Control and Prevention (CDC) in 1985 (Greene 1992). The PATCH protocol outlines a standard process that public health organizations can follow for analyzing a few selected health issues, determining their root causes and key intervention points, and planning effective strategies for addressing these issues. Expanding on this effort, the American Public Health Association developed a protocol to assist public health organizations in creating community health planning and monitoring systems that address a comprehensive range of health-related problems. This protocol, named *Healthy Communities 2000: Model Standards*, was developed in 1991 and explicitly designed to link with the *Healthy People 2000* national objectives (American Public Health Association 1993). It provides a process for public health organizations to develop a plan based on measurable public health objectives that target specific public health outcomes, processes, and population groups. Both process and outcome objectives are emphasized in the protocol. The Texas Department of Health, for example, used this protocol in developing performance-based objectives for local public health departments within the state (Griffin and Welch 1995). Objectives were constructed so that the time frame and quantity of improvement could be specified by each local agency, as in the following outcome and process examples:

- The rate of bicycle-related injuries in children ages 5–14 in *[name]* County will be reduced from *[number]* per 100,000 in FY *[year]* to *[number]* per 100,000 in FY *[year]*.

- By end of FY *[year]*, secure passage of a local ordinance requiring mandatory use of bicycle helmets.

Another assessment and planning tool, the *Assessment Protocol for Excellence in Public Health (*APEX-PH), was developed in 1991 by the National Association of County and City Health Officials with sponsorship from CDC (National Association of County and City Health Officials 1991). This self-assessment workbook for public health officials includes components for assessing the internal capacity of public health organizations as well as the external capacity of other organizations serving the community. The workbook relies on an array of process indicators, including those addressing public health authority, community relations, community health assessment, policy development, financial management, personnel management, program management, and governing board procedures. An expanded version of this protocol, the *Assessment and Planning Excellence through Community Partners for Health* (APEX-CPH) is currently under development. This new protocol aligns the indicators in APEX-PH with the 10 essential public health services identified by HHS, and expands the community capacity indicators to include a broader array of community organizations and activities.

Drawing on these efforts, the U.S. Agency for Health Care Policy and Research developed a planning tool designed specifically to assist local health departments in responding to managed health care systems. This workbook, entitled *Assessing Roles, Responsibilities, and Activities in a Managed Care Environment*, provides health departments with guidelines for assessing budgets, staffing, and service delivery activities; developing managed care contracts and affiliations; assessing community health needs; and monitoring policy and marketplace trends (Bartlett et al. 1997).

Health Assessment and Improvement Tools

Other assessment initiatives formally integrate the tasks of collecting and analyzing community health data with the processes of community health planning, priority-setting, and intervention. In many communities, the hospital industry has become actively involved in these activities.

Following up on pioneering efforts in Pennsylvania, Vermont, and Wisconsin, growing numbers of state hospital associations actively encourage their members to conduct community health assessment and improvement initiatives within their service areas (Gordon et al. 1996). The Pennsylvania association's process, which has served as a model for many assessment initiatives across the country, involves a five-step sequence: (1) compiling a community health profile, (2) identifying priorities for community health needs, (3) developing an action plan, (4) implementing community health interventions, and (5) evaluating the interventions. The assessment initiative adopted by the Wisconsin association draws heavily on the Pennsylvania model as well as the APEX-PH protocol originally developed for public health agencies. California state law now requires its hospitals to conduct periodic community health assessments using an established protocol in order to maintain their not-for-profit status. Hospitals must also demonstrate involvement in community health assessment as part of the accreditation process conducted by the Joint Commission on Accreditation of Healthcare Organizations.

The IOM Model

The proliferation of community health assessment and improvement efforts in the public and private sectors led the Institute of Medicine (IOM) to convene an expert panel to review the many existing processes and recommend a consensus approach for undertaking these efforts. The IOM's work identified several essential characteristics of an effective community health assessment and improvement effort. These characteristics include:

- use of an iterative process that cycles continuously through the tasks of assessment, action, and evaluation
- use of a team approach, through which decisions are made largely by consensus among community representatives
- use of an incremental strategy for improvement, whereby progress is accomplished through a series of small steps rather than through major breakthroughs

The IOM proposed a model for community health improvement processes consisting of two related cycles of implementation (Figure 15–1)

Cycle 1: Problem Identification and Prioritization

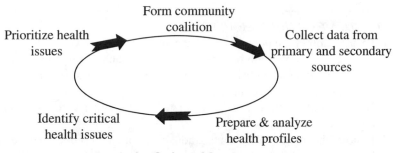

Cycle 2: Analysis and Implementation

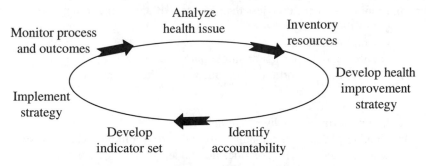

Figure 15–1 The Community Health Improvement Process

(Institute of Medicine 1997). The first cycle consists of three main activities: forming a community health coalition; collecting and analyzing data for a community health profile; and identifying high-priority health issues. Community efforts can begin with any phase of this cycle. As part of activities in this first cycle, the IOM proposed a set of 25 indicators for use in assessing community health status, as shown in Exhibit 15–2 (Perrin and Koshel 1997). These indicators are an expanded version of a consensus set of 18 indicators that the CDC recommended in 1991 to track progress towards achieving *Healthy People 2000* objectives (National Center for Health Statistics 1991). Of course, for any specific community, these general indicators may need to be supplemented with additional measures corresponding to the specific problems and needs of that community. Community improvement strategies may be broad-based—simultaneously exploring a number of health issues, as in the APEX-PH model. Alternatively, strategies may focus on a small number of specific issues, as in the PATCH model.

Exhibit 15–2 Community Health Indicators Proposed by the Institute of Medicine

---

SOCIODEMOGRAPHIC CHARACTERISTICS
1. Distribution of the population by age and race/ethnicity
2. Number and proportion of persons in groups such as migrants, home-less, and the non-English speaking, for whom access to community services and resources may be of concern
3. Number and proportion of persons aged 25 and older with less than a high school education
4. Ratio of the number of students graduating from high school to the total number of students who entered 9th grade three years previously
5. Median household income
6. Proportion of children less than 15 years of age living in families at or below the poverty level
7. Unemployment rate
8. Number and proportion of single-parent families
9. Number and proportion of persons without health insurance

HEALTH STATUS
10. Infant mortality rate by race/ethnicity
11. Number of deaths or age-adjusted death rates for motor vehicle crashes, work-related injuries, suicide, homicide, lung cancer, breast cancer, cardiovascular diseases, and all causes, by age, race, and gender
12. Reported incidence of AIDS, measles, tuberculosis, and primary and secondary syphilis, by age, race, and gender as appropriate
13. Births to adolescents (ages 10-17) as a proportion of total live births
14. Number and rate of confirmed abuse and neglect cases among children

HEALTH RISK FACTORS
15. Proportion of 2-year-old children who have received all age-appropriate vaccines, as recommended by the Advisory Committee on Immuniza-tion Practices
16. Proportion of adults aged 65 and older who have ever been immunized for pneumococcal pneumonia, and the proportion who have been im-munized in the past 12 months for influenza
17. Proportion of the population who smoke, by age, race, and gender
18. Proportion of the population age 18 and older who are obese
19. Number and type of U.S. Environmental Protection Agency air quality standards not met

---

continues

Exhibit 15–2 continued

> 20. Proportion of assessed rivers, lakes, and estuaries that support beneficial uses (e.g. fishing and swimming approved)
>
> *HEALTH CARE RESOURCE CONSUMPTION*
> 21. Per capita health care spending for Medicare beneficiaries
>
> *FUNCTIONAL STATUS*
> 22. Proportion of adults reporting that their general health is good to excellent
> 23. During the past 30 days, average number of days for which adults report that their physical or mental health was not good
>
> *QUALITY OF LIFE*
> 24. Proportion of adults satisfied with the health care system in the community
> 25. Proportion of persons satisfied with the quality of life in the community

Once a specific health issue has been targeted by a community, the health improvement process moves on to the analysis and implementation cycle (Figure 15–1). The steps in this second cycle include analysis of the health issue, an inventory of health resources, development of a health improvement strategy, discussion and negotiation to establish where accountability lies, development of a set of performance indicators for accountable entities, implementation of the health improvement strategy, and measurement to monitor the outcome of efforts by community organizations.

To identify risk factors for problematic health outcomes, organizations can use the APEX-PH model and its process for cause-and-effect analysis (National Association of County and City Health Officials 1991). The State of Florida Department of Public Health and Rehabilitative Services has successfully used this type of analysis, in combination with on-site reviews and team meetings, to help communities identify public health interventions (Speake et al. 1995, 1448–1449).

A critical step in the community health improvement process is to formulate appropriate action based on the results of a community health assessment. The IOM uses the term *accountable entities* to refer to stakeholders expected to achieve specific results as part of the community's strategy for addressing a health issue. Traditionally, communities have viewed the local public health agency as the primary accountable entity. As described earlier, solutions to public health problems require action by many groups within a community, and accountability should be recognized as an issue of shared responsibility. An important part of the community health improvement process is to designate accountable entities, and to establish agreements among entities that specify areas of responsibility, measures of performance, and rewards for successful performance. Performance gaps should trigger problem analysis and a reformulation of each stakeholder's approach to the health issue (Halverson and Mays 1998).

Public Health Practice Guidelines

Practice guidelines are another quality improvement tool that public health organizations are beginning to use. Like their counterparts in medical care, public health practice guidelines provide scientifically based, tailored information regarding optimal methods for implementing public health interventions for specific population groups. Guidelines can be used to reduce unnecessary variation in the implementation of public health interventions, and thereby enhance the effectiveness and efficiency of these interventions. The development of practice guidelines has occurred slowly in the field of public health, principally because of the limited availability of scientifically valid information regarding the outcomes and costs of public health interventions. For many of these interventions, the outcomes accrue over long periods of time, making scientific evaluation methodologically difficult and financially costly. Nonetheless, several important sources of public health guidelines exist for assisting organizations in implementing public health quality improvement initiatives. First, organizations may use externally developed guidelines such as those issued by the U.S. Preventive Services Task Force and the CDC. Additionally, a growing number of organizations implement internally developed guidelines based on evidence collected and analyzed within the organization.

Externally Developed Guidelines

One of the most widely recognized external sources for public health practice guidelines is the *Guide to Clinical Preventive Services*, issued by the U.S. Preventive Services Task Force (U.S. Preventive Services Task Force 1989). Based on an extensive review of scientific evidence, the Task

Force constructed guidelines for the provision of more than 100 primary and secondary prevention services designed to address more than 70 illnesses and health conditions. The evidence used to develop these guidelines included randomized controlled trials, controlled trials, cohort and case-control studies, multiple time series studies, uncontrolled experiments, and expert opinion. For each intervention, guidelines specify the sociodemographic characteristics of the target population, the timing and sequence of component processes, the contraindications associated with each intervention, and the health risks and benefits of each intervention. Originally produced in 1989, the *Guide* was updated in 1996 to reflect new scientific evidence and newly developed interventions (U.S. Preventive Services Task Force 1996). Evidence from randomized controlled trials serves as the gold standard for guideline development, but the *Guide* continues to be heavily dependent on expert opinion and nonrandomized studies due to the limited clinical research in many areas of prevention practice.

Expanding on the process for clinical preventive services, the CDC appointed a U.S. Task Force on Community Preventive Services to develop similar guidelines for population-based public health interventions that target communities, schools, and work sites rather than individual patients. Although still under development, the *Guide to Community Preventive Services* is expected to offer practice guidelines in the following areas:

- changing risk behaviors
- reducing specific diseases, injuries, and impairments
- changing ecosystems, including environmental concerns
- cross-cutting public health activities (Pappaioanou and Evans 1998).

Rigorous outcomes studies are also limited for these types of interventions; therefore, the guidelines for community preventive services rely heavily on expert opinion and nonexperimental studies.

Numerous additional sources for externally developed public health practice guidelines exist. These include specialized task forces and advisory panels convened by the National Institutes of Health and the CDC, such as the Advisory Council for the Elimination of Tuberculosis, which developed guidelines for the implementation of tuberculosis prevention and control programs (Simone 1995). Professional associations such as the American College of Preventive Medicine are also active in developing and disseminating prevention practice guidelines (Patel and Kinsinger 1997; Ferrini 1997).

Internally Developed Guidelines

Increasingly, public health organizations are engaging in efforts to develop their own practice guidelines—either alone or in combination with other health organizations. These tools are based on evidence and experience that individual organizations have amassed in serving specific population groups rather than on the collective knowledge, research, and expertise of national scientific and professional groups. One approach is to begin with a nationally developed guideline and tailor its specifications to the individual needs and capacities of the organization and the community it serves. This strategy blends the concepts of *mass customization* with the more general framework of evidence-based process improvement. The Texas Department of Health used this approach in developing its performance measurement process for district health departments (Griffin and Welch 1995), which drew heavily on guidelines established in the American Public Health Association's *Healthy Communities: Model Standards* and in the National Association of County and City Health Officials' *Assessment Protocol for Excellence in Public Health*. Texas went beyond the generic practices described in these resources by developing specific process objectives tailored to the capacities and policy priorities of its local health agencies.

Similarly, the Denver Health Authority in Colorado developed an internal quality assessment process based on guidelines established in the National Committee on Quality Assurance's (NCQA) *Health Plan Employer Data and Information Set* (HEDIS). Denver added performance elements that were not included in HEDIS but that its key stakeholders, including staff, local and state policy officials, and consumers perceived as important (Halverson et al. 1998). The agency also eliminated HEDIS elements that were not relevant to the organization or that proved to be too difficult to measure accurately. Denver uses the resulting process shown in Table 15–1 to demonstrate accountability for contract funds received from the City and County of Denver, and for Medicaid funds received from the Colorado Division of Medical Assistance.

Some public health agencies adopt practice guidelines developed by other organizations with which they interact. Managed care plans are key

Table 15–1 Quality Assessment Indicators for Denver Health Authority

INDICATOR	*REPORT FREQUENCY*
I. Primary Prevention	
Pediatric immunizations	Monthly
Adult immunizations	Monthly
Family Planning	
Sterilizations	Quarterly
Family planning visits	Quarterly
Teenage births	Quarterly
II. Secondary Prevention	
Infant screening (EPSDT)	Quarterly
Lead screening	Quarterly
Mammography	Quarterly
Cervical Pap smears	Quarterly
Violence intervention/prevention	Quarterly
Cholesterol screening	Quarterly
III. Tertiary Prevention	
Diabetic ophthalmology	Quarterly
Asthma management/admissions	Quarterly
Care of chronic mental illness	Quarterly
Frail elderly	Annually
IV. Perinatal Care	
Early prenatal care utilization	Quarterly
Teenage births	Quarterly
Vaginal births after Caesarean Sections	Quarterly
C-section rates	Quarterly
Low-birth-weight infants	Quarterly
Neonatal ICU admissions	Quarterly
V. Member Satisfaction	
Member satisfaction survey results	Annually
Member grievances: quality of care	Monthly
Disenrollments	Monthly
VI. Access to Health Care Services	
Appointment availability	Monthly
Appointment waiting time	Monthly
Utilization of emergency services	Quarterly
In network/out of network	Quarterly
VII. Appropriateness of Care	
Hysterectomies	Quarterly
Abortions	Quarterly
Patient Transfers	Quarterly

among the organizations helping to disseminate practice guidelines among public health agencies. Public health agencies that contract with plans for the delivery of personal health services adopt many of the same health plan guidelines that medical care providers use. These may include practices for assessing patient health status, delivering clinical preventive services, and making referrals to other health care providers. Agencies participating in health plan provider networks often benefit from the quality improvement processes that these plans maintain, which allows agencies to compare their own performance in a guideline area with that of other providers. The Memphis and Shelby County Health Department in Tennessee, for example, uses the information it receives from health plans to compare its performance with private providers in areas such as childhood and adult immunization, cervical and breast cancer screening, and asthma and diabetes management. The agency uses documentation of its performance to negotiate favorable contracts with health plans and to demonstrate accountability to local government officials and the public (Mays 1998b).

At the same time, public health agencies play important roles in disseminating public health practice guidelines to managed care plans and other health care organizations. For example, following a large measles outbreak, the City of Milwaukee Health Department conducted on-site provider education seminars with community physicians—including those in managed care plans—regarding optimal strategies for childhood immunization delivery. More recently, the health department has sponsored workshops on tuberculosis diagnosis and treatment strategies for physicians practicing in managed care plans (Halverson et al. 1997b). Health plan executives in Milwaukee identify the local health department as an important source of information concerning effective prevention practices. In Vancouver, Washington, the Southwest Washington Health District conducts periodic on-site workshops with community physicians concerning optimal ways for storing vaccines—an effort motivated by an earlier health department study that showed widespread use of inappropriate storage techniques.

In some communities, public health agencies have begun to work jointly with other health care organizations in developing community-wide practice guidelines (Mays et al. 1998b). These efforts represent potentially powerful strategies for improving community health through the coordinated actions of multiple stakeholders, including health care providers, purchasers, insurers, and consumers. In one such initiative in Genesee County, Michigan, a local public health agency is working in partnership with a group of hospitals, health plans, employers, community-based organizations, unions, and the local medical society (Mays et al. 1999b). This coalition has formed working groups to develop a broad range of community practice guidelines in areas such as primary care, clinical preventive services, chronic disease treatment and control, and violence prevention. Once guidelines are developed, each participant encourages adoption and implementation within his or her organization as well as among peer organizations.

Community Health Report Cards

Among the range of performance assessment and evaluation tools, report card systems are emerging as promising strategies for monitoring and improving performance in many areas of health care. Although they vary widely in their structure and content, report card systems typically consist of a set of standardized performance measures that are collected consistently across a group of organizations, individuals, or other entities under study. Using these measures, report card systems employ a metric for comparing and profiling the performance of each entity against its peers on a periodic basis. These systems are distinct from other types of assessment approaches that rely primarily on trend analysis or on comparisons against *a priori* performance standards and goals.

Report cards are being used successfully in other sectors of the health care field to monitor performance and encourage improvement through comparison (Auerbach 1998; Longo et al. 1997; Chassin et al. 1996; Health care report cards 1995; National Committee on Quality Assurance 1995; U.S. General Accounting Office 1994; Pennsylvania Health Care Cost Containment Council 1991). Recent evidence suggests that report card methodologies are also being used to assess community-level health issues in some localities (Fielding and Halfon 1997). These existing approaches appear to vary widely in their purpose, scope, and methodology.

Report cards offer several distinct advantages over these other assessment approaches, including: (1) encouraging continuous improvement in performance rather than establishing specific floors or ceilings for performance; (2) motivating performance improvement through benchmarking and comparisons with peers; (3) enabling aggregate measures of performance across a group of organizations, individuals, or communities using standardized, consistently applied measures; and (4) creating a framework for identifying best practices among the entities under study. In the health field, report card systems are thought to be particularly effective in improving performance among organizations that compete for patients, revenue, or other resources, such as hospitals, physician practices, and managed care plans (Health care report cards 1995). These organizations can use report cards as tools for marketing their services to patients, payers, and purchasers. There exists evidence suggesting that some of these systems have encouraged substantial improvements in health care quality (Auerbach 1998; Longo et al. 1997; U.S. General Accounting Office 1994).

The rationale for using report card systems at the community level relies more on coordination and cooperation than competition. By facilitating comparisons of community-level health measures across local areas, report card systems may serve as tools for mobilizing collaborative, interorganizational efforts in community health improvement. Report card systems can be used to profile the aggregate effects of multiple health organizations and interventions within a community, thereby exposing gaps in performance needing of remedy. To be sure, local public health agencies and other community health organizations already have an extensive battery of tools, protocols, and planning guides for conducting community health assessment (National Association of County and City Health Officials 1991; Greene 1992; U.S. Agency for Toxic Substances and Disease Registry 1992; American Public Health Association 1993). By enabling comparisons among peer groups of local communities, however, report card systems may offer local public health agencies more meaningful and relevant measures of community health performance than other assessment approaches (Gerzoff 1997).

Community health report card systems are attractive tools for organizations other than the local health department (Mays et al. 1998c). If broadly implemented, these systems may assist state and federal health agencies in targeting health resources and services to areas of greatest need, and in evaluating the community-level effects of health-related interventions. These systems may be able to integrate the reporting requirements and accountability systems of multiple federal and state health programs, thereby reducing reporting duplication and respondent burden while enhancing their utility in program evaluation. Similarly, report card systems may help to inform the progress toward performance-based contracting initiatives in public health, which are currently taking shape at both federal and state levels (U.S. General Accounting Office 1997; Nelson et al. 1995; Griffin and Welch 1995; Washington State Department of Health 1996). Under these initiatives, state and local governments may use report card systems to obtain enhanced measures of public health performance at the community level and thereby demonstrate accountability for funds which are appropriated to support public health activities. Finally, report card systems may prove to be valuable tools in the movement toward national performance standards and accreditation programs for local public health agencies (Turnock and Handler 1996). An appropriately structured report card system may provide an ideal framework for establishing performance standards and measuring performance levels among participating agencies.

A frequent criticism of standardized assessment tools and reporting systems in public health is that they fail to account for the unique ways in which public health is organized and administered at local levels. Local public health officials have raised this issue in relation to community health report cards, questioning the local relevance and utility of a standardized system designed for broad implementation. In response to this issue, a research effort has recently been undertaken to explore the extent to which there exists a degree of commonality in the assessment needs and capacities of local public health agencies that might support a standardized report card system (Mays et al. 1998c). The motivating hypothesis for this research is that a core set of community health indicators can be identified. These indicators are scientifically sound, locally available, and widely regarded as relevant and useful for measuring community health status. Early results from this effort suggest that this hypothesis is supported. A representative survey of the nation's local health agencies during 1997 revealed that a strong majority of agencies reports interest in a national report card initiative, and that a core set of community health indicators is available at the local level to form the basis of such an initiative.

Additional research and development efforts are needed to identify relevant, reliable, and feasible indicators of community health that can be used to monitor outcomes and practices at the community level (Halverson and Mays 1998). The set of 25 indicators proposed by the Institute of Medicine (1997) provides an appropriate starting point for this work (Exhibit 15–2). Ultimately, national consensus is needed on a minimum data set that will permit valid comparison of peer groups of local and state jurisdictions, and that will facilitate progress toward achieving state and national health objectives. What is needed is a small number of measures that are vitally important to customers for community health improvement reports. These measures must be readily and uniformly acceptable and understandable; be measurable using easily available data; and indicate specific interventions for public health action as well as broad general measures of community health and program effectiveness. Additionally, strategies are needed for measuring outcomes and practices in small geographic areas, where statistics may not be stable because of small denominators. Valid methods are needed for adjusting community outcomes for the severity of health problems being addressed and the underlying risks that are present in individual communities. Finally, methods must be developed for identifying peer groups of communities for comparison and benchmarking purposes, such as groups based on population size, sociodemographic composition, and/or health resources availability.

Public Health Information Networks

Community health improvement strategies often face the challenge of acquiring and integrating information from multiple sources in order to adequately monitor practices and outcomes at the community level. Several computerized information management systems have been developed to assist community efforts to collect and display data from multiple sources. Two examples are the Michigan and CDC APEX-PH Information Manager, and the Seattle-King County Department of Public Health VISTA PH computer software (Vaughn et al. 1994; Epidemiology, Planning, and Evaluation Unit, Seattle-King County Department of Public Health 1995). These computer programs facilitate display of data, such as demographics, adult death rates, infant death rates, hospitalization rates, and infectious disease rates.

A broad range of other public health information systems are being developed at state and local levels to facilitate public health management and decision making. The CDC's *Information Network for Public Health Officials* (INPHO) program has supported a number of these efforts, which involve the establishment of integrated information networks that can support information sharing and communication across public health agencies within the states. State health data organizations, hospital associations, managed care plans, and health care purchasing coalitions are carrying out other efforts (Mendelson and Salinsky 1997). These state and local resources complement the information systems available at the national level through such resources as the *CDC Wonder* online warehouse of public health data and information, and the National Library of Medicine's online databases of health sciences literature (National Library of Medicine 1999). Public health managers at state and local levels need to identify the information needs of their programs and services, and to understand the array of information resources and systems that may be tapped in addressing these needs.

Performance-Based Contracting Systems

Another strategy for achieving continuous improvement in public health practice is through the use of performance-based contracting mechanisms. By making contract awards and financial payments contingent on measurable attributes of performance, these mechanisms potentially create powerful incentives for improvement both in the processes and in the outcomes of public health practice. In the domain of medical care, managed care plans have pioneered numerous strategies for performance-based contracting, including risk-adjusted capitation payment rates, payment withholds and bonuses based on provider performance, and payment formulae based on performance in specific clinical areas (such as immunization rates). In the field of public health, performance-based contracts are currently being applied on at least two levels. First, federal grant-making agencies are using performance-based contracting principles as part of the grants they issue to state and local public health agencies. Much of this activity is occurring in response to the *Government Performance and Results Act of 1993*, which requires federal agencies to be more accountable for the public funds they administer. The U.S. Department of Health and Human Services (HHS) is rapidly moving toward implementation of "performance partnerships" grants with state health agencies, which would require these agencies to establish action plans and measurable performance objectives as part of their contracts with HHS for federal public health funding (U.S. General Accounting Office 1997).

Second, many state and local health agencies have begun to integrate aspects of performance-based contracting in their relationships with other health organizations. Many of these efforts are being adopted as part of public health privatization efforts that transfer responsibility for certain public health functions from public agencies to private (or quasi-private) contractors (Halverson et al. 1997). For example, the local health department in Milwaukee, Wisconsin, contracts with a network of community health centers to provide specified clinical services to health department clients. Similarly, in Mecklenburg County, North Carolina, the county health department contracts with a hospital-based integrated delivery system for the provision of most personal health services traditionally provided by the health department (Keener et al. 1997). Performance-based contracting mechanisms offer public health agencies promising strategies for ensuring the quality of services and activities that are purchased from private providers.

Several implementation characteristics of performance-based contracting efforts warrant attention. First, these efforts require a clear definition of the public health functions and activities to be carried out under the contract, and a clear delineation of responsibilities to be assumed by each party. Without these elements, contract provisions can be difficult if not impossible to enforce. Second, these efforts require accurate, reliable systems for measuring public health performance. Initiatives based on measures that are self-reported by the contractor introduce a clear moral hazard for "up-coding" these measures in order to receive higher payments. Effective performance-based contracting strategies therefore require substantial investments in measurement systems that are resistant to these types of gaming. Third, performance-based contracting initiatives must be supported by effective plans for enforcing contract provisions and payment rates. Barriers to effective contract enforcement include a lack of alternative contractors, the risk of reducing the financial viability of contractors, and the political influence maintained by contractors. Public health agencies must anticipate these barriers and incorporate contract mechanisms that offer alternative methods of enforcement.

Several state health agencies have initiated performance-based contracting efforts as part of their public health quality improvement efforts. Rhode Island's Department of Health delivers personal health services and community health services exclusively through contracts with private providers, such as community health centers and voluntary health associations, since the state is not served by a system of local health departments. Currently, the state relies primarily on process-based measures of performance in developing and enforcing contracts with private providers. These measures include elements such as waiting times, appointment availability, service volume, and consumer-initiated complaints. The state is in the process of developing strategies to link contracts with measurable public health outcomes—particularly those that are emphasized in the *Healthy*

People 2000 national health objectives (Mays et al. 1998a, 63–78). Similarly, Washington State's Department of Health is exploring the feasibility of developing performance-based contracting mechanisms linked to an 84-indicator performance measurement system for local health departments, based on the Institute of Medicine's (1988) framework. The Utah Department of Health is phasing in performance-based contracting mechanisms in four core areas: services provided under the federal *Preventive Health Services Block Grant*; services provided through the federally supported *Children with Special Health Care Needs* program; services provided through the federal *Special Supplemental Food Program for Women, Infants, and Children* (WIC) program; and services provided through state HIV and tuberculosis prevention and control programs. Utah develops individually tailored action plans with each contractor, which specify both short-term process objectives and long-term outcome objectives. Objectives are developed through a process that includes input from contractors as well as consumers, and that links with the national *Healthy People 2000* objectives.

Public Health Performance Measurement Systems

Proposals for measuring the adequacy of public health performance have been offered repeatedly in the U.S. for the past 70 years, since shortly after the establishment of local health departments became widespread. The conceptual bases for many of these proposals are reviewed elsewhere (Turnock 1997). Even as the need for evaluating the adequacy of public health practice became well established, no consistent plan of evaluation was put into practice. Licensure of public health agencies and workers, based on some presumed national standard of performance, was often discussed but never implemented. Public health agencies justified their efforts largely through reports on encounter tallies such as the number of immunizations rendered, prenatal visitations, and septic tanks inspected. These reports seldom included population-based denominators, or data on unmet need. The presumption was strong that if public health agencies increased their encounters each year, the population's health was well served and further support for the agency was justified.

Efforts to measure the performance of public health organizations have grown substantially over the past decade. These efforts have emerged as public health practitioners face growing pressures to improve their systems for ensuring community health and to demonstrate the value of these systems to policymakers, payers, providers, and the public at large. The Institute of Medicine's 1988 report on public health, which delineated three core functions for public health organizations, provided a rationale and a framework for many of these efforts (Institute of Medicine, Committee for the Study of Future Public Health 1988). In 1990, HHS formalized the need for public health evaluative efforts in its *Healthy People 2000* objectives for the nation, challenging agencies to "increase to at least 90 percent the proportion of people who are served by a local health department that is effectively carrying out the core functions of public health." (American Public Health Association 1992).

To monitor progress toward this objective, public health researchers, practitioners, and policymakers have begun to implement approaches for measuring local public health performance. Performance assessment survey instruments include those developed by researchers at the University of North Carolina at Chapel Hill (Miller et al. 1994a) and by researchers at the University of Illinois (Turnock et al. 1994, 653–658). Both of these are based upon the Institute of Medicine's three core public health functions and upon an associated list of 10 public health practices identified by a work group convened by the CDC (Dyall 1995). Other performance assessment approaches have developed around a set of 10 essential public health services identified by the HHS and the Essential Public Health Services Work Group (Baker et al. 1994; Eilbert et al. 1996; Eilbert et al. 1997; Grason and Guyer 1995). Additionally, many public health organizations have developed their own approaches for monitoring performance.

Performance Measurement Surveillance Efforts

The performance measurement approach developed by Miller and colleagues has received considerable attention because it focuses on the contribution to public health practice by all providers in a jurisdiction—both public and private—rather than limiting performance measure to the role of the local health department. The organizing framework for this surveillance system consists of the three core functions formulated by the IOM and linked to the 10 practices previously described. A group of indicators was developed for each practice drawing on materials from many sources, including *Healthy People 2000* and the *APEX-PH* process. Eight to ten indicators were selected for each practice, yielding a total of 84 indicators. Local health department directors responded to the survey.

Results yielded scores for the surveyed jurisdiction with regard to adequacy of performance for each practice, the proportional contribution to performance by the local health department, and the identification of other providers contributing to the coverage of each practice within the jurisdiction. Schematic representation of the results is illustrated in Figure 15–2. Note that the top graph line for each public health jurisdiction illustrates the extent that it is served by all providers according to each of the 10 practices. The bottom graph line illustrates the contribution to each of the practices by the local health department. The decimal notations in the line immediately under the graphs show scores representing performance within the jurisdiction for each of the three core functions, and the proportion of each function performed by the local health department. The alphabetical key at the bottom of the graphs identifies providers other than the local health department that contributed to each of the 10 practices. The

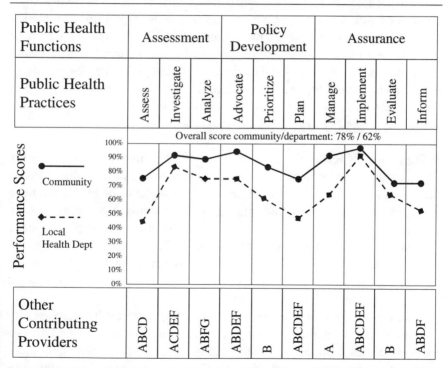

Other provider codes: A = state agencies; B = local agencies; C = nonprofit agencies; D = hospitals; E = community health centers; F = universities; G = other.

Figure 15–2 Public Health Performance Profile for a Sample Community and Local Health Department survey protocol and scoring methods that yield these data are available in the source document for this method (Mays et al. 1999b). A shortened version of the protocol (26 indicators) was tested in all local jurisdictions in six states. It correlated reliably with scores obtained from the longer protocol for overall public health performance, as well as for performance of each of the three core functions and for some of the 10 practices (Griffin and Welch 1995). A subset of four indicators reliably predicted the overall score (Bartlett et al. 1997).

Most recently, the Miller and Turnock measurement protocols were combined into a set of 20 public health performance indicators, again linked to the three core public health functions that the Institute of Medicine identified in 1988. During 1998, these 20 indicators, shown in Exhibit 15–3 (Turnock et al. 1998) were used in a national survey of all local health departments serving jurisdictions of at least 100,000 residents (N=496) (Table 15–2). Results confirm that wide variation in performance persists despite many public health improvement efforts implemented at national, state, and local levels during the 1990s. On average, 64 percent of the 20 public health indicators were performed in local public health jurisdictions. The average local health department performed 24 percent of these services directly, or 38 percent of the total community effort.

Other Performance Measurement Systems

Public health agencies use a variety of other approaches for measuring organizational performance. A survey of the nation's state health agencies during 1997 revealed that 88 percent had some level of involvement in local public health performance measurement systems (Mays et al. 1998a). Of these departments, 50 percent maintained an ongoing performance assessment process that was currently active, 30 percent were engaged in developing a new or revised performance assessment process that was not yet active, and 20 percent reported past involvement in a performance assessment process that was no longer active.

When queried about how performance assessment results were used by state agencies, 39 percent of the agencies having involvement in assessment processes reported that their results were used for state-level planning and policy development activities. These activities included developing new training and technical assistance projects for local health departments; modifying state contract requirements and programmatic objectives to

Exhibit 15–3 Twenty Indicators of Local Public Health Performance

1. In your jurisdiction, is there a community needs assessment process that systematically describes the prevailing health status in the community?
2. In the past three years in your jurisdiction, has the local public health agency surveyed the population for behavioral risk factors?
3. In your jurisdiction, are timely investigations of adverse health events conducted on an ongoing basis—including communicable disease outbreaks and environmental health hazards?
4. Are the necessary laboratory services available to the local public health agency to support investigations of adverse health events and meet routine diagnostic and surveillance needs?
5. In your jurisdiction, has an analysis been completed of the determinants of and contributing factors to priority health needs, the adequacy of existing health resources, and the population groups most affected?
6. In the past three years in your jurisdiction, has the local public health agency conducted an analysis of age-specific participation in preventive and screening services?
7. In your jurisdiction, is there a network of support and communication relationships that includes health-related organizations, the media, and the general public?
8. In the past year in your jurisdiction, has there been a formal attempt by the local public health agency to inform officials about the potential public health impact of decisions under their consideration?
9. In your local public health agency, has there been a prioritization of the community health needs that have been identified from a community needs assessment?
10. In the past three years in your jurisdiction, has the local public health agency implemented community health initiatives consistent with established priorities?
11. In your jurisdiction, has a community health action plan been developed with community participation to address priority community health needs?
12. In the past three years in your jurisdiction, has the local public health agency developed plans to allocate resources in a manner consistent with community health action plans?
13. In your jurisdiction, have resources been deployed as necessary to address priority health needs identified in a community health needs assessment?

continues

Exhibit 15–3 continued

14. In the past three years in your jurisdiction, has the local public health agency conducted an organizational self-assessment?
15. In your jurisdiction, are age-specific priority health needs effectively addressed through the provision of or linkage to appropriate services?
16. In your jurisdiction, have there been regular evaluations of the effects of public health services on community health status?
17. In the past three years in your jurisdiction, has the local public health agency used professionally recognized process and outcome measures to monitor programs and to redirect resources as appropriate?
18. In your jurisdiction, is the public regularly provided with information about current health status, health care needs, positive health behaviors, and health care policy issues?
19. In the past year in your jurisdiction, has the local public health agency provided reports to the media on a regular basis?
20. In the past three years in your jurisdiction, has there been an instance in which the local public health agency has failed to implement a mandated program or service?

respond to areas of low performance; and developing new state-sponsored public health programs and policies in areas of low performance. Agencies that maintained centralized and shared administrative relationships with local health departments appeared more likely to use assessment results for these purposes. Twenty percent of agencies with performance assessment processes reported that results were fed back to the local public health agencies to assist them with local planning and policy development activities. Agencies with decentralized administrative structures appeared somewhat more likely than other types of agencies to use results for this purpose. Agencies in seven states, or 16 percent of the states with performance assessment processes, indicated that results were used to allocate state agency funds among programmatic areas and among local public health jurisdictions. Three other state agencies (seven percent) reported that performance results are used to inform the budgetary decisions made by their state legislatures. Finally, two agencies (five percent) indicated that performance results were used to evaluate the effects of public health programs, policies, and services on community health.

State health departments cited financial, staffing, and methodological issues as the greatest challenges for state health departments in conducting local public health performance assessment activities. More than two-

Table 15–2 Average Public Health Performance Scores for Local Public Health Jurisdictions Serving Populations of at Least 100,000 Residents—United States, 1998

Indicator	N	Community Performance	Performance Scores			
			Adequacy of Community Performance [a]	Health Dept. Contribution [a,b]	Health Dept. Contribution as % of Community Performance [a,b]	
1 Needs assessment	335	73%	36%	21%	58%
2 Behavioral risk factor survey	331	47%	22%	11%	52%
3 Adverse health events investigatio	336	99%	75%	57%	76%
4 Laboratory services	336	96%	73%	37%	50%
5 Analysis of health determinants	333	63%	30%	16%	54%
6 Participation in preventive service	333	29%	13%	8%	61%
7 Support and communication	333	79%	43%	21%	48%
8 Inform elected officials	335	82%	38%	29%	77%
9 Prioritization of health needs	335	67%	35%	21%	61%
10 Implementation of initiatives	333	83%	35%	21%	61%
11 Community action plan	333	42%	16%	9%	54%
12 Plans to allocate resources	335	27%	11%	7%	63%
13 Resources for priority needs	333	50%	19%	10%	54%
14 Self-assessment	333	57%	32%	29%	89%
15 Provision/linkage of services	332	76%	36%	19%	51%
16 Evaluation of services	333	35%	16%	12%	71%
17 Process/outcome measures	331	47%	22%	16%	75%
18 Public information	334	76%	33%	20%	61%
19 Media information	335	76%	40%	31%	78%
20 Mandated programs/services	323	92%	92%	92%	100%
Assessment (#1–#6)	336	67%	41%	25%	60%
Policy Development (#7–#12)	336	63%	29%	18%	61%
Assurance (#13–#20)	336	63%	36%	28%	78%
Total Score	335	64%	35%	24%	67%

Note: Performance scores represent the proportion of communities/departments that perform the selected public health activity.

[a] Scores adjusted for perceived adequacy of performance (five-point scale)

[b] Scores adjusted for proportion of effort contributed by the local health department (five-point scale)

thirds of respondents agreed that the cost of conducting performance assessment activities is a major challenge for their organization. By comparison, approximately 60 percent of respondents agreed that securing qualified staff to conduct performance assessment activities is a major challenge for their organization. Fifty-eight percent of respondents reported the lack of appropriate methods for assessing the performance of local public health systems as a major challenge. Somewhat surprisingly, only a minority of respondents (27 percent) indicated that securing the participation of local health agencies was a major challenge to their department's performance assessment activities. Agencies with decentralized administrative structures appeared no more likely to report this barrier than other types of agencies.

A review of written protocols from 18 (51 percent) of the agencies reporting existing or planned performance assessment systems reveals several important design characteristics that may warrant further attention as these systems are refined and expanded over time (Mays et al. 1998a). First, relatively few of the systems reviewed here include measures of health outcomes, especially those that are sensitive to local public health interventions. Most of these activities are constructed around indicators of public health structure and process, such as measures of service availability, capacity, and accessibility. For example, a structural measure that one agency used indicates whether or not the local health department has a publicly available policy agenda and strategic plan. Several other agencies use a process measure to indicate whether or not the local health department has conducted a community health needs assessment. By contrast, outcome measures indicate the extent to which public health interventions are having a desired impact on health. Only three of the assessment systems reviewed here incorporate these types of measures. All three systems use community-level measures of health status, such as the prevalence of behavioral risk factors or the incidence of vaccine-preventable diseases within the community. One of the assessment systems also uses outcome measures, which are targeted at specific public health services, such as the proportion of family planning clinic clients who become pregnant. Whether community-wide or service-specific, outcome measures enable performance assessment systems to inform resource allocation decisions at both state and local levels, based upon the effectiveness of alternative public health interventions.

Another prevalent design characteristic of state assessment systems is a focus upon local health department activities and performance (Mays et al.

1998a). Recent studies have documented the substantial public health contributions made by organizations other than the local health department (Halverson et al. 1996). Nonetheless, few of the assessment systems examined in this study include public health performance measures for other organizations, such as hospitals, community health centers, private physician practices, and managed care plans. Public health performance assessment systems should strive to measure the contributions made by these other organizations, especially in light of the growing responsibilities being transferred to them through contracts, managed care programs, and other privatization initiatives.

A final and related design characteristic of performance assessment systems involves the ability to evaluate the roles that public health agencies play in monitoring and enforcing public health responsibilities carried out by other organizations in the community (Mays et al. 1998a). In many communities, public health agencies are reducing their involvement in direct service provision, and acquiring expanded responsibilities in monitoring and evaluating the services provided by other organizations. Despite these trends, most of the performance assessment systems examined in this study include only cursory measures of activity in monitoring, evaluation, and oversight. Performance assessment systems need to place added emphasis on these roles, which are becoming critical responsibilities of public health agencies in the current health care environment.

QUALITY IMPROVEMENT AND PUBLIC HEALTH: KEY IMPLEMENTATION ISSUES

A variety of methods, tools, and approaches are now available to assist public health organizations in implementing quality improvement initiatives at local, state, national, and international levels. Nonetheless, public health organizations generally have not been as quick or as successful in adopting CQI methods as have other health care organizations (Scutchfield et al. 1997). Public health organizations face several unique challenges in implementing quality improvement efforts, which must be addressed to ensure success. First, public health organizations frequently confront severe resource constraints that limit their ability to devote human and financial capital to improvement initiatives. Funding streams for public health organizations are often limited and inflexible, consisting mainly of governmental appropriations, categorical grant programs, and charitable contributions. Nonetheless, it is critical that public health organizations secure an initial supply of available human and financial resources that can be devoted to the improvement effort. A large and permanent funding stream is not essential, since successful improvement efforts often become self-sustaining as early successes lead to resource reallocation and an expanding base of support from core organizational resources. Start-up resources, however, are essential, and may be patched together from sources such as demonstration grants from local health care foundations, volunteer labor, and in-kind donations.

Second, governmental public health agencies often function under stringent operational requirements concerning activities such as hiring, salary and benefit determination, purchasing, and contracting. As a result, these organizations seldom have full and immediate control over their own operational processes. Effective quality improvement efforts may require greater administrative flexibility than is typically available within these organizations. Several strategies may be used to address this constraint. Public health agencies may collaborate with private organizations that have fewer administrative constraints, and allow these private partners to assume responsibility for those tasks that are difficult for a public agency to undertake (Mays et al. 1999b). Alternatively, public health agencies may cultivate sufficient political support for their quality improvement efforts in order to secure exemptions from administrative requirements— at least on a temporary demonstration basis. As an extreme example, the public health agency and hospital system in Denver, Colorado, successfully achieved local and state approval to convert from a county agency to an independent health care authority chartered by the state government. This change substantially enhanced the agency's ability to undertake quality improvement efforts (Mays et al. 1999b).

Third, adoption of CQI methods is made difficult by the fact that public health practice is inherently a multiorganizational activity, with no single entity within the community being wholly responsible for population health processes and outcomes. To be optimally effective in improving community health, CQI methods must be implemented across multiple organizations—a daunting task for many public health organizations. Nonetheless, multiorganizational efforts for community health improvement have become increasingly common in recent years, fueled by marketplace and policy developments that have created shared incentives for improving health at the population level (Lasker 1997; Mays et al. 1998b; Institute of Medicine 1999). These developments have also created new opportunities for using CQI methods as part of multiorganizational public health processes. To capitalize on these opportunities, public health agencies must assume a leadership role in identifying shared interests and incentives among community organizations, developing effective mechanisms of communication and information-sharing among organizations, and motivating collective action to address shared interests.

A final reason for the limited uptake of quality improvement processes by public health organizations has been the lack of sufficient external pressure to do so (Scutchfield et al. 1997). Public health organizations historically have not faced the same pressures—from competitors, consumers, purchasers, and regulators—to improve quality, efficiency, and value in service delivery as have medical care providers. Public health organizations are no longer protected from these market and policy forces. Many agencies now must actively compete for patients, negotiate relationships with managed care plans and other private health care organizations, and demonstrate accountability for the public funds they receive from government sources for their activities. In this environment, many public health organizations are turning to quality improvement processes as strategies for surviving and thriving in the evolving health system.

CHAPTER 16

Applying and Supporting CQI in Academic Health Centers

Susan I. DesHarnais and Curtis P. McLaughlin

Academic health centers (AHCs) play a central role in health care delivery. They deliver a significant portion of the nation's direct health care. They educate virtually all of the country's physicians as undergraduates and postgraduates and a significant number of other health professionals. They conduct much of the nation's basic health care research, especially clinical research. Some, such as the University of Utah (James 1989), Henry Ford Health System (Griffith et al. 1995), and the University of Michigan (Gaucher and Coffey 1993) and Case Western Reserve (Headrick et al. 1998) have also taken the lead in implementing, evaluating, and adapting total quality management (TQM) to the health care setting. Furthermore, AHCs can take a much more active role in justifying the use of continuous quality improvement (CQI), in conducting research relevant to the issues uncovered in CQI efforts, and in disseminating the results of clinical quality efforts throughout the health care system. The purpose of this chapter is to review the CQI roles that an AHC could and should play and to recommend ways that the AHC can incorporate CQI into its teaching, its research, its patient care, and its outreach. Outreach in continuing education is especially important to the dissemination of CQI.

TEACHING

The education of health professionals has been slower in taking up CQI as a topic than the practice environment (Baker et al. 1998). A 1993 survey showed that only 17 percent of medical schools included continuous improvement methods and concepts in their curricula (Headrick et al.

1995). A symposium announcement associated with the 13th Annual Conference of the Association of American Medical Colleges (November 12–13, 1991) stated that "the state of development of quality improvement in medical education at the present time can be characterized as embryonic. There is much to be done in the area of theory development and application. In addition, as educational institutions, medical schools have a responsibility to educate future physicians about continuous quality improvement." The proposers of the symposium mention work at Harvard University on continuous improvement applied to curriculum development and at the Cleveland Asthma Project at Case Western Reserve Medical School. Their assessment appears to be correct. Interest in CQI as a model seems to be centered much more in hospital administration than in medical school teaching. This is possibly because hospitals, under diagnosis-related groups (DRGs), have felt the impact of rising costs much more so than faculty practice plans. Also only they are subject to the Joint Commission on Accreditation of Healthcare Organizations' (Joint Commission) requirement of having a CQI process in place by the next accreditation visit. Furthermore, faculties are much more likely to acknowledge excellence in research and excellence in teaching than excellence in clinical care.

In response to this slow educational start, the Institute for Healthcare Improvement (IHI), with assistance from the Bureau of Health Professions and the Pew Health Professions Commission, launched an initiative in 1992 to develop and demonstrate models for education about interdisciplinary continuous improvement in health care. This became known as the Interdisciplinary Professional Education Collaborative with working groups at four university clusters. Their efforts resulted in a series of suggestions about how to overcome the barriers to CQI teaching and learning among health professionals, which is summarized in Chapter 10 (Table 10–1) and is particularly applicable to applying and supporting CQI in academic health centers.

When To Teach CQI in the Medical Curriculum

Managers often ask when and how physicians should be trained in TQM. It seems unlikely that specific TQM training will be effective when added to the undergraduate medical curriculum as a discrete topic. That will just be another session that many students will cut. The place where CQI training is most likely to be effective is in residency programs. There the learners are interacting with the hospital system with great intensity. Some residents and fellows, especially the chief residents, are coming into contact with the governance process, sitting on committees such as pharmacy and therapeutics. Their education should include the results of team studies in their field in order to demonstrate that CQI is legitimate clinical research, participation on teams applicable to their area of specialty, and using the residency program as a CQI project in and of itself. This is the time in their careers that they begin to see the strengths and weaknesses of their departments in systems terms. They are also sensitive to the fact that the system is poorly designed to meet their needs and that their approach as "short-timers" affects their motivation to fight for change in the many "Kafkaesque" situations in which they find themselves. Using their program as an object lesson might do a lot to enhance their interest and to motivate them to devote their scarce time and energy to participating in the CQI process. Weingart (1998) reports that efforts to utilize house officers on CQI team can be successful when supported by the institution's hierarchy and institutional purpose. This active leadership and faculty support is needed to stabilize the residents' roles through rotations and to counterbalance competing demands for effort, sleep and personal time.

An alternative time to train physicians in AHCs is when they first begin teaching. If they have not been a chief resident, the committees and the governance structure of the school, the teaching hospital, and the department are all new to them, and they are again sensitized to the system, or nonsystem as the case may be. This is a critical time to involve young physicians because once they learn how to manipulate the system, many of them detach themselves from it and thus become harder to engage in systems issues.

The University of Michigan and the University of Rochester, for example, are involving faculty in research on clinical pathways and clinical guidelines and are offering financial support for research, including faculty time, to support the development of clinical pathways, recognizing the traditional routes of motivation through professional recognition. Improvements in clinical pathways are likely to be reflected quite rapidly in the clinical behavior of new learners. This approach, however, teaches little about the CQI process and philosophy and may take a long time to have an impact on the experienced physicians working in other settings.

Continuing Education

Those responsible for continuing medical education and Area Health Education Centers (AHECs) can contribute by making sure that the results of CQI efforts, including illustrations of the CQI philosophy and process, are included in a broad spectrum of continuing education courses. There has been some demand for CQI training in AHEC programs, but the likelihood of reaching a wide cross section is greater when CQI outcomes are included in a variety of continuing education offerings. Therefore management must develop CQI champions in continuing education as well as in clinical practice and research.

Practice Management

Faculty practice plans under the resource-based relative value scale must become more involved in issues of cost and quality than in the past if they are going to fulfill their financial commitments to faculties. Initial efforts include improved outpatient care facilities to attract patients, participation in HMOs and preferred provider organizations (PPOs), outreach through satellite centers, and more aggressive marketing of services. With that, however, will have to come concerns about customer-oriented quality of care measures. This is not likely to happen rapidly, given the current emphasis on selecting faculty practice plan executives based on their ability to do accounting, billing, and collections. They will get involved in quality of care issues only when the dean, department chair, or medical director becomes very active in practice management and emphasizes quality improvement.

A likely reason for a teaching group to become involved in practice standards is the utilization of a quality improvement program in a competing HMO. Gottlieb et al. (1990) report the development of a number of algorithms for use by the Harvard Community Health Program (HCHP) staff and their incorporation into continuing medical education programs and into information gathering systems. They suggest that the criteria for developing algorithms should include:

- frequency, involving commonly seen clinical conditions

- unexplained variability in clinical practice, resource utilization, or referral patterns
- conflict with internal resource constraints
- apparent risk management problems
- perceived quality of care issues with patients, clinicians, or managers
- introduction of new technology
- uncertainty about use or about cost implications

These appear to be the criteria that should be of interest to the faculty of a medical school as well. Yet it seems that HMOs are leading the way, presumably because the expectations of autonomy in practice activity are much less strong in a staff-model HMO such as HCHP (Madison and Konrad 1988).

Competitive stimuli, however, can force medical school staff into quality studies. For example, the faculty of an academic family medicine department became truly interested in continuity of care only when the largest employer in the community threatened to cancel its workers' compensation/ industrial medicine contract with the department because of time costs related to lack of physician continuity. There had also been many complaints about continuity of care from individual patients, but the staff became involved only when threatened with the loss of this major account. Most of the time, lost patients disappear one at a time without a ripple.

Because of the insulation of academic departments from such information through the hospital and the practice plan, improvements in care will come about when the faculty decides that the learners in the institution must experience practicing the right way. Quality will result when the faculty, as well as the teaching hospital management, decide that students (undergraduate and residents) must see exemplary practice in action. It will take medical leadership within the faculty to make that an organizational objective. In doing so, the leadership must also deal with the fact that faculty in a teaching setting are significantly less efficient than their competitors who are not teaching. As Garg et al. (1991) point out, this means facing up to some of the true costs of teaching in the clinical setting, especially in the increasingly important outpatient clinic.

Inclusion in Curriculum Development

Headrick et al. (1991) report on the four-year educational project at Case Western Reserve University School of Medicine to introduce CQI into the curriculum. It is part of an eight-week clerkship at one of a number of urban and suburban clinic sites. The application was highly constrained by time, multiple sites, and poor cost and patient information systems. Each student's assignment focused on outcomes of both costs and symptoms and then on process improvement. The strength of the reported barriers to these future physicians' learning about costs at all was amazing. The students did seem to absorb cost gathering and process improvement, but the curriculum still lacked the skills development necessary to work well in or to lead group processes.

The authors reported that:

> While still rudimentary in terms of what physicians need to be leaders in process improvement, the degree to which hospitals, business leaders, and doctors are committed to CQI or TQM sends a signal to medical students about how important such efforts are. If students, residents, and physicians find indifference all around them about costs, outcome, and process of care, they will promptly forget what was taught. . . . The project has made us realize that good care must be provided in partnership between providers, payers, and patients. That parts of the process lie beyond the physician's office or emergency room should have come as no surprise, but we have failed to act on this knowledge. With a close ongoing partnership, perhaps we can do so in the future (Headrick et al. 1991, 260).

We owe a debt of gratitude to the Case Western team for making this start, but it is damning of academic medicine if this remains the current educational state of the art in continuous improvement. As the above quote indicates, the concepts of quality, with or without continuous improvement, will permeate medical practice only when they permeate the medical school and its teaching settings.

Affiliation Agreements

Much that the students, residents, fellows, and faculty learn about CQI takes place in the teaching hospital, which may or may not be under a common management with the medical school. One important step that the medical school can take to enhance the CQI knowledge is to emphasize affiliations with those hospitals that have or are working on a CQI climate and culture. It would be nice if the medical school had that culture too, but it is more important that the training sites do. All hospitals are involved with CQI in one way or another with the impetus from the Joint Commission, but to varying degrees. The criteria that are set up for affiliations and the concerns of those visiting sites and managing the affiliation relationship should reflect a bias for quality and for a CQI climate and culture. If all or most of the training sites are involved with CQI, it is only a matter of time before the medical school is too.

Cost Consciousness

Control of costs can be taught both directly and indirectly. For example, Durand et al. (1991) report that third-year medical students who are best able to organize hypotheses about patients' problems are more likely to order the appropriate diagnostic tests. The ordering of necessary tests is not affected by this factor, but the ordering of inappropriate tests is. There is, however, much more to be studied about the correlates of lower cost behaviors.

For example, Feinglass et al. (1991) report that costs go down significantly in teaching settings as autonomy in medical decision making allowed by attending physicians goes up. These authors suggest that this reflects the busy residents' inherently conservative practice style that favors moving patients out. One might also interpret it as reflecting defensive medicine directed against one's attendings. At least it indicates the large amount of variability introduced into the treatment system by lack of commonly accepted treatment processes (protocols) even within specific teaching institutions.

Multilevel and Multidisciplinary Teams

As the Cleveland Asthma Project indicates, the medical education environment has significant problems in finding ways to give medical students and residents theoretical and experiential tools to work with in the multilevel and multidisciplinary teams. One of the reported findings of that study was the insight that the process of care is much more complex than the medical teachers had assumed and that an effective outcome depends on factors outside the clinic setting as well as inside it (Headrick et al. 1991).

Hellman (1991) notes similar problems within the university in terms of bringing to bear the many relevant disciplines of the university on modern health care problems. He argues: "Despite this impressive panoply of opportunities for better health care, the system has disturbing maldistribution with little organized preventive medicine. All these changes have vexing ethical and social policy considerations. At such times there are unique opportunities for scholarly thought and discussion involving much of the university, with the possibility that changes may be directed by such considerations" (248).

Residency and fellowship program directors should be encouraged by AHC leadership to motivate participation of their charges in CQI team efforts. They will learn a lot. It is often easy for them to opt out of CQI efforts because of existing heavy workloads and the short-term nature of their commitments. They will require the encouragement of their mentors to put in the added effort and learn the ropes of this new approach to health care quality improvement.

Practice Model Assumptions

Perhaps the most important impact of service delivery in AHCs is the model of practice that it develops in the minds of its learners. Many physicians tend to stay with what they learned during that period of their lives, and many values are internalized there. What are the implications of the emphasis on income generation in many teaching clinics? What is the impact of that experience on future attitudes toward process improvement? What is being learned about how variation in the treatment process is viewed and dealt with? How is process analysis to go forward in the practice setting, with its ruthless time pressures? Clearly, AHCs must continue to address these issues. Academic health center management has a number of possibilities, the most powerful of which is to support champions as they emerge among opinion-leading clinicians. As these people teach, practice, and publish, they will attract the attention of new and old learners far faster than any program.

Fear of looking bad may be one of the barriers to CQI efforts in academic medicine. As Gaucher and Coffey (1993) point out, AHC management often does not recognize the presence of fear in their systems. Professionals would rather define quality than measure it. AHCs do not necessarily have much to fear about quality, however. Current practice results at AHCs may be favorable as well as unfavorable. Caper (1988) shows that the conservative admission pattern of university/teaching hospitals may more than offset the higher technology and costs of such institutions. Johnson (1990) makes a similar argument concerning quality of care. He argues that teaching institutions have something to crow about. The U.S. Congress's Office of Technology Assessment's 1988 meta-study gives no indications that teaching institutions have poorer quality results than nonteaching institutions (U.S. Congress Office of Technology Assessment 1988). Certainly, as Caper (1988) argues, "the time for stopping stonewalling and for taking the lead in quality issues is at hand" (61).

RESEARCH

In their capacities as contract research establishments, medical schools are among those doing most of the research affecting health care quality. The Health Care Financing Administration (HCFA), National Institutes of Health (NIH), and other government health agencies understand that the way to get studies undertaken is to offer to fund them. The already extensive capacity to do clinical trials of new technology can be turned toward both prospective and retrospective studies of the older technologies that account for most of the cost of care. There is also a core of expertise available to participate actively in the development of national and specialty guidelines and a research capacity to conduct new research aimed at resolving gray areas in current theory and practice.

National Guidelines and Standards

At present, the two loci for studies of practice guidelines are (1) the government, through the Agency for Health Care Policy and Research (AHCPR) and its Forum for Quality and Effectiveness in Health Care, and (2) medical specialty organizations.

One might well ask whether AHCs are already taking the lead in this process. Some might argue that they are. The specialty groups that are setting practice guidelines, such as the American Society of Anesthesiologists, the American College of Physicians/American Heart Association

Task Force, and the American College of Obstetrics and Gynecology, include many academics. AHCs are also the loci of the AHCPR studies. The government's grants and contracts system, however, emphasizes individual investigators. Institutional leadership seems neither to speak out very decisively nor provide leadership in many situations.

PORT Studies

Key AHCPR activities have included many studies by Patient Outcomes Research Teams (PORTs), which use administrative databases, epidemiological methods, and outcome evaluations by patients and health services researchers to look at the relative effectiveness of alternative ways of diagnosing and treating high-volume conditions, including low back pain, stroke, benign prostatic hyperplasia, bedsores, urinary incontinence in adults, and depression. Medical school researchers play major roles in these large retrospective studies. Presumably, their results will be used as inputs into local consensus-building approaches and effective practice guidelines. Medical schools could and should play a major role in disseminating as well as developing such guidelines.

Consensus Conferences

Consensus conferences would seem to be the most natural of activities for academic health centers to conduct. When called together by NIH or other agencies, the renowned medical specialists from many medical centers gather and freely offer their opinions on the assigned subject. It would seem that most decisions at an AHC would come about through local, internal consensus conferences. Yet that seldom happens. There seem to be a number of factors involved:

- There is honor in being asked to a national conference, with its recognition as a noted expert as well as opportunities to network with international "peers."
- The local consensus conference would imply constraints on future behavior in a way that an extrainstitutional consensus would not.
- There is no central authority to enforce a consensus in an AHC, and the faculty would just as soon maintain their individual autonomy. Main-

taining professional autonomy is a key issue in the implementation of quality programs.

A precursor to consensus conferences is development of clinical process analyses within the organization. These can stimulate recognition of the need for practice guidelines and standards. A good working description of practice guidelines is: standardized specifications for care developed by a formal process that incorporates the best scientific evidence of effectiveness with expert opinion. Such effects should show whether experienced effectiveness approaches potential effectiveness. Any set of measures of experienced effectiveness should include components of customer satisfaction.

One of the places where academic health center leadership should be active is in encouraging local consensus conferences as an appropriate collegial activity carrying credit both in research and in teaching. Where there are not sufficient data to support a consensus, that should be a signal for an opportunity for high-impact clinical research.

Epidemiological/Small Area Studies

The Minnesota experience indicates that epidemiological studies based on small area data can also be the basis of research on quality (Chassin et al. 1986; Borbas et al. 1990). Individual investigators or organized medicine in a geographic area can perform these. But the academic studies, though interesting, may not be applicable to the rest of the medical community. Leape (1990) and Leape et al. (1991) outline a number of methodological criteria that should be applied to these retrospective studies, starting with automated insurance records.

These small area studies should not only deal with methods of treatment (technical management), but should also examine issues of accessibility, interpersonal process, and continuity of care. For example, Hand et al. (1991) report that the degree of compliance with technical standards (omission of hormone receptor tests and radiation therapy) varies by hospital and drops off with urban location and a higher proportion of poorly insured patients. Likewise, Lazovich et al. (1991) report that breast-conserving surgery among women with Stage I and Stage II breast cancer increases with education and income.

Implementing TQM/CQI

The AHC's quality assurance activities can adopt a number of strategies, one of which involves adopting a research or continuous improvement attitude rather than a compliance one. This process often starts with the collection and comparison of clinical indicators, even though they deal with disease and provide little information on the processes producing the reported results (Linder 1991). As Marder (1990, 60) argues, however: "Indicators and practice guidelines have a symbiotic relationship. Each adds value to the other, and their development is performed simultaneously, rather than sequentially. The result is a continuing cycle of measurement and analysis leading to the knowledge necessary to develop the tools for quality management in health care needed in the 1990s." Work at Latter Day Saints Hospital by faculty of the University of Utah medical school indicates great promise for the combination of carefully designed treatment protocols and computer-based expert systems in complex ICU cases where the number of variables to be manipulated is beyond individuals' limited information-processing capabilities (Morris 1992).

PATIENT CARE

AHCs are the institutions that set the standard for health care quality. There are real questions about the quality of that care. A major study indicates that three to four percent of hospital admissions suffered adverse events due to negligence or medical mismanagement (Brennan et al. 1991). This study does not report the error rates for teaching institutions separately, but even if they are lower than the mean, it still indicates that there is great room for improvement in the technical quality of health care. When one adds the negative experiences of the patient while being served and billed, there are opportunities for improvement.

As AHCs go about their work of serving numerous client publics, they have many opportunities to educate the public and professionals about CQI, its concepts, its values, and its philosophies. The CQI story can be told in many ways as the AHC responds to its various publics in its mission statement, in its treatment of its constituencies and client populations, in its organization of care, in its governance processes, and in its continuing education efforts.

As Linder (1991) points out, organizations that try to influence the image of quality through public relations and marketing are likely to end up badly. The public's perception of quality depends on its comparison of expected quality versus experienced quality. If one works hard to convince someone that quality is there, one is as likely to raise expectations as to bias perceptions favorably. Therefore if the quality is in fact not raised but the expectation of it is raised, the perception gap is being widened. Any attempt to bias that perception favorably is likely to backfire.

On the other hand, there is merit in educating the public about how to judge quality. This involves managing expectations by helping the public determine what to look for and where to find it. There is a wealth of new information available on outcomes that is raw data which must be interpreted. Here the public could use some unbiased expert help. Many states are requiring the disclosure of patient care quality indicators, patient care outcomes, and medical staff qualifications. Despite hospitals' reluctance to share this information, the data will get out to the public and to the press. So will information from the National Practitioner Data Bank. Both hospitals and physicians, however, will have to explain what this means to themselves and to their patients. AHCs can take a leadership role in this area by defining quality and by educating the public and the professionals about this new area.

Many hospitals have statements about the importance of quality in their mission statements. Some go further in seeing to it that all employees are aware of the quality content of that mission statement and can communicate it when asked to do so. Even with these broad statements, there are differences about operational meanings. For example, the 1991 Andersen study shows that there is still a difference of opinion between hospitals and physicians about the relative importance of cost-effectiveness (Arthur Andersen & Co. 1991). The physician attributes most valued by hospitals, as seen by hospitals and by physicians, are shown in Table 16–1. After the listed attributes, the percentages fall off. Note that by far the greatest disagreement between the hospital CEOs and the physicians is over the importance of cost-effectiveness. Yet cost-effective care has to become part of the expressed mission of teaching institutions unless they wish to become niche players in health care.

Cost-effectiveness represents a serious threat to most academic medical centers. One of our colleagues has pointed out that what the payers expect is not care by the most expert provider, but rather care by a qualified provider—by the least credentialed, least specialized provider who is still

Table 16–1 Physician Attributes Prized by Hospitals, as Seen by Physicians and Hospitals

	Percent Reporting "Very Important"	
Physician Attribute	Among Hospital CEOs	Among MDs
Clinical quality/technical competence	97	93
Relationship with patients/reputation	94	94
Cost-effectiveness in hospital practice	92	78

qualified. The academic setting operates in almost the opposite way, emphasizing the greatest possible specialization, and steers patients in that direction. Any attempt to focus on gatekeepers or generalists as the primary mode of care cuts off the financial lifeblood of the institution and with it the patient flows necessary for teaching and research. In the long run, teaching institutions will have to find room for care by the least qualified person who is still qualified rather than by the most qualified person who is still qualified, or they will see their patient flows dry up.

OUTREACH/ACCESS/POPULATION BASE

Lewis and Sheps (1983) argue for an alternative role for academic health centers. They should take responsibility for a specific population base in order to address issues such as prevention and access (and perhaps cost-effectiveness). As care moves in the direction of capitation payments, most academic health centers will be faced with such a choice again and again. Only then are basic issues such as prevention, perceived quality of care, and access likely to be addressed fully. Until then, the faculty will continue to choose autonomy over accountability.

The AHC must have a philosophy about whether it will be responsible for a population base above and beyond that sporadically attracted by the reputation of its specialist faculty. This decision will center on the nature and purpose of the primary care that the faculty deliver. The AHC must decide whether the primary care that it delivers is the core of its undertaking or merely an appendage. Vinten-Johansen and Riska (1991) characterize the choices here and the debate over them as being over how to maintain professional autonomy between "Oslerians and Flexnerians." Those value systems have to be reconciled if the institution is to pull itself together to agree on quality of care in its fullest sense. This will come out of work on a mission statement and a core set of values, should the AHC embark on a CQI process at levels above the teaching hospital.

Organization of Care

Quality is both a value and a cooperative process in an AHC. Therefore the governance processes of the institutions involved must reinforce it. Faculty do pay attention to quality in the tenure and promotion processes of the medical school. They must, however, also become intensively involved with it in the governance of the teaching hospital. Shortell (1985, 1990) outlines a hospital's mechanisms for involving the physician staff in its governance processes, including many quality activities such as the various peer review activities and the board of trustees. He also points out that this process has to be managed carefully to bring younger staff along in the skills necessary to maintain an effective governance process over time.

Even though Shortell emphasizes the need to integrate or bond physicians operating in a private practice, fee-for-service mode, his points are still relevant to the AHC. Physicians on a faculty must still be courted so that they are induced to buy into and conform to institutional norms, including those of quality and process analysis and change.

The introduction of cost control measures, such as DRGs, has created both new motivations for quality improvement and new areas of potential conflict as caregiving organizations move toward a single package price for services such as a normal obstetrical delivery. The medical school faculty and the hospital have a community of interest in having a safe and efficient process that attracts and satisfies patients. If obstetricians are losing patients because the care is traditional, not attractive, and costly, the hospital and the obstetricians can cooperate to develop a competitive process. But there can be other situations, such as the interaction between radiologists and the hospital administration, where the motivations of fee-for-service physician payment and DRGs put the two in an adversarial position on cost and perhaps on quality of care.

In the managed care setting, there is less apparent conflict between management and the caregivers than in a fee-for-service setting. Pressures for productivity and reduced costs, however, can still lead to conflict between the two. Somehow, the governance process has to allow these issues to be brought to light, discussed, and settled if the AHC is to maintain momentum in the quality arena. There are also possible conflicts within the roles of the caregivers. On one hand, the primary caregiver is expected to be an advocate and facilitator for the patient. On the other hand, the primary physician is expected to control costs by being a gatekeeper to specialists and an auditor of their performance. The governance process must address these issues squarely if the patient and the physician are to feel comfortable with the process. True early involvement should occur at the medical student or residency stage, not when one gets into practice. Instead of being sheltered from knowledge of the costs of care, including the cost of quality, students and residents should become knowledgeable about the cost issues involved as they learn about the technical alternatives.

CONCLUSION

As the producers of future physicians and other health care providers and the current producers of research, AHCs are the first line of offense in health care quality. They must assume responsibility for quality in their own operations, in their research, and in their teaching. To the extent that they continue to move cautiously in this area, they are likely to find their competitive position further eroded. The patients and payers will demand that health care be delivered in a cost-effective manner. They will remove their business from institutions that cannot deliver such care.

CQI efforts raise many challenges for AHCs. First, AHCs must ensure that their learners practice in institutions with a good quality climate and culture. They should encourage champions among their learners and faculty to undertake or participate in CQI efforts. They should support research that leads to quality improvement and reduction in unnecessary variation and waste, including setting up a modest research grants system. Their governance system and their marketing and public relations efforts should be aimed at increasing public and professional awareness of quality and of the CQI process and philosophy.

CHAPTER 17

CQI and Patient-Centered Care

David Levy, William Thar, and Curtis P. McLaughlin

Chapter 1 introduced terms such as process enhancement, mass customization and co-configuration. Now it is time to examine the significance of these in the light of the future of the quality movement in health care. If continuous quality improvement (CQI) is a way station on the way to something, what is that something? What might it look like? Certainly, the patient will have a much greater role in the care process. Patients and their families are already empowered with an increasing amount of medical information available to patients and their families in various media . In fact, they may be beset from information from so many sources that they need the help of professionals to sort things out. Therefore, it seems likely that patients will demand a caregiving relationship that is interactive and responsive, that is efficient, but customized to fit their needs and values.

As an example, we can look toward what is called patient-centered care. Levy (1997) has pointed out that most care today remains site-centered; that is, when presented with a patient everyone does his or her job, but optimization of the resulting experience from the patient's point of view is often lost as a succession of professionals sequentially focus on the illness. He cites the case of a terminal cancer patient (Levy 1997).*

> What they exemplify is a health care delivery system focused on treatments and treatment sites, not on the needs of a sick human being. The patient should be important. Illness should be tangential.
>
> Let us examine all aspects of this patient's journey with his illness to test the assertion that his medical management did not

Source: Reprinted from D. Levy, Disease Management in Patient-Centered Care, in *The Physician's Guide to Disease Management*, J.B. Couch, Ed., pp. 274–276, © 1998, Aspen Publishers, Inc.

necessarily represent his best interests or those of the treating physicians or the health benefit plan that paid for the care. For example, a patient may have an outpatient versus an inpatient procedure. In this situation a 23-hour admission is negotiated and a "real" admission avoided, reducing the payer's admission and bed-day rates. However, there is at least an equal chance that this outpatient procedure cost more than its equivalent inpatient stay, particularly in light of acute care hospitals' cost shifting to less controlled outpatient environments. It is hard to say whether this patient would have been more comfortable not being shuffled in and out so quickly or whether he would have preferred to be at home.

Once the diagnosis was made, the patient was offered a treatment plan proffered by a leading specialist. Alternatives were not explored, and the patient accepted the plan "as is." He also gave up his relationship with his primary care physician. Most probably, no extensive discussion occurred regarding the patient's long-term view of his illness. The patient's participation in the decision making was minimal. . . .

As the treatment moved along, there were several conversations between [the] utilization management nurse and both the patient and oncologist. The nurse had never met the patient or his family. When the tumor recurred and a new regimen was suggested, the utilization management nurse referred the case to the medical director. The discussion around the new plan with the medical director and the oncologist related to coverage and medical appropriateness. The focus was the care plan and the benefit plan, rather than the care plan and the patient with an illness. . . .

With the deterioration of his condition and the reduction of the quality of his life, the patient wanted to reevaluate his situation. He made his wishes clear to his wife, but the only physician with whom he had a relationship was not available for guidance or support. It is no surprise that when he became septic in a downward-spiraling clinical course, he landed in an intensive setting, where he expired. . . .

The insufficiencies of the current paradigm as described above can be reviewed from the perspectives of the patient, physicians, and payer. The patient never had any real informed choice upon which he could base a treatment plan suitable to himself, and thus was not a part of the decision-making team. He had many interactions with a utilization management nurse, none of which changed the course of the treatment and illness. Worse, these represented lost opportunities to help the patient with his needs. Trying to change the course of treatment late in the illness required support and execution from his providers of care, but the requisite time, and perhaps interest, of his physician was not available. Finally, the terminal care events, once launched, were irrevocable.

The primary care physician was taken out of the equation early. Little or no feedback was forthcoming from the oncologist on the course of treatment. Home care was not coordinated through the primary care physician's office. It is difficult to assess whether this was a matter of lack of interest or lack of confidence on the part of the primary care physician. The oncologist was distracted on several occasions with interactions with the utilization management nurse and the medical director of the benefit plan that involved negotiating for the site of care, with no tangible effect on the patient. Perhaps the oncologist's time would have been better spent with the patient and his wife. The oncologist, as a member of the benefit plan network, certainly had her fee discounted, but not nearly as much as the extra cost generated by the treatment the patient did not want. All the specialists during the terminal event did their jobs. All organ and physiologic systems were treated correctly and, as the utilization management company verified, at the right site.

The payer was generally blind to the actual course of treatments paid for by its benefit plans. Others were retained to determine eligibility, ensure coverage for specific services at specific sites, and pay claims. The payer received data on cost by provider type and service site utilization. In the managed care world, "report cards" on a variety of measures almost never address the conduct and content of care (274–276).

Can we build a system that is patient-centered? Franklin Health, Inc., a disease management company, specializes (or should we say generalizes) in the one percent of truly complex, catastrophic health care cases with average annual claim costs in excess of $70,000 that account for approximately one-third of the cost of medical care—terminal cancer, spina bifida, hemophilia, AIDS. These patients are the traditional outliers in any insurance benefit program and represent an important challenge for managed care organizations. Furthermore, they are growing in number as participants in new health plans age and as plans begin to handle Medicare and Medicaid populations. No two patients in this group seem to have exactly the same set of co-morbidities and severities nor do they want to be treated the same. Benefit plans are not written with them in mind and usual measures of limiting utilization through optimal disease protocols and closed networks seem to fail them and to generate considerable backlash in the process. These cases are also most likely to present practical and ethical problems for the patient-physician relationship. Services that these cases require may be outside the attending physician's capabilities and actually require out-of-network resources. Furthermore, the seriousness of the issues, especially death, involve a number of troubling personal, family, cultural, religious, and community issues that tend to be unknown to decision-regulators inside a large managed care system.

A PATIENT-CENTERED APPROACH

In response to these issues, Franklin Health, Inc. is developing a patient-centered approach to the care of these cases that uses community-based case management nurses who work with local primary care physicians, the patients, and their families. They are backed up by information technology linking them to databases and epidemiological studies, and to the advice of world-renowned clinical researchers. These individuals perform a nursing assessment and discuss options with the patient and family and primary caregivers. Instead of being like a case manager in the hospital, who is mostly concerned with finances and outplacement, they deal with all types of community and family resources from hospital to pharmacy to hospice to home.

At the same time, due to the automation of records and reports, Franklin Health supervisors and physicians review the cases and treatment plans as often as weekly with an eye to ensuring that best practices and relevant treatment choices as identified by Franklin Health epidemiologists, and clinical consultants are available to physician and patient alike. The challenge is for Franklin Health and other disease management companies to aggregate data on these rare events from the many insurance plans providing coverage and build comprehensive databases to better manage complex cases.

Relationships with the employer-payers center on early identification of complex cases to allow early, close management. Polypharmacy in patients and unnecessary lab tests can be avoided. The patient has an ally in avoiding pressures from family and friends to go to yet another famous medical center in hopes of a miracle or a death-denying opinion. On the other hand, when invasive procedures are called for, patients can be moved from lower-quality to higher-quality centers (based on current outcomes data) where total-episode fees are negotiated, allowing length of stay to become a quality of life issue and not a reimbursement one.

Patient-Centered Care Pilot Study

In 1996, Franklin Health and Oxford Health Plan conducted an extensive study of this co-configuration prototype, called the Patient-Centered Care Pilot. The Patient-Centered Care Pilot showed that two-thirds of all severely ill patients in the program reported an enhanced quality of life as a result of patient-centered care management, when surveyed by an independent group. At the same time costs were significantly reduced. A comparison of 1,313 cases in the pilot study involving 10 medical diagnostic groups (MDGs) compared with claims data from HCIA Inc. and severity adjusted showed an 11.7 percent savings in adjusted claims expenses with the average savings per case approaching $20,000.

What this experiment also showed was that patient-led, patient-centered case management that fully informs patients about options for care and their consequences and ensures the effective implementation of the choice made can lead to better satisfaction with the plan, subjectively improved quality of life, and reduced costs. Furthermore, physicians were relieved that they were fulfilling their roles as patient advocates rather than being caught between their instincts and time spent overcoming insurers' standard procedures.

The nurses in the field who support this system are co-configurers with the primary care physicians, the supervisory physicians at Franklin Health, the patient, and the patient's family.

A legitimate question, however, is whether or not this situation is merely a successful application of the old craft mode of delivery with a new orientation or really represents an application applying the concepts of mass customization. Each situation that they face is virtually unique, the situation to which the craft approach is best suited. On the other hand, many of the conditions of performance enhancement followed by mass customization obtain. Data on each case are carefully collected and maintained over the Word Wide Web in a proprietary database. which is also compared with existing databases at HCIA for benchmarking. Epidemiological studies are regularly performed to identify the most effective treatments and most effective timings of interventions. Consultants at major medical centers are retained to provide information on new treatment profiles and mounting outcomes experience and summaries on the effectiveness of existing choices. For the more commonly encountered diagnoses such as prostate cancer and breast cancer these can be packaged in an up-to-minute presentation of alternatives that are also available to nurses, patients, families, and physicians over the Web. In essence, the company uses intensive searches for organizational knowledge from centers of excellence all over the world and then rapidly disseminates it to its supervisors and field nurses to apply to new and ongoing cases. This frees the cognitive capacity and the time of the staff to focus on local matters and on the preferences of the patient and the patient's primary care physician.

The models of the evolution of health care identified in Chapter 1 can be seen as exhibiting two parallel movements. The first is the addition of science and medical technology to the art of medicine and the second is the addition of organizational learning mediated by information technology. What the caregiver can and should provide is modified by both of these movements. Since the early craft days, laboratory information and imaging and testing devices have added to the physician's diagnostic skills and more drugs and procedures become available for treatment. The clinician still senses things about the patient face-to-face, but adds to that the objective data of tests and images and then expends the time and effort saved in selecting and customizing treatments to deal with the patient's specific needs. The digital age can bring the world-class consultant to the practitioner instead of sending the patient to the local specialist, but the process is still essentially the same. The consultant adds to the range, currency, and depth of the primary care physician in treating his or her patients, and the local nurse case manager extends the range, currency, and depth of the primary care physician in dealing with local institutions, financial issues, and personal and social issues. Has the primary physician lost control? No. Has the primary physician lost autonomy? To some extent yes, since that physician is now accountable for responding to the recommendations of the consultants, the patient, the patient's family, and the local case manager. Many physicians left solo practice, however, to join practice groups for the support, quality, and accountability that those groups can provide. Patient-centered care is still another collegial group but with a wider variety of degrees, backgrounds, and skills. The adjustment may be difficult, but not insurmountable.

PATIENT-CENTERED CARE FOR NONCATASTROPHIC CASES

Because the individual cost of noncatastrophic cases is much lower, the cost of developing a mass customization system must be either reduced or spread over a much larger number of cases. For the more expensive of these—chronic diseases such as asthma, diabetes, hypertension, congestive heart failure, hypercholesterolemia, colitis, and specific procedures such as childbirth, cardiac catheterization, knee injuries, and early-stage neoplasms—there is a need to ensure that treatment is timely, economical, and effective.

Managing these cases means making sure that best practices are understood and implemented in a way that motivates appropriate patient and provider behavior. The key to that is in the physician-patient relationship. The physician must motivate behavioral change on the part of the patient and also use the support of the disease management process to keep up with best practice in both treatment and patient motivation. This disease management process may often involve financial risk-taking by the primary care physician or a disease management firm. In either case, there is technical and behavioral support for the process that is based on organizational learning and a disciplined approach to education and treatment. Again the physician is the configurer, one hopes, in a cooperative venture with the patient and the family. There is likely to be less variability induced by co-morbidity and the seriousness of the episode, however, so a more standardized approach can be followed.

This is the type of situation that the insurance systems and HMOs are currently designed to control. If the practices were able to control them effectively, however, they could accept the risk of capitation and be free of the hassle factor that is so much a part of the current clinician-payer relationship. Utilization control is warranted in many cases, but the process can be so much more responsive when the delivering organization self-regulates. When physicians talk about "taking back control," they must understand that they are not talking about a return to the old days, but about a new self-regulating system that demands conformance when it is warranted by knowledge about best practices.

Standard CQI team approaches can be used to develop these processes. One can start with clinical guidelines available from a number of professional sources. The organization's quality council or its equivalent, however, needs to decide which clinical conditions warrant intervention based on undesirable outcomes including unnecessary variability and cost. These also tend to be high-volume, high-total-cost clinical conditions. The CQI team usually starts with a review of the scientific literature and of similar clinical guidelines developed elsewhere. Clinician members or support staff may conduct this search, but it must end up selling the clinicians enough to buy into the constraints that the guideline inherently imposes. Then the CQI team compares this ideal approach with the current approach and identifies the steps necessary to change habits and behaviors to implement it. Then it proceeds to set up procedures to identify patients that the clinical guideline covers, train and motivate personnel to use it, and monitor its performance. One must soon recognize, however, that there are steps necessary to support patient-centered aspects of the clinical guideline.

The guideline should be reviewed from the patient's point of view and adjusted, where possible, to improve the experience. If the team did not include patients who experienced the old procedure, then the first few patients that go through the process should be interviewed about their feelings and perhaps even meet with the team to make suggestions.

The next steps, however—the ones that are totally missing in the literature—relate to how to support the process with information technology. The questions asked would be: How can we support the current process with information technology to free up the clinicians to make the process more customized for the patient? How might the patients vary? What are the likely co-morbidities that were not included in the clinical guideline and its implementation into a clinical pathway and/or clinical protocol? How can we capture patient attitudes and preferences efficiently and effectively? How can we use that information in motivating better compliance and self-care? How can we make the patient feel empowered? How can we elicit the best health behaviors from the patient's point of view? Where should a case manager intervene, if at all? How can we capture data that cue the case management function to enter the picture? What information about local institutions, social services, patient's family setting, and cultural factors should be available to assist the case managers? How can we gather data on the cost-effectiveness of such interventions to help with such decisions?

What patient-centered care would seem to imply is an attempt to mass customize the service, to adapt to patient needs with a system for providing personalized service economically on a large scale. At every level the organization should be thinking about how to build on the platforms produced by CQI and reengineering efforts to move in the direction of making the face-to-face interaction responsive to patient needs and values. This means freeing up the cognitive capacity and time of clinicians and case managers to elicit and respond to those needs directly and indirectly.

Specialized systems may be necessary to handle areas where either the clinicians are inexperienced or slow to respond or the benefits systems that are meant to control utilization are unable to respond. Today these specialized systems are called *disease management* companies. They focus carefully on a narrow range of disease entities with a specifically designed approach applicable to both the treatment of the problem and the utilization control. One feature of these organizations is that they develop highly specialized databases that are relevant to the management of their caseload based on numbers aggregated from many practices and even multiple insurance pools.

CONCLUSION

So far we have focused on the approximately 10 percent of patients—the complex catastrophic cases and the more severe chronic cases—who represent two-thirds the cost of health care. The remaining 90 percent of patients represent acute illnesses treatable in the outpatient setting, self-resolving problems, and the worried well, as well as routine preventive care. Here the volume is high, the cost is low per episode, and co-payments and deductibles have a notable impact. Here again information technology can provide support in making the process efficient and effective. Nelson et al. (1998) focus on the clinical microunit and its flow and information requirements. Their list of processes that need rationalization includes enrollment and assignment to a provider; orientation to the practice and its services; first visit, initial assessment, and care planning; care delivery; an information environment to support work of clinicians and knowledge of patients; and support tasks to gain knowledge of the patients and populations, measure health status, costs, and outcomes, and to measure microunit performance. The transition to this state requires a massive CQI and reengineering effort to build the platforms necessary to make such a system responsive and reliable. (See Chapter 9.) Moreover, this information must be made relevant to people in need of health care, as described by Nelson and his colleagues (1998), "relevant information that can help a person take actions that will increase the odds of good health; access to highly competent clinicians and the latest biomedical breakthroughs; timely expert knowledge on emerging health problems and information on different treatment approaches that might be considered; shared decision making with a competent health professional who knows them, cares about them, and can help them get what they want and need . . ." (12–13)

All of these require the development or the purchase of platforms to get to the point where that level of service can be delivered at a reasonable cost. Capital investment of this magnitude at a time when profit margins in health care are shrinking must come out of reduced waste and improved clinical performance. For a while, there was hope that physician practice management (PPM) organizations would provide that technology and capital for such a transition, but that now seems questionable. Therefore, the CQI route to this ideal is perhaps the only feasible way to go. Once again, the knowledge, skills, and intelligence of the health care work force, its existing intellectual capital, must be enhanced and activated to move toward such objectives. CQI has a promising future, so long as those implementing it understand where it is headed in building a platform for a client-centered system of care throughout medicine.

PART V

Illustration

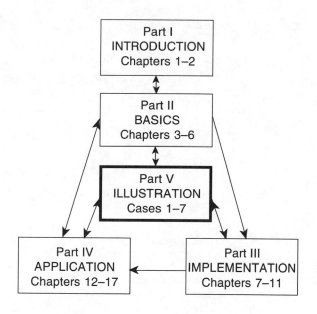

CQI Principles for a Personnel Problem

Michael McDade

In the fall of 1996 the Mandelsohn Laboratories of the Midstate University Medical Center Hospital consolidated its administrative functions into a single financial services unit. Typical of laboratories in many large hospitals, the shift of laboratory functions from a revenue generation mode to that of a cost center led to staff downsizing. Clerical and purchasing functions that had utilized 14 FTE [full-time equivalent] personnel scattered through the various discipline-based laboratories (anatomic pathology, cytogenetics, molecular pathology, chemistry, hematology, transfusion medicine, and coagulation) were now performed by 8 FTEs. This reduction in force had been accomplished so far through attrition, but not without considerable turmoil among the staff.

BACKGROUND

Midstate University Medical Center Hospital is the primary teaching hospital for the Midstate University Medical School. Both are located on the Centerville campus of Midstate University. The medical center hospital and the medical school are separate institutions with separate management and procedures, although both are subject to state government

---

purchasing and personnel rules. Many of the senior professionals in the Laboratories also hold faculty appointments in the medical school and have research grants and contracts administered by the medical school as well as clinical income collected through the medical school faculty practice plan. Therefore, a senior pathologist might travel one week to look at new hospital equipment on a trip charged to a hospital budget and the next week present a research paper at a conference with the expenses charged to her research grant through the medical school. Most technician-level and administrative personnel in the Laboratories were hospital employees, but occasionally would be charging travel and purchases to medical school accounts.

The Purchasing Unit*

Mr. Harold Banes, budget administrator for the Laboratories, was placed in charge of the purchasing function which now involved three experienced individuals who previously had worked in three separate laboratories. Ms. Marjorie Yarborough had worked in the chemistry laboratories, while Ms. Anna Anatoli had worked in transfusion medicine. Both were classified as accounting clerk III. Ms. Cherzina Zololak, an accounting clerk IV, had worked previously for the associate laboratory director for research. All were hospital employees.

Harold's interviews with the three clerks indicated that there were serious staff problems in the unit. There was lack of trust among the three clerks, feelings that job classifications and pay scales were arbitrary and unfair, and little or no consensus as to what was an appropriate quantity and quality of work in these newly formed positions. The conflicting work styles and expectations of each employee in this unstructured work environment resulted in multiple personnel clashes every week. Given that there was no common sense of mission or culture among the work force, he decided to initiate a "customer-focused" view of the purchasing unit.

He first developed a customer survey form, based on a marketing textbook (Kotler 1997), that was sent to key personnel in the laboratories that relied on the purchasing unit. (See Exhibit 1.1.) The summarized results showed that customer expectations were very high for all responses, while the perceived performance of the unit was quite variable. The survey was highly suggestive that personnel in the unit were trying "to

---

Source: Marketing Management: Analysis, Planning, Implementation and Control, edited by Kotler, © 1997, pp. 480–481. Adapted by permission of Prentice-Hall, Inc., Upper Saddle River, NJ.

Exhibit 1.1 Performance Survey

This section is a performance survey. Your input on the statements below is needed!! We would like you to rate our services by giving your opinion on the statements below. There are two responses for each statement (1–20). The statement on the left is equivalent to a "1" on the scale. The statement to the right is equivalent to a "4" on the scale. Indicate your opinion by circling or placing an "x" in the appropriate boxes.

1. The group does not put much emphasis on improving its service.

how things are now
[1] [2] [3] [4]
how things should be
[1] [2] [3] [4]

The group places a great deal of emphasis on improving its service.

2. The staff in this group are almost never approachable.

how things are now
[1] [2] [3] [4]
how things should be
[1] [2] [3] [4]

The staff in this group are almost always approachable.

3. The amount and scope of work for this group is not appropriate.

how things are now
[1] [2] [3] [4]
how things should be
[1] [2] [3] [4]

The amount and scope of work for for this group is very appropriate.

4. Work flow for this group is not organized to maximize productivity.

how things are now
[1] [2] [3] [4]
how things should be
[1] [2] [3] [4]

Work flow for this group is organized to maximize productivity.

5. The lines of authority in this group are unclear to me.

how things are now
[1] [2] [3] [4]
how things should be
[1] [2] [3] [4]

The lines of authority in this group are clear to me.

6. The policies, procedures, and standard practices set by this service make it hard to get the job done.

how things are now
[1] [2] [3] [4]
how things should be
[1] [2] [3] [4]

The policies, procedures, and standard practices set by this service do not get in the way of the job.

7. People in this group are reluctant to take action to get the job done.

how things are now
[1] [2] [3] [4]
how things should be
[1] [2] [3] [4]

People in this group gladly take action to get the job done.

8. The productivity of this service often suffers from lack of organization and planning.

how things are now
[1] [2] [3] [4]
how things should be
[1] [2] [3] [4]

This productivity of this service rarely suffers from lack of organization and planning.

9. The turn-around time for work submitted to this group is unacceptable.

how things are now
[1] [2] [3] [4]
how things should be
[1] [2] [3] [4]

The turn-around time for work submitted to this group is exceptional.

10. The quality of service by this group is unacceptable.

how things are now
[1] [2] [3] [4]
how things should be
[1] [2] [3] [4]

The quality of service by this group is exceptional.

continues

Exhibit 1.1 continued

	how things are now	
11. This group does not exhibit high standards of professionalism.	[1] [2] [3] [4] how things should be [1] [2] [3] [4]	This group exhibits very high standards of professionalism.
12. This group is almost never accessible.	how things are now [1] [2] [3] [4] how things should be [1] [2] [3] [4]	This group is almost always accessible.
13. This group almost never offers personalized service.	how things are now [1] [2] [3] [4] how things should be [1] [2] [3] [4]	This group almost always offers personalized service.
14. Services provided by this group are rarely convenient.	how things are now [1] [2] [3] [4] how things should be [1] [2] [3] [4]	Services provided by this group are almost always convenient.
15. The process to request services from this group is almost always difficult.	how things are now [1] [2] [3] [4] how things should be [1] [2] [3] [4]	The process to request services from this group is almost always easy.
16. Appropriate follow-up is almost never provided by this group.	how things are now [1] [2] [3] [4] how things should be [1] [2] [3] [4]	Appropriate follow-up is almost always provided by this group.
17. People in this group put very little effort into making their performance the best it can be.	how things are now [1] [2] [3] [4] how things should be [1] [2] [3] [4]	People in this group put a lot of effort into making their performance the best it can be.
18. Lab staff are left in the dark regarding changes that may affect their use of this service.	how things are now [1] [2] [3] [4] how things should be [1] [2] [3] [4]	Lab staff are kept up to date about changes that may affect their use of this service.
19. The policies and procedures set by this service are confusing to me.	how things are now [1] [2] [3] [4] how things should be [1] [2] [3] [4]	The policies and procedures set by this service are clear to me.
20. This service sets many unnecessary procedures.	how things are now [1] [2] [3] [4] how things should be [1] [2] [3] [4]	This service keeps unnecessary procedures to a minimum.

do a good job," but lacked direction and efficiency. Poor communication and a lack of policy and procedures were noted in a number of the specific customer comments.

Although Harold was quite busy with his budget and planning duties, he decided to hold weekly "team meetings" with the purchasing group. They started out with "brainstorming" sessions that produced three pages of issues of concern to them and to customers in the survey. They then summarized these into six categories: (1) work flow, (2) customer service, (3) communication, (4) personnel, (5) policies/procedures, and (6) training/continuing education. Because these meetings had been quite contentious, Harold then suggested that the group develop a mission and vision statement as a "foundation of understanding" for the group. This effort took several weekly meetings and resulted in the following:

> Purchasing Unit Vision Statement: We strive to be an integral part of the Laboratories' team and deliver high quality support and services by being innovative, efficient, informed, and informative.
>
> Purchasing Unit Mission Statement: We provide (1) Financial services and support functions, (2) Procurement of supplies and services, (3) Travel support—through effective customer service.

In the meantime, interpersonal relations in the unit did not improve. Cherzina no longer wanted to back up Marjorie after they clashed over a group assignment. She suggested that Marjorie and Anna cover for each other and that she be given special assignments when university purchasing and travel did not fill her time. She was ending up covering for one or the other at least half of the days that she worked and still felt unfamiliar with their procedures. Marjorie felt that Cherzina was "not pulling her weight" by doing only travel and university purchasing and not taking responsibility for the heavy volume of hospital laboratory purchasing. Marjorie and Anna complained to Harold that their hospital purchasing workload was overwhelming and was the vast majority of the workload for the financial services unit. Cherzina told Harold that at times she felt she wasn't busy enough, but that she didn't like spending half her time "backing up" for Marjorie and Anna. It had reached the point where "team" members were only communicating when necessary.

Work Flow Issues

The group then moved on to work flow issues. Harold explained the principles of continuous quality improvement, focusing on emphasis on the customer and data-driven decision making. Then they began to flow-chart the major processes in the unit. Cherzina processed travel requests and reimbursements for laboratory personnel that went through either hospital or medical school processes. The two processes were quite different. Her other primary duty was processing purchasing requests that went through the medical school purchasing process. Flowcharting showed that both travel paperwork processes and both purchasing processes were quite different. In addition, she served as backup for Marjorie and Anna when they were absent.

Marjorie and Anna had nearly identical job responsibilities, purchasing the Laboratories' $7 million annually of supplies, equipment, and services. Flowcharting showed that various lab areas submitted requests for supplies and services using many different methods–cards, forms, letters, slips of paper. Each clerk dealt with a different set of vendors. One took the front half of the alphabet and the other the back half. This had led to complaints from laboratory personnel that they had to deal with two different clerks when they had questions about deliveries, contracts, inventory usage, budget information, especially on high-volume items for which multiple vendors were used.

Harold then suggested that each clerk use a "Daytimer-like" form to keep track of the following by hour of the day:

Type of Work	Direct Customer Interaction (minutes)	Orders Requested Completed	Phone Calls In Out	E-Mail Messages In Out

This effort was conducted for three weeks, the period requested by the staff. Disbursement records for the preceding year were also reviewed to identify the number of travel requests and medical school purchase orders processed.

Of the work normally assigned to Cherzina, the unit had processed 87 medical school purchase orders, 64 medical school travel requests, and 106 hospital travel requests during calendar 1997. During the three-week period, April 6–24, 1998, the total number of hospital purchase order requests received was 461 and the number placed was 444. Of these, 240 orders were processed by Marjorie, 164 by Anna, and 57 by Cherzina. During the same three-week period, 595 phone calls and e-mails were placed: 400 by Marjorie, 113 by Anna, and 82 by Cherzina. The timing of these demands on the clerks was quite variable with about half of the orders coming in on Monday and Tuesday, especially Tuesday when 39 percent of the orders were received. Travel tended to be heaviest during the spring and fall and medical school purchasing at the end of both the fiscal and calendar years.

The steps in each purchase were similar: Price the requisition against a contract; encumber the funds in an account; place an order under the contract or negotiate a contract if one does not already exist; follow up on the order, if not received when promised or when the lab needs it; compare the receiving slip with the order and invoice; debit the account for the amount of the invoice; and then authorize the writing of a check to pay for the merchandise. Many major contracts were negotiated at the statewide, university-wide, or hospital-wide levels, since the state operated a number of health care institutions and the university also purchased materials for use in a number of laboratories on a number of campuses.

Cherzina estimated that medical school purchase orders required 0.5 to 1.0 hours to process, while each travel request took from 0.5 to 5 hours to process. There were also a number of collateral duties that ended up in this unit as well, including processing requests for parking permits once a year, handling return of purchased goods, handling time sheets for grants administration, media billing, and costing of tests for budgeting and pricing. Cherzina also served as supervisor in Harold's absence and performed special studies as requested.

Several other factors were also relevant to this process analysis. The administrative manager of the department of pathology in the medical school felt that his staff were underutilized and wanted all medical school travel and purchasing routed through that office. The hospital was in the process of buying and installing a new hospital-wide financial information system that would have the capability of performing inventory control on laboratory supplies and automatically generating purchase requisitions when inventory levels reached specified reorder points.

Armed with this information, Harold presented to the group two proposals for workload allocation in the group. In both cases the medical school purchasing and travel would be shifted to the department of pathology offices. In Proposal One, the hospital purchasing was equally divided among the three clerks with each taking a third of the contracts according to the assigned section of the alphabet. In Proposal Two, the various laboratory units were designated by laboratory cost center and each assigned to one of the clerks. In each proposal, laboratory cost centers assigned to a worker who was absent were specifically and consistently reassigned to one of the remaining two.

Harold was personally in favor of Proposal Two for the following reasons:

- It was customer- and cost center-driven rather than vendor-driven.
- Each laboratory unit would have one clerk to go to with all of its requirements and an identified backup during her absences.
- Once the new hospital financial information system was in effect with its purchasing component, the assigned clerk could work with specific laboratory cost centers in setting maximum and minimum inventory levels for specific items.
- The clerks would better understand the needs of the individual laboratories for financial analysis services to assist with budget preparation and monitoring and test costing. This would enable the clerks to develop their skills at fiscal analysis rather than concentrating only on order processing.

The unit staff was in favor of Proposal Two and Laboratories management welcomed it enthusiastically. It was scheduled for implementation during June 1998.

Future Issues

Discussion of the implementation of this new system identified a number of issues that needed further consideration:

- developing a clearer understanding of "customer service" expectations among unit staff
- developing expected turn-around times for placing orders from the labs
- developing standards for consistency in filing and documentation
- designating one of the staff to be in charge of training lab personnel in policies and procedures
- developing a scheduling system consistent with the hospital's personnel and leave policies
- planning how to maximize the utility of the "inventory control" features of the new system

Harold was interested in deciding how to use the CQI process to deal with these issues once Proposal Two was implemented.

CASE ANALYSIS

This case illustrates how an individual can use the CQI approach within a work unit context. All of the other cases in this book tend to be multidisciplinary. We see him using this approach to attempt to hold together a dysfunctional work group and build a new set of work norms within the group.

Introduction

Mr. Banes used a fact-based approach where there had been much blaming of each other by his newly assembled staff. It did not necessarily change the interpersonal dynamics of the group, but it allowed them to focus on a clear discrepancy in workload and performance. He also looked at customer responses to his group's performance as an input to the design of the new system.

Basics

Data collection was a basic part of this effort and it told a clear tale. There was little need to use most of the other tools, given the frequency distribution of the workloads. He did, however, use the customer information as an additional point of view to focus on. Given that the issue was unavoidable, group members—especially Mr. Banes—began to generate alternatives.

Implementation

Mr. Banes attempted to keep as much of a participatory view as possible, even though the employees were likely to try an end run to get him to take responsibility for change. He kept pushing the team to make joint decisions as much as possible. What he brought to the table was the knowledge of what others in the institution were thinking and the ability to generate alternatives that required interaction with other departments. He was very fortunate in that the medical school's administrative staff wanted to take over the functions that Cherzina had been doing, allowing him to bypass her preferences. However, it gave him the opportunity to reallocate the work. What was not clear at the end of the case was whether or not the staff could now be reduced to two clericals.

Applications

It is not clear here that Mr. Banes did accomplish anything lasting in terms of the institutionalization of CQI in the laboratory. He did not publicize the results for obvious reasons. Therefore, it is not clear that the institution has benefited from his efforts as much as he has squeezed out of a difficult spot.

CASE 2

The Family Practice Center

David C. Kibbe and Curtis P. McLaughlin

The Family Practice Center (FPC) is the home of the 35-physician group practice of the department of family medicine at the School of Medicine, University of North Carolina (UNC) at Chapel Hill. In July of 1991 the faculty was discussing the possibility of expanded evening and weekend office hours for patients. Two points of view were being expressed about faculty and patient attitudes toward continuity of care. There typically is a trade-off between offering patients (1) the convenience of being seen the same day they call in and (2) the opportunity of being seen by their own physician (i.e., continuity of care). Some staff argued that there was a trend in patient attitudes toward convenient appointment times and away from concerns about continuity with the same physician, while others disagreed.

Mr. Tony Galiani, MBA, the FPC manager, had recently come to Chapel Hill, North Carolina, from the Harvard Community Health Plan, where fact-based management and continuous improvement methodologies had been pioneered under Dr. Donald Berwick. At UNC, however, no system of customer satisfaction surveys had been in place at the FPC, so [Mr. Galiani] instituted a policy of "listening to the customer." Any customer expressing dissatisfaction was referred to him by the staff and he recorded their complaints. On reviewing his records, he found that there had been over 200 unsolicited complaints about continuity of care between November 1, 1990, and August 1, 1991. Approximately 75 percent of the com-

Source: This case was prepared as a basis for classroom discussion rather than to illustrate the effective or ineffective handling of an administrative situation. Copyright © 1993 by the Kenan-Flagler Business School, University of North Carolina, Chapel Hill, NC 27599-3490. All rights reserved. Not to be reproduced without permission.

443

plaint records contained a reference to continuity problems. Patients' dissatisfaction about continuity could be captured by either one or both of the following patient statements: "I can't see my own (i.e., primary, usual) physician often enough when I want to," and "I don't see the same doctor often enough for the follow-up of an acute problem."

The continuity issue came to a head when another "customer," a large employer that referred its employee workers' compensation and industrial medicine cases to the FPC, threatened to withdraw from its contract on the grounds that follow-up visits were made infrequently with the same physician who initially evaluated the patient. An employer representative stated, "We believe patients seen in your practice are out of work longer than those seen by other doctors' practices, and we believe this is due to lack of provider continuity at your facility." The message was clear: "Either fix it or lose our business." Loss of this customer would mean a significant financial loss to the practice.

FORMING A TEAM

Mr. Galiani had already discussed the possibilities of starting a total quality management (TQM) process in the department of family medicine with David Kibbe, MD, MBA, who was beginning a faculty development fellowship and studying quality management in medical practice. The approach they agreed on was the FOCUS-PDSA cycle, a Deming-based approach, that usually follows these steps:

- Find a process to improve.
- Organize a team that knows the process.
- Clarify current knowledge of the process and its variation.
- Understand the causes of process variation.
- Select the process improvement.
- Plan the improvement.
- Do the data collection, analysis, and improvement effort.
- Study the data for process improvement and customer outcome.
- Act to hold the gains and continue improvement.

They decided to put together the initial quality team to study the continuity problem that had now become so evident. The team was made up of seven staff volunteers with functional knowledge of the continuity problem. There were three physicians—Dr. Kibbe; Dr. Bob Gwyther, the FPC medical director; and Dr. Sam Weir—plus Mr. Galiani; Ms. Eleanor Benz, MSPH, the quality assurance coordinator; and Ms. Beverly Spencer, RN, a nursing supervisor. This group then chose Ms. Donna Harrison, MBA, of the University Hospital's department of management engineering to act as the group's TQM/CQI consultant.

At its first meeting the team adopted as its project objective "to improve continuity of care in the Family Practice Center." Specific goals of the team included:

1. to define the problem of continuity from the patient's point of view
2. to examine in depth relevant aspects of the problem of continuity of care at the FPC using a CQI process
3. to learn and apply some of the tools and analytical methods of TQM/CQI as a means of evaluating real problems of importance to medical practice in the FPC
4. to document the effort and methods used in order to share the process with others in the FPC at the end of the project period

CONTINUITY OF CARE

Although research studies have produced conflicting results about the ability of continuity of care to improve the quality of health care outcomes, most physician observers have included continuity as one of the principles of family practice, one worth preserving (Ware and Snyder 1975). In October 1991 the team surveyed the department's faculty. A large majority of the 25 surveyed agreed or strongly agreed with the statement "Continuity of care improves the quality of patient care" and all agreed or strongly agreed with "We should retain continuity of care as a principle of family practice in the FPC and teach medical students and residents its value." In the October survey of faculty preferences the majority responded that the FPC should strive to make it possible for patients to see their regular physician some 70 percent of the time. Figure 2.1 summarizes their objectives.

Next, the team decided to assess the actual degree of discontinuity in the practice. A chart audit was performed to provide information on usual

"We should strive to attain a usual provider continuity level of..."

Figure 2.1 Faculty Survey on Continuity of Care, UNC Department of Family Medicine

provider continuity, which is simply the percentage of total visits a patient sees his or her regular physician. A random sample of 125 charts was audited for the period July 1, 1990, to June 30, 1991, and the visits were classified into three categories: health maintenance, chronic illness, and acute care. The "usual provider" was determined by noting the physician named on the face sheet as the assigned physician of record or, when this was not available or was inaccurate, by the chart auditor's assessment of the clinical notes as to which physician most regularly saw the patient. These results were compared with a similar audit of 265 charts performed in this practice in 1984 (Fleming et al. 1986). The comparison showed that usual provider continuity had dropped significantly in the intervening period.

	% Usual Provider Continuity	
Type of Visit	*1984*	*1991*
Health maintenance	86%	74%
Chronic illness	76%	61%
Acute illness	55%	29%
Overall, all visits combined	61%	45%

Therefore the team concluded that there had indeed been an actual loss of continuity in the practice that justified the perception among customers of a problem of continuity.

What the Customer Wants

The team wanted to understand what its customers wanted in terms of continuity and to establish the precedent of going directly to the customers to find out what their preferences were. Therefore in December they conducted a two-week survey of clinic users in which 229 out of the 769 visitors during the period completed the questionnaire shown in Exhibit 2.1. Given a choice between seeing their regular physician for each visit or seeing any physician at the time that suited them best, 79 percent of the respondents chose continuity over convenience. The respondents were further asked to choose between seeing their regular physician with a one-week wait versus coming in when they wanted to come for a variety of situations. Seventy percent or more preferred to wait for their annual physical, for treatment of chronic conditions, for work-related physical exams, and for situations where the medicine did not seem to be working or when a hospital stay might be required. Seventy percent or more preferred immediate care by any available physician for a painful problem, a cut or sprain, or a problem that would result in missing work. There was less agreement on preferences when the symptom was frightening or had lasted three days or more or had kept the patient awake all night, or when the medication was causing "bad effects."

The team concluded that there was little difference in attitudes concerning continuity between patients and physicians, but that neither group was having its expectations for continuity met. One team member described this situation as "an unexpected problem of alignment between professional principles, patient preferences, and group practices having to do with continuity." At this point the team felt that efforts to improve continuity were justifiable and likely to improve patient and provider satisfaction.

Understanding the Causes of Process Variation #4

Now the basic question became, "Given that patients have complained about discontinuity, that providers are desirous of a level of continuity around 70 percent, and that the practice attained a level of continuity above 60 percent in 1984, what has caused the decline to an overall level of 45 percent, which includes the especially sharp decline in the acute illness category, from 55 percent to 29 percent?" A key concept of TQM/CQI is

Exhibit 2.1 Family Practice Center (FPC) Patient Survey

We want to improve our scheduling of doctors' appointments. Will you help us by answering the following questions? Your answers will be confidential. There is no way for anyone to know how you or any other patients answered.

Please CHECK (✔) your answers:

How long have you come to the FPC for care?
_____ less than 1 year   _____ 1–2 years   _____ 3 or more years
_____ Before today, how many times in the last 3 months have you been to the FPC?

	YES	NO	UNSURE	
1.	____	____	____	Do you usually get a checkup or physical exam at least once a year?
2.	____	____	____	Do you think you should get a yearly checkup?
3.	____	____	____	Do you have a regular doctor at the FPC? (If no, skip to 6)
4.	____	____	____	Would you ever send a friend to your doctor?
5.	____	____	____	Have you ever thought of changing doctors?
6.	____	____	____	Would you like to have a regular doctor if you have none?

NONE	SOME	VERY	
____	____	____	How IMPORTANT is it for you to have a regular doctor when you visit the FPC?
____	____	____	How IMPORTANT is it for you to get an appointment at the times you want?

At the FPC we have different types of patients: men, women, older patients, younger patients, parents with children, single patients. We need to know how these different types of patients feel about our services and how we can meet their different needs. Would you help us by answering a few questions about yourself? Please CHECK (✔) the type that best describes you.

____ Man	*Age:*	____ Never married
____ Woman	____ 18–29 yrs.	____ Married
Years of School:	____ 30–39 yrs.	____ Divorced or separated
____ 1–6 yrs.	____ 40–49 yrs.	____ Widowed
____ 7–12 yrs.	____ 50–59 yrs.	____ Special friend
____ Technical School	____ 60 or older	
____ College		____ Black
____ Postgraduate		____ White
		____ Other

Are you now: ____ employed full time? ____ employed part time?
____ unemployed? ____ retired?
____ other? (describe) _____

How would you describe your health? ____ Poor   ____ Average   ____ Good

_____ Number of people who live with you? (Don't count yourself.)

continues

Exhibit 2.1 continued

To help us set a time for you to see a doctor, tell us which is more important:

(1) to see a REGULAR DOCTOR even if you must wait a week, or
(2) the TIME you need or want to come.

Read each question below and CHECK (✔) either column (1) or column (2).

(1) Regular Doctor	(2) Time	Reasons for Seeing the Doctor
——	——	Yearly physical exam or checkup
——	——	Physical exam for school, work, or insurance
——	——	A problem that will make you miss work today
——	——	A problem that is very painful
——	——	An injury like a cut finger or sprained ankle
——	——	Something you think may lead to a hospital stay
——	——	A problem that kept you awake all night
——	——	A problem you've had for 3 days and not getting better
——	——	A condition that needs regular visits such as high blood pressure, diabetes, arthritis, heart problems
——	——	You are having bad effects from a medicine
——	——	You think your medicine is not working
——	——	You have a problem that frightens you

In October, we added evening hours. Patients can now make appointments to see a doctor from: 8:30 a.m. to 7:00 p.m. Monday through Thursday;
8:30 a.m. to 5:00 p.m. on Friday;
8:00 a.m. to 12:00 noon Saturday.

What are YOUR BEST TIMES to come to the FPC? _____

CHECK ONLY ONE: If you HAD TO CHOOSE, would you rather
____ see your regular doctor for each visit
     OR
____ come to see any FPC doctor at a time that best suits you?

What DO YOU LIKE about the Family Practice Center? _____
_____
_____
_____

What DON'T YOU LIKE about the Family Practice Center? _____
_____
_____
_____

THANK YOU. PLEASE PUT THIS SHEET IN THE BOX ON THE COUNTER.

that any problem is likely to have multiple causes. Unfortunately, managers often waste time trying to find "magic bullets," that is, simple solutions to try to fix complex problems. TQM/CQI offers a number of methods, such as brainstorming, cause-and-effect (Ishikawa) diagrams, Pareto diagrams, and flowcharts to help identify and define the various and often complex causes of a systems problem. The team used several of these approaches to better understand what had been causing discontinuity to occur. Using these methods helped the team make rapid progress in a relatively short time in determining why a patient was or was not able to see his or her physician of choice.

Although it is normal for everyone to have an opinion and to think that his or her opinion should form the basis of the solution, the TQM/CQI process requires that the team members suspend their personal judgments, especially at this stage, and simply try to enumerate as many possible causes as they can think of. During an early meeting the team brainstormed to develop a complete list of possible causes that enabled them to construct the cause-and-effect or fishbone diagram shown in Figure 2.2. That cause-and-effect diagram organized the various theories under four major headings: procedures, people, policies, and databases.

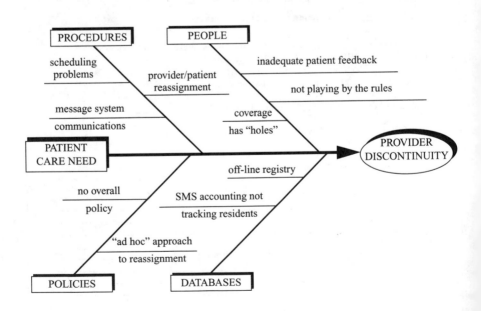

Figure 2.2 Cause-and-Effect Diagram

The exercise of developing the cause-and-effect chart encouraged team members to see connections between disparate parts of the process that might otherwise have been overlooked. Insights were expressed with statements like "You mean that's the way we have been doing things?" or "I didn't know you changed that procedure!" For example, during the August 21 meeting when the diagram was constructed, the team observed the following:

- Under procedures:
  1. Many patients did not know who their primary physician was because the formal reassignment of patients to residents had not taken place in July 1989 and July 1990.
  2. Medical records personnel had stopped transferring the name of the assigned physician into the chart in 1989.
  3. The patient scheduling system was not able to schedule patients into provider schedules more than one month in advance, due to persistent delays in getting out the provider schedules.
  4. The team approach by faculty and residents had been changed a year earlier when the FPC moved into a new building, reducing the level of communication between providers.
  5. The clerks handling patient call-ins for appointments did not have a written procedure to follow for making appointments.
- Under people:
  1. Several faculty physicians had adjusted their schedules to allow overbooking outside the routine scheduling system, possibly in an attempt to improve continuity.
- Under policies:
  1. There had not been a formal policy of promoting continuity, even though it had been a shared value. Front office staff were not aware that continuity was a priority.
- Under databases:
  1. There were three databases used in the FPC to track patient information. The one that included data on physician/patient assignments was not online and could not be readily accessed by staff when patients did not know or remember their physician's name.

Selecting Specific Causes To Address

At the next meeting the team was asked to assess which were the most important causes of discontinuity. At this stage the usual approach is to develop a Pareto chart of the causes of the problem. This chart presents the causes in order of descending frequency, which usually illustrates the Pareto Principle that whenever a number of individual factors contribute to some overall effect, a relative few of those items account for the bulk of the effect. In most cases the causes of each adverse event are identified and the frequencies of the causes charted. In this case there were no data on the specific causes of observed discontinuity. Therefore the committee was asked to vote on the importance of 11 identified causes. The five committee members present were each allowed 10 points to divide among the possible causes. The results are displayed in Figure 2.3.

Just three of the items—1, 3, and 4—gathered 55 percent of the available points. Although item 4 is a policy item ("Lack of an overall policy re: operationalizing continuity"), the first two pertained to scheduling problems. The conclusion of this exercise was that scheduling system problems were a major root cause of the discontinuity problem.

This was a surprise to several team members who thought that the assignment of patients to providers would be the area of intervention most likely to help improve continuity. Others had started out believing that the computer-assisted assignment process that matched physicians and patients would be a primary target. The dialogue around the Pareto diagram resulted in a change in some people's minds about the interactions between assignment, scheduling, and continuity. They now saw assignment, while perhaps an important issue in its own right, as having less impact on continuity than scheduling problems. Everyone involved was impressed with the efficiency of this approach. Several of the "solutions" that people brought with them to the table might have turned out to be dead ends in terms of their adverse impact on continuity.

Understanding the Scheduling System

The team decided to focus on the call-in appointment process, where most appointments were made for chronic and acute care visits. Ms. Donna Harrison assisted the team in making a flowchart of the current call-in appointment process (Figure 2.4). It was obviously a complex process in which the patient might talk to two or more FPC desk clerks or nurses before obtaining an appointment. This complexity alone might affect continuity adversely.

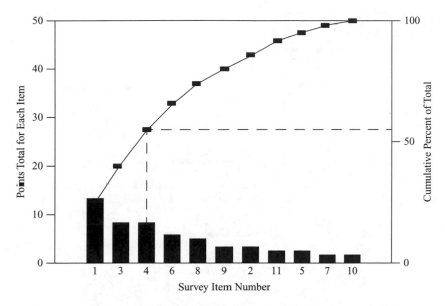

A Pareto diagram is a means of capturing and displaying the root causes, or "critical few" causes, leading to a problem, in this case provider discontinuity. The survey item numbers correspond to the following causes for provider discontinuity suggested by team members.

1. Not enough open provider appointment slots per session.
2. Not enough open appointment slots per physician, i.e., physicians not assigned enough clinic time per week.
3. Problems associated with scheduling system, e.g., too complicated, no callback system, clerks making errors.
4. Lack of an overall policy re: operationalizing continuity.
5. Conflict within the department between the goals of the residency program and those of the FPC practice.
6. An "ad hoc" approach to patient/physician assignment.
7. Problems with the process of assignment of providers to patients.
8. Not enough feedback from patients and staff when problems occur.
9. Problems due to having to use the hospital's computer database.
10. Not enough team identity in the FPC.
11. People breaking the rules and policies.

Figure 2.3 Pareto Diagram: Causes of Discontinuity, UNC Department of Family Medicine

The team meetings identified that the front desk clerks were a major influence on continuity, depending on how they would elicit patient preferences when their first choice of physician and appointment time was not available. They could offer the patient other options for times in their

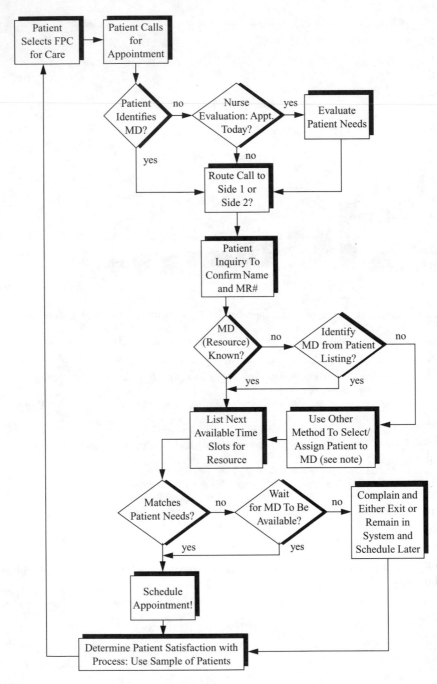

Figure 2.4 Call-In Scheduling Flowchart

regular physician's schedule (continuity), or offer the patient a different physician at the desired time (convenience). Direct observation and interviews with the clerks showed that in most cases the four clerks assumed that the patient wanted to see the first available physician (urgency) and offered the patient an appointment at his or her preferred time (convenience). This systematically biased physician scheduling against continuity.

In the absence of the specific instructions from practice management to offer the patients the continuity option, the clerks took the route most convenient and less time-consuming to themselves. Given the current system, it was much easier and less disruptive of their other tasks to schedule call-ins on the basis of the next available provider at a given time than it was to identify the primary physician and then try to fit the patient's time preferences into the available openings in the provider's schedule. Because the patient reassignment had not been done properly in the past three years and because there was no easy way to access the assignment information online, on many occasions it was impossible to identify the patient's primary physician during the course of a phone call.

Specific Recommendations

In its last three meetings the team developed specific recommendations to the department and the FPC on ways to improve provider continuity. The recommendations were grouped into five categories of potential improvement: call-in provider scheduling, provider resource planning and scheduling, provider/patient identification, information systems, and staff education and development. They called for establishing a position of "resource scheduling clerk" that would handle all call-in appointments. All four clerks would be trained for this assignment and rotate through it. This would simplify the scheduling process, especially when the scheduler had the recommended up-to-date list of patient-physician assignments and had the recommended training in procedures that would promote continuity. Figure 2.5 shows the recommended process flowchart that the TQM/CQI team developed.

Provider availability was to be expanded by increasing the number of available physicians and leaving gaps in their schedules to see acute care patients. Since it was common to tell chronically ill patients to "call in for an appointment in three months," the team recommended that the sched-

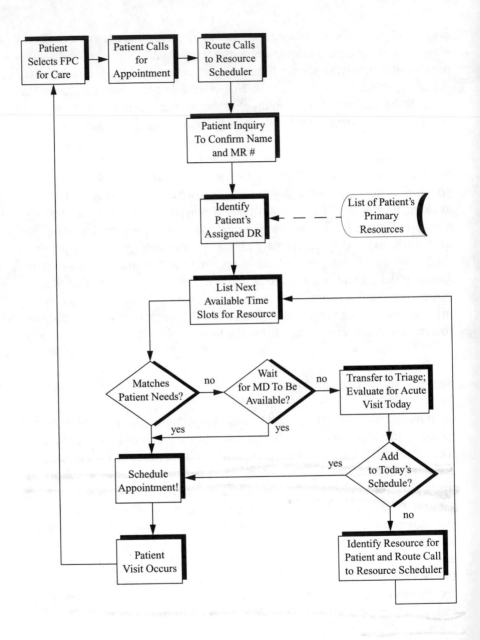

Figure 2.5 Recommended Call-In Appointment Process: Revised Flow Using Resource Scheduler

uler have physician schedules available for assignment at least three months in advance so that these patients could be scheduled with their physician before they left the building.

To promote easier identification of the primary physician, the team recommended that the practice be reorganized into four groups located on specific, color-coded hallways to assist with patient/provider identification and promote provider-to-provider communication. Once that was implemented, patients were to be given the physician's business card, which would include the names of other members of the physician's small group or "team." New patients would have labels with the physician's name affixed to their charts and to their plastic clinic registration card.

Longer term, the committee recommended a new FPC online information system to replace the existing three inflexible systems. They also made extensive recommendations concerning training, which are presented in Exhibit 2.2.

Implementation

Recommendations for changes, usually small and incremental changes, were discussed with key leaders, and some were implemented as early as the third month of the project. The formal recommendations were included in the team's December 1991 report that Dr. Kibbe prepared. It was 33 pages long plus appendices and was designed to explain TQM/CQI to the faculty and staff as well as provide a history of the process, present the data gathered, and justify the recommendations. Then the team presented its findings and recommendations to departmental grand rounds in January 1992. The presentation was well received. Most of the questions centered on the TQM process (e.g., "Why were there no clerical personnel on the original team?") and on the implications of the team system for the providers.

The FPC went ahead with the training recommendations to raise everyone's level of awareness of the need to improve continuity. The faculty and residents were organized into small practice groups located on specific, color-coded hallways to facilitate patient-provider identification, and the call-in appointment and triage procedures were changed to simplify patient and staff decisions about whom the patient would see. The FPC is planning to adopt a computerized clinical database that will integrate the

Exhibit 2.2 Recommendations in Staff Education and Development

Before initiating a program for staff education and development, a central question needs to be answered: Who is considered staff? In a TQM/CQI context, ALL individuals in the Department should be considered staff and should be educated on the processes at work in a TQM-oriented operation. The levels of participation will vary according to the activities performed (e.g., people involved in scheduling versus clinicians), but the commitment to improve should be equivalent. For the purposes of this discussion, the term "staff" will denote members of the Department, specifically the FPC, who are involved in nursing care, laboratory services, telecommunications, finances, and scheduling. However, it is important to recognize that the "top" of the organization needs to participate in the same training and education activities. Staff Education also needs to be Staff Reeducation for all those who have been operating under the current ineffective system.

It is recommended that all individuals receive training in the basic philosophy and methodology of TQM/CQI. In this trial program new and current members need to subscribe to the notion of providing *continuously improving and innovative* quality care to our primary customers, that is, the patients. Secondarily, in the context of the organization's "new" philosophy, the operational staff of the FPC should also receive an enlightened perspective towards the other major customers, the FPC clinicians.

Once adoption of the new FPC (or, alternatively, Departmental) philosophy occurs, everyone should recognize (and be recognized for) his or her contribution to the system, and become much more aware of the impact they have on efforts to improve the quality of our project (continuity of patient care) on a continuous basis. When problems occur in the system, each individual staff person should have a sense of investment to help identify, analyze, and resolve these problems. Similarly, staff should have the support and encouragement of upper and mid-level management of the FPC to accomplish this.

It is recommended that the education provided have as one of its main goals that each staff member form a clear understanding of his/her role, responsibilities, and specific duties associated with his or her position, and how it relates to the mission of the FPC and the Department as a whole. An active Mission Statement must be developed, adopted, and continuously reviewed to be of value to such a system. Adequate time must be set aside for detailed education (and continuous reeducation) of each staff member. New members of the Department, particularly staff members, cannot be

continues

Exhibit 2.2 continued

trained by coworkers who do not have a command of the "big picture." Supervisors at all levels, who will have been oriented and trained in the TQM philosophy and methods, must take initiative to develop processes to ensure that everyone has received an adequate level of training prior to beginning work. Supervisors must also create an environment where staff can achieve their maximal potential without interference or barriers. Similarly, if facts and data are used as major factors in the management of the TQM-oriented system, then this information must be made freely available to staff for continuous improvement to occur. It cannot stop there. Education and training must be a continuous process for the FPC to improve and innovate in the future.

three sets of information and relate outpatient data with hospital specialty clinic data, laboratory results, and pharmacy services in the near future.

Outcomes and Holding the Gains

The last stage of the FOCUS-PDSA cycle calls for steps to hold the improvement gains and to continue to collect data that identify the new baseline for improvement. A second chart audit on 125 randomly selected charts was conducted covering the period July 1, 1991, to June 30, 1992. The levels of continuity were up considerably from a year earlier and even above the 1984 study, as Figure 2.6 indicates. The overall continuity had increased to 74 percent from the prior year's 45 percent and was now in the range that the faculty had targeted in the TQM/CQI team's survey. Even more significantly, there were no patient complaints about continuity during the months of June, July, and August 1992.

Continuing Development

As of September 1992, there were two additional TQM/CQI teams in the FPC working on improving the timeliness of filing patient laboratory reports into patient charts and on reducing the number of charts lost or misplaced en route to and from [the medical records department]. These teams had already developed flow diagrams to clarify the processes

Visit Type	1984	1991	1992	% Change, 1991–1992
Health maintenance	0.86	0.74	0.95	+28%
Chronic illness	0.71	0.61	0.84	+38%
Acute care	0.55	0.29	0.57	+97%
Overall UPC	0.61	0.45	0.74	+64%

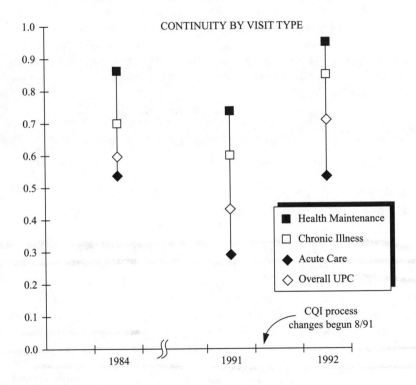

Figure 2.6 Family Practice Center: Provider Continuity Levels Pre- and Post-CQI Project Interventions. Department of Family Medicine, University of North Carolina at Chapel Hill.

involved and had collected data to obtain base-line performance figures. Faculty/resident teams now routinely included representatives from nursing, reception, and medical records in their bimonthly meetings. "Talking with data" had become much more common in committee meetings, and the tools of brainstorming, flowcharting, and cause-and-effect diagrams had become accepted tools of group work.

In conjunction with the UNC Hospitals, all employees would receive basic training in CQI methods during a half-day workshop in October, and third-year family practice residents would devote seven of their senior seminar sessions during the upcoming year to study of CQI in clinical settings. These sessions were being coordinated by Dr. Kibbe and would be open to residents in other specialties throughout the university.

CASE ANALYSIS

This effort has been successful in that the problematic indicator has been improved markedly. The staff have been sufficiently convinced of the value of the approach that new teams are being formed and are receiving cooperation and support. The reader will want to review the case to see why it was a success in an environment that many believe to be more difficult than most, a teaching faculty in a medical school.

Introduction

The approach used to assess and attack the continuity of care issues was one based on the experience of the National Demonstration Project and the Harvard Community Health Plan, where Mr. Galiani had previously worked (Berwick et al. 1990). Dr. Kibbe also espoused a Deming approach like the one outlined in Chapter 1.

This case is unusual in that a single, very simple performance measure was used, namely, the proportion of the time that the patient saw the same physician on a return visit. This issue generated a number of complaints that were recorded but not acted upon until a major customer threatened to refer its industrial medicine patients to another institution. One must wonder why the rest of the complaints had gone unheeded, although with the communication gaps uncovered by the team, that problem should not be any special surprise. The achievement in terms of the improvement in continuity of care was sufficiently significant to warrant reporting in the medical literature (Kibbe et al. 1993).

Basics

The team consisted of a mixture of clinicians and administrative staff personnel with a facilitator from the hospital's management engineering department. Many of the principles on CQI teams outlined in Chapter 6 were violated. There were no clerical staff or any residents on the team, and many of the solutions considered affected both groups. The reason for this was the educational purpose of the exercise. The team consisted of opinion leaders in the department who, once the team was successful, could provide the support for further efforts within the department involving all levels of personnel. The resistance was considered to be most likely to occur among the faculty, so they were heavily represented on the team.

Later on, the team and/or the team's staff interviewed the telephone schedulers and found out what their decision rules had been for assigning patients to available physicians and investigated the idiosyncrasies of the clinic's information systems.

The team designed a special questionnaire to assess both staff and patient interest in continuity of care. This showed that the patients had a relatively sophisticated view of continuity of care contingent on the circumstances. The staff handling the telephone calls and doing the scheduling had a unidimensional approach focused on convenience rather than factoring in the type of encounter or the issue of continuity. The questionnaire was not the kind of general satisfaction questionnaire emphasized in Chapter 5, but it is another tool typical of what a team might choose to use from time to time to get base-line data for a critical analysis.

Implementation

This case shows how the leaders of a CQI process will often choose to tailor their approach with an eye toward implementation. The team was composed of individuals who might facilitate implementation as well as process analysis. Because of this weighting, additional help was obtained from the hospital's management engineering department. Administrative staff also helped serve on the team, many of whose members would not spend large amounts of time on data gathering. Careful attention was paid to the types of professional autonomy and pride issues and the issues of physician time concerns and styles of decision making discussed in Chapter 7. When senior medical staff members missed meetings, no attempt was made to try to make them feel guilty. The work proceeded without them. Thus they remained on board to approve the findings and sanction the implementation.

Applications

The results of the team's efforts were presented at grand rounds in the department, which gave the effort academic legitimacy in the teaching setting. Then the results were written up in article form and submitted to an academic journal. The publication of those results was intended to enhance the acceptance of CQI efforts and concepts as a part of the array of approaches relevant to academic medicine (see Chapter 16).

CASE 3

Holston Valley Hospital and Medical Center

Curtis P. McLaughlin and Kit N. Simpson

After five years of training and team projects, Mr. Paul Bishop, administrator of Holston Valley Hospital and Medical Center (HVHMC), was seeing the positive results of his quality management program in many ways in administrative areas, but he was still concerned about how to make more headway with the clinical use of resources.

Quality improvement had become a community-wide effort in Kingsport, a thriving industrial town of 36,365 in northeastern Tennessee. Quality management was a community-wide concern, involving employers, the Chamber of Commerce, the school system, the community college, and both hospitals in town. Most people agree that this concern began in 1982 with Eastman Chemical Company (Eastman), a subsidiary of Eastman Kodak employing over 11,000 at its Kingsport plants. Faced with stiff foreign competition in its markets, Eastman adopted a program that included a customer focus, employee empowerment, statistical methods, performance management, continuous improvement, education, and training management leadership. This program received an all-out push in 1985, and in 1988 Eastman was one of the nine finalists for the Malcolm Baldrige National Quality Award. Exhibit 3.1 outlines the sequence of quality events at the hospital and in the community.

QUALITY FIRST

In 1986 Eastman executives were instrumental in having the Chamber of Commerce sponsor a QUALITY FIRST training session for community

Exhibit 3.1 Quality Events Time Line

The Community/Hospital Partnership	
Community	**Hospital**
	Quality Assurance Trained
	In Quality Improvement Tech.
Iowa Headquarters of 1991	
Heritage Started with MFE	Quality Assurance Merged
	with Quality Management
Area Hospitals Working Together	
To Sponsor Quality Management	
Seminar 1990	Hospital Board Instructed
	in MFE
Heritage HMO Started	
Improvement Project	Administrative Team
	Started Training
Kingsport Area Healthcare	
Improvement Process Formed 1989	
National Center for	Hospital Introduced to
Quality Established	Managing for Excellence
MFE Consulting Training	MFE Consulting Training
Offered to City	Offered to Hospital
	The Sixth Project Team
City of Kingsport	to Quality First Training
Started with MFE 1988	
School System Introduced to	Admission Process
Performance Management	Redesigned and Shortened
1987	
Quality First Started at	Patient Satisfaction
Northeast State. Tech.	Instrument Implemented
Kingsport Foundry	
Started Effort 1986	Hospital Introduced to
Chamber of Commerce	Project Improvement
Researching Quality	
Customer Focus 1982	
at Eastman Chemical	
—Holston Valley Hospital and Medical Center—	

leaders at Northeast State Community College (then called Tri-Cities Community College). Mr. Bishop and a team of Holston Valley Hospital executives attended it. The program was taught by two professors from Jackson Community College in Michigan, where the QUALITY FIRST program had been developed with assistance from the Ford Motor Company. QUALITY FIRST is a 16-week, project-focused program for teams of four or more from a firm. It emphasizes data collection and analysis, control charting, and prevention of error methods, all generally based on the precepts of W. Edwards Deming. Mr. Bishop, trained as a hospital administrator, was impressed with the approach and continued to send teams, more than 20 teams with approximately 90 participants. Documented savings at HVHMC from these team efforts included $72,000 in lower costs of linens, reductions in nurse turnover (costing $10,000–20,000 per nurse) of six percent, and reductions of medication delivery lead time from the pharmacy to the nursing floors from 3 to 1¼ hours.

The executives on that first team in August 1986 had trouble translating Deming concepts like a "single supplier" into the hospital context. Since they did not directly supervise service delivery, they took as their project the development of a patient satisfaction survey. Yet they sent four more teams that year, mostly on the basis of the reported successes of the industrial teams. Then they began to see results like the following:

- Admitting wait and processing times were reduced from 30 minutes to 5.6 minutes.
- Preadmission lab testing went from 30 percent to 75 percent.
- Length of stay dropped one day, mostly due to the efforts of the discharge planning team.

In some ways the QUALITY FIRST program was ideal for the hospital. People were gone only one day every other week for 16 weeks. The course was project-oriented, so people could see the effects in the workplace.

Partnerships for Excellence

Seven major projects were completed by the end of 1988, but Mr. Bishop wanted to speed up the process. So did the city manager of Kingsport. He went to Eastman Chemical, which agreed to donate the services of Mr. David J. McClaskey, a quality management coordinator, to help adapt and use his "Managing for Excellence" training course to allow

HVHMC to bring quality training "in-house." David McClaskey was an examiner for the Malcolm Baldrige National Quality Award and helped develop the examiner preparation course. One assistant administrator at HVHMC, Mr. Dale Richardson, received more than 100 hours of training. Then the management team and two potential in-house facilitators—a nurse and a business manager—went through the initial 80 hours of training over about seven months. During this initial run the participants found that about 30 percent of the material required modification to replace industrial illustrations with health situations. With Mr. McClaskey's cooperation they modified the material, which they now call "Partnerships for Excellence." By June 1991 the hospital was staffed with six full-time facilitators. The hospital had some 23 "natural teams," which included direct reporting relationships from the administrator through assistant administrators to department directors and to their supervisors. By June 1991, 80 percent of the natural teams had completed the "Partnerships for Excellence" process, with the remainder scheduled to complete the process within eight months.

The total quality management (TQM) program consisted of four training modules. The first 80-hour module was for natural teams (groups with common supervision). It was an introduction to Deming's (1986) 14 points, the Red Bead Experiment, team-building exercises, listening skills, managing customer expectations, developing process measures, flow-charting, statistical thinking, and the whole QUALITY FIRST process, followed by an exercise in developing a performance management plan for the unit and planning the rollout of quality improvement in the department. There were also two modules on process teams and one on quality improvement projects, averaging 40 hours each. Process and project teams were both responsible for multifunctional issues, with the process teams intending to maintain their oversight of a process and the project teams having more of an ad hoc nature.

An example of a quality improvement project was the one concerned with nursing turnover, which had been averaging 25 percent annually. The initial task had been to define turnover, measure it, and then set a goal of reducing the rate. The target for reduction was set at 6 percent, with the new target at 19 percent. Figure 3.1 illustrates the run chart developed by the team before and after its efforts started in August 1990 with four-hour meetings every other week. The project team decided not to deal with nursing recruitment, with anyone working less than 32 hours per month, with issues of absenteeism, or with non-nursing employee turnover. Turn-

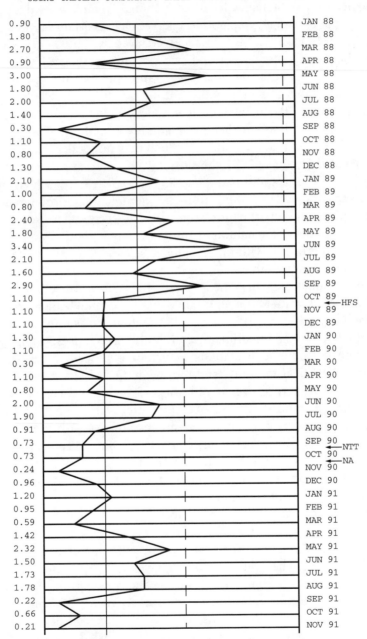

Figure 3.1 Run Chart of Nursing Turnover

over was defined as the number of full- and part-time equivalents (FTEs) transferred/terminated/resigned monthly, divided by the budgeted number of full- and part-time RN, LPN, nonlicensed, and clerical personnel FTEs. There was always a tension over whether to focus on total employee turnover or RN turnover only. There was a tangible need to benchmark HVHMC against other comparable hospitals to test the target of a six-percent annual turnover reduction that some had presented. The costs of recruiting and training a new RN-level nurse had been estimated at $10,000 to $20,000.

Not all groups received the full 80 hours, since the program can be modularized, especially the process teams. A process team works together for an extended period of time to study an important patient care process. An example might be the "heart process" involving open heart and cardiac cath patients. Process teams were started most recently, require a well-trained facilitator, and generate the most conflict. Mr. Bishop noted, "We are still developing the process team framework. It is very hard for managers to stay out of the business of the process team long enough for them to produce results—we have found that we have had to limit participation of managers unless they are specifically assigned to the team." Exhibits 3.2 and 3.3 show how the roles of the natural teams and process teams have been defined to deal with the ownership role, called the role of *process steward* at HVHMC.

Exhibit 3.2 Relationship of Process Teams and Natural Management Teams (Owners)

- Process Teams regularly report progress/accomplishments to Natural Team.
- Owner and the Process Team member communicate to all departmental employees information regarding changes to the process.
- Priorities of what to work on are discussed and negotiated with Department Natural Team.
- In determining what to work on, Process Team considers input from:
  −customers of process
  −team members
  −"Owner's Team"
- Major decisions and changes to process should be discussed with Departmental Natural Team.

—Holston Valley Hospital and Medical Center—

Exhibit 3.3 Responsibilities of Process Teams*

1. Understand customer needs and define customer requirements.
2. Determine where the process stands in relation to customer requirements.
3. Study/analyze process:
   A. Flowcharts
   B. Discussions with people involved with process
   C. Analysis of data
   D. Benchmarks
4. Determine measures of process:
   A. Results/output measures
   B. In-process
5. Determine and list areas for improvement.
6. Feedback to Natural Unit Management Team.*
7. Work on improvement projects agreed on by Natural Unit Management Team.
8. Routinely manage the overall process by:
   A. Monitoring process measures.
   B. Detecting and appropriately responding to process upsets that cannot be handled routinely within the process.
   C. Receiving and listing ideas to improve the process.

*When appropriate, the "team" can be just the process steward.

—Holston Valley Hospital and Medical Center—

When a team completes the program, its members receive certificates, called licenses (implying the need for renewal), at a celebration ceremony in front of all the managers, including first-line supervisors. Often a figure from the community and/or the hospital board is asked to hand out the certificates.

HVHMC has also adopted the "Service Excellence" modules developed by the Einstein group of Philadelphia.

Of the hospital's 1,800 employees, 1,500 have received this training, with the rest slated to receive it by the end of 1991.

Community Competition

The Tri-Cities area, involving Johnson City, Kingsport, and Bristol, Tennessee, and Bristol, Virginia, represents the nation's 82nd largest Metropolitan Statistical Area (MSA), with a 1990 population of 436,047.

It ranked 31st out of the 281 MSAs in manufacturing earnings as a percent of total earnings in 1988. During the first quarter of 1991, when the national unemployment rate was 7.1 percent, Kingsport's rate was 3.8 percent, Johnson City's 5.6 percent, and Bristol TN-VA's 5.4 percent. It is heavily doctored. There are four substantial hospitals, two in Kingsport, and a medical school as part of East Tennessee State University in Johnson City. By mid-1991 Kingsport had 18 obstetrician-gynecologists with two more coming soon. Hospital lengths of stay, despite managed care, were above the national average. Advertising for hospitals and physicians abounds in the press, on billboards, and in local business periodicals.

Both HVHMC and Indian Path Medical Center, owned by Hospital Corporation of America (HCA), operated well below their licensed bed level. HVHMC was licensed for 540 beds, after giving up 50 beds to help bring in a for-profit rehab hospital, but operated 350 to 375 beds, having converted its wards and semiprivate rooms to all-private room status. Most community-based physicians practiced at both hospitals. Most of the physicians in the town belonged to the Kingsport Independent Practitioners' Association (IPA), which contracted to deliver services to Heritage National Healthplan (an HMO established and owned by John Deere, initially founded to service its own employees). Sixty-two percent of Eastman Chemical Company's employees were covered under contracts with Heritage. The rest were covered by Blue Cross-Blue Shield of Tennessee under a contract that covered a wide range of services, including some preventive care. Table 3.1 provides a financial and statistical statement of operations for fiscal years ending June 30, 1988 to 1992.

HVHMC was structured with a parent holding company, Holston Valley Health Care, Inc. (HVHC). The hospital was one of three separate divisions, together with a foundation for endowment and the for-profit HVS Company, which managed a home health agency, respiratory therapy services, weight loss programs, psychiatric counseling, laundry, and other services to physicians' offices, and a number of joint ventures, including diagnostic imaging. HVHMC included a trauma center, a neonatal intensive care unit, an open-heart surgery team, and a cancer center. It was one of the larger servers of the medically indigent in the state.

Indian Path Medical Center administrative team had also participated in the same initial QUALITY FIRST training program. They also had gone through HCA's Deming-based quality management training in 1989. One project there had reduced outpatient registration wait time from 35 minutes to 5 minutes.

Table 3.1 Comparative Statement of Operations

	Year Ended 6-30-88	Year Ended 6-30-89	Year Ended 6-30-90	Year Ended 6-30-91	Est. Year Ended 6-30-92
FINANCIALS ($)					
Patient serv. revenue	100,184	118,130	137,970	164,926	193,738
Revenue deductions	24,992	30,551	41,629	51,562	68,195
Other operating revenue	2,438	2,457	4,672	5,781	4,407
Net revenue	77,630	90,036	101,013	119,145	130,950
Operating expenses	74,857	86,849	97,935	113,356	129,470
Nonoperating revenue	963	768	1,922	1,867	3,271
Nonoperating expenses	512	601	130	39	58
Net nonoperating income	451	167	1,792	1,828	3,214
Net gain (loss)	3,224	3,354	4,870	7,617	4,693
STATISTICS					
Adult admissions	15,202	15,804	15,718	15,432	14,970
Adult patient days	111,803	110,459	105,498	106,304	103,368
Newborn days	4,982	4,594	4,444	4,889	4,657
Open heart cases	469	498	496	556	547
Surgical procedures	7,949	8,266	8,872	9.657	10,291
Same day service visits	5,637	5,563	5,344	6,961	7,931
Emergency room visits	52,943	55,725	56,294	57,086	58,324
Radiological procedures	75,959	77,797	78,963	81,318	84,662
CT scan procedures	6,784	7,098	7,523	8,263	8,941
Lab procedures	824,391	903,724	978,338	1,020,393	1,108,309
Cath lab procedures	2,416	2,010	2,103	2,224	2,428
MRI procedures	1,742	2,839	3,889	4,113	3,968
Length of stay	7.3	7.0	6.7	6.9	6.9
Average FTEs	1,578	1,707	1,666	1,820	2,323
FTEs/avg. occup. bed	4.3	4.7	4.7	5.0	5.3

Community Cooperation

Despite the intense competition, Kingsport also became involved in a cooperative effort to improve the community's health. In 1988 the Midwest Business Group on Health, after studying health purchasing and quality assessment tools, received funding from the John A. Hartford Foundation of New York to develop three demonstration sites for community cooperation to stress teamwork and reduce variation in health. Kingsport became the first demonstration site. Someone at HCA, which itself invests heavily in Deming-based quality management programs, suggested Kingsport and the request was finally brought to the attention of Mr. Rob Johnson, manager of benefits coordination at Eastman. He coordinated the development of the Kingsport Area Health Improvement Project (KAHIP), which involved representatives of the Kingsport Area Business Council on Health Care (KABACH), HVHMC, Indian Path Medical Center, Indian Path Pavilion (psychiatric), the IPA, and Heritage. After going through an intensive quality training session, the KAHIP members' representatives reviewed the health problems affecting Kingsport's population and finally selected the area of respiratory diseases as their focus. Four improvement projects were undertaken:

- reducing the number of readmissions for chronically ill respiratory patients, whom the group dubbed "frequent flyers"
- developing a more effective process for transitioning respiratory patients to nursing homes
- developing a process to encourage youth to quit/not start smoking
- determining the most appropriate means of conducting third-party utilization review

Three of the teams attended the QUALITY FIRST program with their tuition paid for by the Midwest Business Group on Health, and the four worked with an individual facilitator. In retrospect, Rob Johnson noted that this process was frustrating. "We didn't do a good job of using our project selection criteria. The projects we selected were difficult to deal with. They were too broad or aimed at a system instead of a process. Our data system wasn't effective enough to narrow the projects down to processes." Ownership was also a problem in this type of organization. "Everybody has ownership or nobody has ownership. Because KAHIP is a community-oriented project, no one organization could claim ownership." Three of the four teams have continued to meet, and the superintendent of schools is trying to reorganize the youth and smoking team. The team working with nursing home placements has had some concrete successes, and the other teams continue to collect and interpret data.

The Heritage National HMO has also started its own quality management program in Kingsport and at its Illinois headquarters, assisted by facilitators from Eastman and HVHMC. Under the leadership of the physicians in the IPA and a team from the IPA, the HMO and the hospitals studied the resources used for postsurgical care of gallbladder removals. They found that there were about as many processes as there were physicians and developed a standard process. The net result has been to reduce the average length of stay for this procedure by two days. Dean Anderson, operations manager of Heritage, says, "Ultimately we hope to have improvement teams in physician's offices. Potential improvement areas we've identified include pediatric office scheduling, lab work, and billing processes. We want to spread the quality virus and get all physicians involved. Physicians develop different practices, but through quality we hope to combine the various procedures into one formalized process."

Dr. Paul Pearlman, president of the IPA, comments, "As physicians, we have to be interested in promoting health care. Physicians have varied backgrounds, so everyone manages problems differently. What we're trying to do through KAHIP is find out why there are variations and how we can reduce them to make our processes better. It shouldn't make a difference which emergency room a person goes to. What's important is that they get quality care wherever they go." One fact that encouraged Rob Johnson was the physicians' choice of low-cost California managed care group practices as their cost and length of stay benchmark for their gallbladder study.

KAHIP has also become the task force on health for the Kingsport Tomorrow project, a community-wide program to envision Kingsport in the twenty-first century. Rob Johnson observed that "we're reassessing teams, poring over new data systems and targeting physicians' offices for facilitators. If we can't zero in on the problems with our present projects, then we'll discontinue them. There are a lot of resources yet to be tapped. We feel we haven't accomplished a great deal, but others looking at Kingsport and KAHIP from the outside see what we're doing here and are amazed. While it's natural for us in Kingsport to cooperate, it is not in other communities."

Community cooperation was the style in Kingsport. Eastman and the other employers wanted a happy, attractive community to attract skilled personnel to their expanding businesses. On the other hand, if health care costs had to be cut, they could and would act unilaterally. Eastman had made a study of medical admissions for low back pain and had severely restricted payments for that service. The number of admissions and their length dropped sharply, especially the admissions by primary care physicians. Eastman was aware that it could achieve the lowest health care costs by selecting a subset of physicians in the town and forming a closed-panel HMO, but Rob Johnson did not want anything that confrontational yet. "That just is not Eastman's style." Besides, he felt that it was best to work with the total system rather than minimizing Eastman's share, since cost shifting one way or another ended up saddling employers with the costs of uncompensated care throughout the community.

National Center for Quality

Another cooperative venture of the quality management community in the Tri-Cities area, building on the QUALITY FIRST program, is the National Center for Quality. This is a nonprofit corporation formed by the three chambers of commerce in 1988 that is dedicated to promoting a national interest in quality and productivity improvement. It has established a core set of courses for organizations to call on. Exhibit 3.4 shows the board membership as of January 1990. In June of 1989, Jim Wallin, community programs coordinator for Eastman, was loaned to the center as its interim director. In January 1990 the board approved handing over the operation to Northeast State Technical Institute, and Al Thomas, director of the QUALITY FIRST program, was asked to serve as part-time executive director of the center.

The center offers a number of courses:

- Seizing the Quality Initiative
- Leading the Quality Transformation
- Survey Techniques
- Quality and Performance Management for Educators
- Malcolm Baldrige National Quality Award
- Managing for Excellence in Healthcare

It currently has under development programs on Quality for Small Business and Quality Consultant Training. On August 5–6, 1991, the center in cooperation with the four area hospitals offered "A Competitive Healthcare and Quality Management Conference." The conference coordinator was Ms. Esther Luster, an assistant administrator at HVHMC. Paul Bishop observed, "Our psychological contract with the supporters of quality management includes our making a special effort to disseminate

Exhibit 3.4 National Center for Quality: Members of the Board

R. C. Hart Eastman Chemical Company *(Chairman of the Board)*	Bill Ring Kingsport Foundry and Manufacturing Corp.
Curtis Burnette Aerojet Ordinance Tennessee *(President)*	Don Royston Kingsport Chamber of Commerce
Will Hutsell Eastman Chemical Company *(Vice President)*	Dennis Wagner United Telephone System
Dr. R. Wade Powers Northeast State Technical Community College *(Treasurer)*	Marie Williams Greater Bristol Area Chamber of Commerce Jerry Moeller Bristol Regional Medical Center
D. Lynn Johnson Eastman Chemical Company *(Secretary)*	Tim Jones Johnson City Chamber of Commerce
Al Thomas National Center for Quality *(Executive Director)*	Ed Fennell City of Johnson City Dr. James Hales East Tennessee State University
Vic Dingus Eastman Chemical Company	Ann Peace Kingsport, TN
James R. White Eastman Chemical Company	Reneau Dubberly Johnson City, TN
Paul Bishop Holston Valley Hospital and Medical Center	Jim Wallin Eastman Chemical Company
	Dick Wetherell Texas Instruments
John Andersen First American National Bank	Dr. Allan Spritzer College of Business, East Tennessee State University

—Holston Valley Hospital and Medical Center—

our story." The second conference was held April 23–24, 1992, and included such well-known presenters as Dr. Paul Batalden, vice-president of medical affairs at HCA, and Dr. James Roberts of the Joint Commission on Accreditation of Healthcare Organizations.

Activities at HVHMC

Paul Bishop was genuinely pleased with the hospital and the community efforts, which were attracting national recognition. For example, he had been asked to prepare and give a presentation at the 1991 *Business Week* Symposium of Health Care CEOs, Rockefeller Center, New York City, June 20–21, 1991, which he entitled "Innovation as a Team Sport: Solutions Through Partnership" (Bishop 1991). Yet when asked about issues to be worked on, he replied, "There are hundreds of them. In health care the average time that people are satisfied with an improved service is half an hour. They immediately internalize the new achievement as the new standard and complain about how poor the service is." Over time, however, he felt that people were beginning to realize that the quality of care had genuinely improved.

His major concerns beyond day-to-day implementation were: (1) how fast to change the organizational structure and the human resource infrastructure to adjust to quality management and performance management, (2) how to increase the emphasis on quality management in clinical decision making, and (3) how to get his vision of the future of this change process across to people. Early on the quality assurance (QA) effort was merged with and made subordinate to the quality management program. The existing QA staff, two medical records specialists who had been doing physician utilization review, were assigned to the new head of quality management, a former nursing supervisor. They then received quality management training. The quality management department grew rapidly with the addition of the six quality management facilitators with the titles of Quality Management Consultant. Their backgrounds included nursing supervision, clinical laboratory support, financial office support, quality management with the telephone company, undergraduate training in statistics, and medical records experience. Dale Richardson, the assistant administrator responsible for quality management, had worked as a consultant with SunHealth, a hospital consulting firm in Charlotte, North Carolina, before coming to Kingsport and still took occasional quality management assignments with them.

The performance appraisal system had been modified somewhat to include contributions to quality management, and so had the job descriptions. Yet Paul Bishop was still concerned about how fast to move away from the periodic appraisal system and toward performance management. Some senior managers who had been successful under the old style of management and believed that "the cream rises to the top" would probably resist such a move. This didn't mean that institutionalization of the concepts of quality management wasn't pretty far along. People had internalized the concepts and terms throughout the organization. A number of physicians were quite interested in some of the projects. Some people who had complained about their supervisors' passiveness were actually saying that they saw positive changes in management, while others sometimes complained about too much time spent in meetings.

The original heart process team had not been terribly successful because the individuals responsible for spearheading the process review had come from outside it. "We went to school on that one," one of the internal consultants said. "Since then the process stewards have all come from within the process. That cuts down on barriers and defensiveness." During the past year, the team and a consulting company—APM—from New York that specializes in service line development have made great strides with the heart process. The key has been in getting commitment from the physicians for improvement of the process, including cost control.

The Linen Management System

The eighth group sent to Tri-Cities Tech, for example, was a team composed of four members of nursing staff, the director of linen and laundry services, and a hospital buyer. The project assigned to them by the administrative staff was the frequent set of complaints from the nursing units about the shortage or excess of laundry delivered by the in-house laundry to the floors. The laundry department had tried to project the daily nursing usage on each unit, but there was little communication or coordination between the laundry and the nursing units. The existing system provided no linen accountability or control and poor utilization of personnel.

When the team first met, there was little agreement on the perceived cause of this lack of coordination. Through the use of brainstorming sessions, the group reached a consensus on improving the linen distribution system. They developed the system flowchart shown in Figure 3.2. The team identified all the units involved in the process, which involved the purchase of linen, its processing by the laundry, and its distribution over two miles of hospital corridors to 22 nursing unit linen closets. They then prepared the cause-and-effect (fishbone) diagram relating to inadequate linen distribution shown in Figure 3.3.

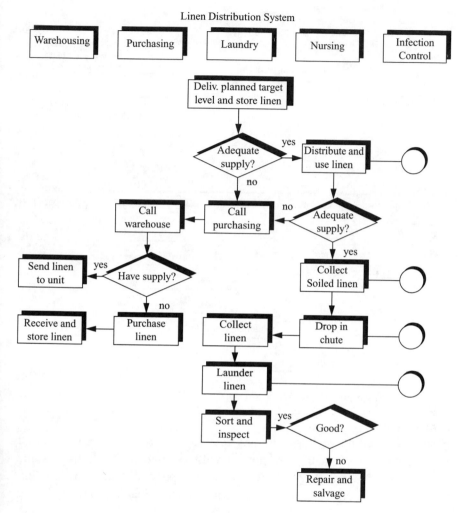

Figure 3.2 Flowchart for Linen Distribution

The group realized that they were still dealing with rather broad generalities and knew little about the specifics of linen utilization. With the cooperation of the 22 nursing units, a linen inventory was conducted. On February 8, 1989, the nursing staff arrived at work to find that their first task was to count each clean piece of linen in patient rooms and linen closets. Then for the next two days all soiled linen was sent to the laundry in bags color-coded by the unit of origin so that the laundry could do a usage count. These counts are shown as Figures 3.4 and 3.5. A tour of the

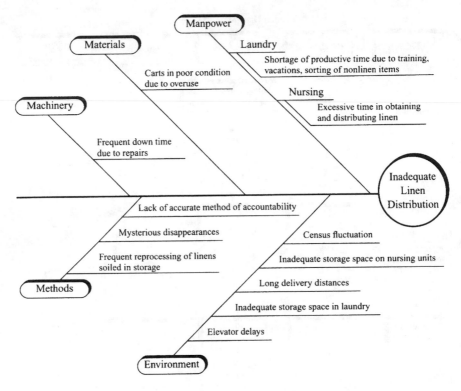

Figure 3.3 Cause-and-Effect Diagram for Linen Distribution

hospital left team members agreeing that there were adequate supplies of linens but they were distributed poorly, with too many washcloths on some units and too few on others. Crowded storage spaces did not allow enough room for storing enough pillows on most units, also leading to linen falling on the floor and needing to be reprocessed. If a unit could not store enough pillows in the linen closet, housekeeping then arranged to store some in the closets of the patient rooms.

The team then decided to conduct a pilot test of linen control on the Neuro-Orthopedics Unit. Control charts were developed based on data on usage over a 16-day period. Linen closets were rearranged and shelves labeled and marked with red tape to meet planned levels. Figure 3.6 contains an example of these control charts. Target inventory levels were set at the upper control limits on these C-charts. Since each day the closets were stocked neatly up to the specified amount, there were few shortages necessitating trips to the laundry and no excesses. The team calculated that

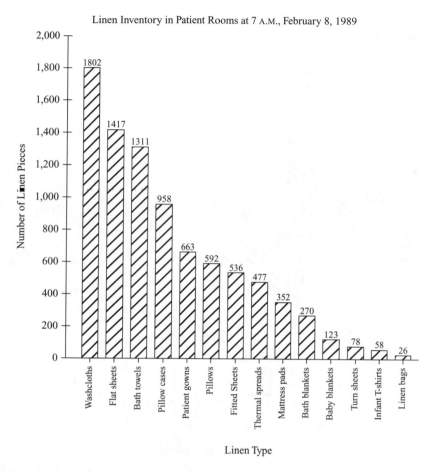

Figure 3.4 Sample Clean Linen Inventory Report

the saving in inventory investment on the pilot floor was more than 50 percent. Extrapolated to the whole hospital, the reduction in investment was estimated at $72,000.

An unexpected benefit resulted from the fact that the pilot unit was going to be renovated and the new plans called for inadequate linen storage space. The team went to the architect and the hospital administration and arranged to have the storage space increased.

The team reported that there were additional savings in personnel time and energy that were difficult to quantify. They suggested that the amount of linen stored could be reduced even further if the laundry had more

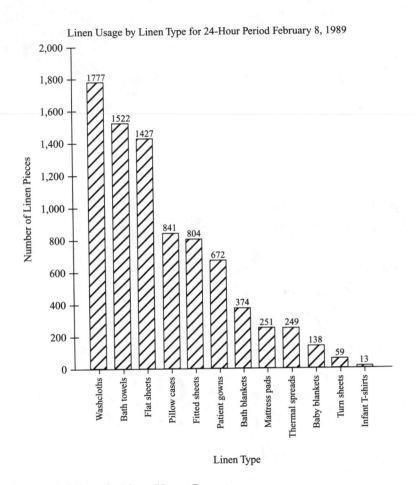

Figure 3.5 Sample Linen Usage Report

storage space, if laundry equipment reliability was improved, or if "mysterious disappearance of linen inventory" could be countered.

The linen team decided to stay intact to expand the approach to all nursing and ancillary departments, to expand the system to additional items such as scrub suits, and to monitor and adjust the system to changing requirements.

Radiology Transport Team

The radiology process team attended the QUALITY FIRST Project training a little after the linen team. The radiology process team met with

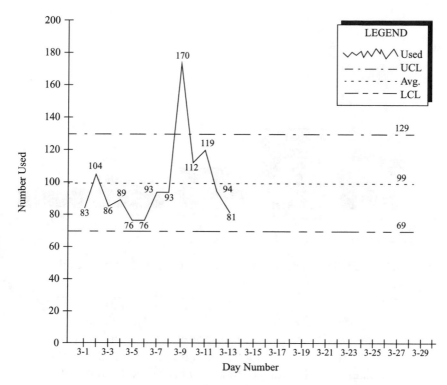

Figure 3.6 Sample Control Chart for Bath Towel Usage

the administrative management team to discuss major improvement opportunities (MIOs) and selected (1) financial viability, (2) high touch, and (3) decreased length of stay. Various subgroups were asked to develop a priority listing for improvements. The one developed by the radiology technologists is shown as Figure 3.7. Their priorities were representative, so the team went to work on processes used to transport inpatients. Patients were constantly complaining that it took too long to get back to their rooms after an exam; in some cases waits of up to two hours were noted. Staff members complained of delays in sending for patients. If a patient was sent for at 10:00 a.m., he or she might not arrive until 2:00 p.m. or 3:00 p.m. Then work flow was disrupted, schedules were delayed, and referring physicians were upset with the total wait time. These delays could hold up other tests and procedures and have a negative impact on the length of stay.

The team decided to focus on patient delays in radiology and the wait time after a procedure was complete on an inpatient. The first piece of data collection was to determine the amount of time it would take an able-

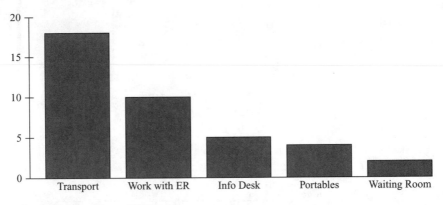

Step 1: Why Choose This Improvement Project?

Developed during February 1990 Meeting

Figure 3.7 Radiology Improvement Projects: Priority Listing Developed by Techs

bodied transporter (orderly) to walk from the furthest point in the hospital to the radiology department. The transporter team member reported 15 minutes. Therefore the team set its standard for a wait for transportation as 15 to 30 minutes. A technologist team member asked each patient over a period of several days what he or she felt was a reasonable wait after a procedure. Patients appeared to consider less than 10 minutes a reasonable time and 20 minutes to be the maximum. Given a focused definition of the problem, the team then decided to find the root cause. They started with a flow diagram (Figure 3.8). With the aid of their facilitator, the team then developed a cause-and-effect diagram (Figure 3.9). Based on this understanding of the process, the team conducted a survey of the transporters about the causes of the delays they encountered. They confirmed the importance of a lack of wheelchairs and stretchers, the subject of another team's analysis that was already underway.

An initial survey showed that the system was meeting the target less than 50 percent of the time. However, there were some questions about the times reported under the "honor system," so a new study was conducted using a Simplex clocking device on which the technologist clocked in when the patient was sent for and the transporter clocked in when he received the card and when he left the radiology department. With the new data system, the figures improved, but still were unsatisfactory 32 percent of the time.

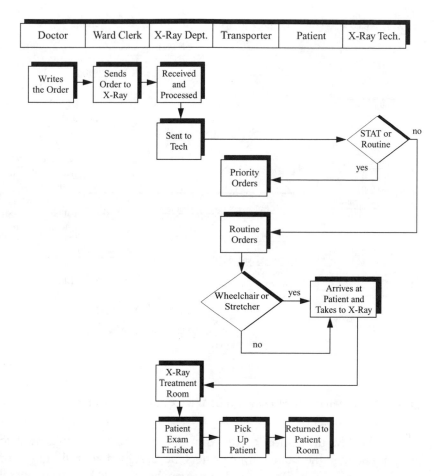

Figure 3.8 Radiology Transport Process

Further study identified the fact that seven radiology transporters all worked various areas of the imaging section. Furthermore, they reported not to a radiology manager, but to dispatch services, a source of territorial battles and attitudinal problems. The head of dispatch service was asked to join the team. The other team members suggested that the radiology transporters should be pooled.

At the transporters' suggestion, each transporter kept a detailed log of how time was spent, accounting for transport travel time (TP.T.), travel to and from the patient (T.T.), and dead time (D.T.). Over half of the time was dead time, raising questions about the perceived need for more transporters (Figure 3.10).

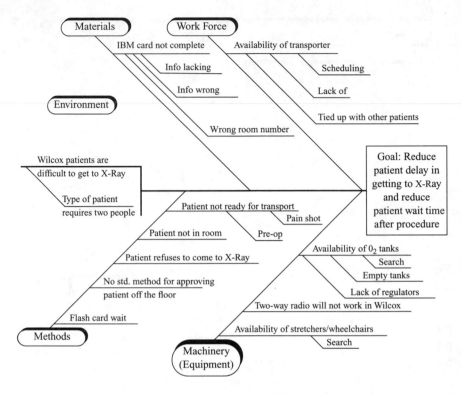

Figure 3.9 Cause-and-Effect Diagram of What Causes the Delays

Given the low utilization of the transporters, the team suggested to management that the seven transporters be assigned to radiology for supervision, solving the issues of "Who is my boss?" and be retrained and upgraded to the position of Radiology Assistant so that they could perform duties such as developing film and obtaining reports. This would help solve the attitude problems since it would expand the job and increase the pay.

During the implementation phase a radio base was purchased, an area was set up for the transporters, and the six months of retraining commenced. At the time of the team presentation, nursing administration was putting pressure on dispatch services to cover weekend shifts without overtime costs. Radiology and administration worked this out in radiology by adding one person to be a dispatcher. The team report noted that, "In all there will be cost in a radio base, carpentry work, raise in pay, and one full-time employee. Sounds like a lot of money and not very financially viable."

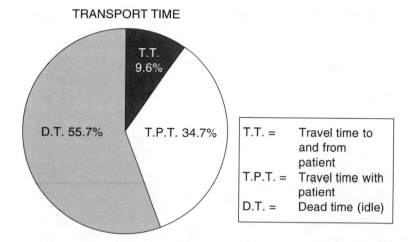

TRANSPORT TIME

T.T. =	Travel time to and from patient	
T.P.T. =	Travel time with patient	
D.T. =	Dead time (idle)	

Figure 3.10 Radiology Transporter Time Breakdown (Seven-Day Average)

The original seven [transporters] covered shifts from 6:00 a.m. to 8:00 p.m., Monday through Friday, and overtime shifts from 7:00 a.m. to 4:00 p.m. on Saturday only. Upon implementation, the shifts covered will be 5:30 a.m. to 11:00 p.m., Monday through Friday, and 7:00 a.m. to 11:00 p.m., Saturday and Sunday. At the addition of one employee, 53 additional hours will be added to the transportation schedule. Overtime has been reduced, the overall utilization of transportation has been increased, and we are projecting this to be at no cost. Now that is financial viability that even Sam Walton would be interested in.

Moving on to Clinical Quality

The hospital had recently received its initial set of SysteMetrics/McGraw-Hill IMPAQ III reports, one of the first sets sent out, providing internal resource utilization, mortality, and complications by diagnosis, by payer, and by physician. Paul Bishop saw two major issues right now: (1) how to adjust them for patient risk, and (2) how to transmit the information to the physicians in a way that would maintain the spirit of cooperation that existed, but still motivate review and action. HVHMC looked good on mortality and not as good on resource utilization. Tables 3.2 and 3.3 show some sample statistics from that report, which, except for the mortality

Table 3.2 Resource Demand Information by Payer, October–December 1990

	Cases	Percent Cases	Mortality Ratio	Days Exceeding Expectation	Charges Exceeding Expectation
All cases	4,197	100		0	
Medicare		47.8	1.263	2,347	616,185
Medicaid		10.3	1.444	−1,185	−146,910
Commercial		19.1	1.091	−471	−281,633
Blue Cross		9.5	0.667	−273	−132,976
HMO		3.8	3.0	−297	−185,562
Self pay		6.7	0.667	−35	212,526
Workers' Comp.		2.8	0.5	−86	− 85,944

data and average DRG [diagnosis-related group] weights, were based entirely on internal comparisons. The same data were available by individual physician. The variable "payer mix index" was based on the amount that the hospital was actually paid after contractual discounts and allowances, claims denials, and bad debts. Other definitions are shown in Exhibit 3.5.

In some situations Paul Bishop was not sure whether the discrepancies were due to coding errors or biases or rooted in physician behaviors. He wanted to use this new information in a way that would enhance HVHMC's effectiveness and financial viability. The hospital was currently operating in the black, and he wanted it to stay that way. On the other hand, he had been careful so far to have the quality program avoid issues that might upset physicians enough to take more of their cases to competing hospitals.

Rob Johnson had suggested sharing the data with the IPA and letting them take ownership for the quality improvement process. "Our experiences with medical backs and gallbladders show that changes in physician practice patterns show up immediately in both hospitals. Why should Paul pay all the costs of the change when Indian Path will get just as much benefit?"

CASE ANALYSIS

Eastman is convinced of the value of TQM and is trying to get all major organizations, including the town government, the schools, and the hospi-

Table 3.3 Resource Demand Information by Product Line, October–December 1990

	Cases	Efficiency Ratio	LOS Ratio	Avg. DRG Scale	HVHMC Resource Demand Index	Payer Mix Index
Cardiac—med.	651	84.9	1.2	1.0752	0.853	66
Cardiac—surg.	162	93.5	1.1	1.0799	4.670	69
Cancer—med.	158	112.3	1.2	1.0677	0.891	64
Cancer—surg.	45	89.2	1.1	1.0044	1.125	66
Neuro—med.	222	76.8	1.0	0.9673	0.730	70
Neuro—surg.	110	96.2	1.1	0.8965	1.894	73
Renal/Uro—med.	98	102.6	1.1	0.9996	0.639	65
Renal/Uro—surg.	61	82.0	0.9	0.9169	0.673	69
Women's health	573	111.3	0.4	0.9665	0.397	67
Ortho	238	94.1	1.2	0.9580	1.229	67
Respiratory	310	82.3	1.1	1.0569	1.276	64
Medicine	530	99.2	1.3	1.0055	0.623	66
Gen. surg.	225	101.0	1.0	0.9895	1.310	69
Other surg.	265	97.5	1.2	1.1616	1.521	68
Newborn	341	153.0	0.8	1.0696	0.302	65
Psychiatry	80	70.1	1.0	1.0484	0.900	66
Ophthal.	7	89.2	0.8	0.8457	0.622	70
Trauma—med.	69	120.6	1.2	0.9907	0.535	61
Trauma—surg.	9	126.1	1.1	1.2811	1.224	62
Dental	2	84.1	0.6	1.0000	0.422	64
Substance abuse	11	73.7	0.9	1.0436	0.826	59
All cases	4,197			1.0261	1.000	66

tal to adopt it. Given the stature of Eastman in this town, Mr. Bishop would have been foolhardy to dismiss it out of hand. But he is not just going through the motions. He is sold on the concept, and he has invested heavily in it, with a staff of four assigned to it, plus an assistant administrator who is also providing overall direction.

Exhibit 3.5 Definitions of Terms from Systemetrics Report

The product line efficiency ratio measures the extent consumption exceeds demand. The higher the ratio, the greater the inefficiency. . . . Demand is set by the clinical criteria of patients, consumption is determined by charges which constitute cost to the buyer or payer. . . . Because the efficiency calculation is specific to each patient, and because the efficiency norm is derived from typical practice patterns of physicians utilizing services in your hospital, the ratio is a reasonable estimate of how average overall product line performance compares to average overall performance in the hospital. . . . In other words, to the extent average clinically adjusted charges in a product line exceed average clinically adjusted charges in the hospital, to that extent charges are inefficient either due to payer mix pricing strategy, a greater use of ancillary charges, longer lengths of stay, or some combination of these. . . .

LOS Efficiency Ratio recognizes aggregate variation from legitimate demand for resources. It answers the question, from the buyer's point of view, that is to say, with all things considered—price, use of ancillaries, length of stay—how efficient is the hospital in a particular Product Line, DRG, payer, or at the physician level? . . . [It] is a unique, discrete analysis of how favorably your actual length of stay compares with the LOS you should expect, given patient clinical condition and discharge habits at your hospital compared to those in the national database.

For example, a ratio of 1.15 means that actual LOS exceeds expected LOS by 15%. More specifically, it means that discharge policy and procedures affecting the PL, coupled with physician disposition practices, result in a 15% longer length of stay in the Product Line than would be expected given overall hospital policy, procedures and practice patterns and their comparison to national norms specific to identical disease categories.

* * * * *

Once senior management has drawn conclusions about Product Line utilization and efficiency, and their effect on limited, acute resources, the next logical place to turn is to the possible improvement of net patient revenue across payers. . . . As with product lines, this analysis begins with an assessment of legitimate payer resource demand relative to total hospital acute demand. Number of cases is often a poor proxy for estimating resource allocation across payers. The legitimate need is not only dependent upon volume, but also in illness severity; and ultimately dependent

continues

Exhibit 3.5 continued

upon resource efficiencies which would increase or lower the allocation requirement.

Mortality—a special "mortality scale" has been developed to predict mortality based on risk of death associated with the stage or progression of disease, and the effect of the interaction of comorbid conditions upon that risk. Ratios greater than 1.0 indicate the extent (percent) actual deaths exceed the national norm for the specific clinical conditions exhibited across the payer population.

Introduction

One of the hospital's primary customers, the town's major employer, is sold on TQM and has helped the hospital implement an approach based on its experience. This allows the reader to think about whether there are differences between TQM and CQI. The hospital did find that the industrial training materials were relevant, but that almost half of these materials required new examples from the health care setting. Is there more difference than that?

The approach used by Eastman and by Holston Valley Hospital and Medical Center is based on the work of Deming that is reviewed in Chapter 1. The trainers at the local community college came from the auto industry milieu.

The exhibits in the case give extensive trend data on the financial and operating performance of the hospital. The reader is encouraged to analyze those data for trends and for signs of the impact of CQI on the hospital's reported results. Chapter 2 gives some examples of the types of savings that hospitals are achieving. These should be compared with the efforts undertaken and the results achieved at Holston Valley.

Basics

The techniques of TQM used by Eastman were easily adapted to this health care setting. The tools and concepts stayed the same, but many of the examples were changed to fit the CQI setting. With the company's assistance in setting up the courses at the local community college and the use of company personnel to develop the training programs, the hospital avoided extensive investments in consultants and course development. As the exhibits indicate, the seven tools as outlined in Chapters 1 and 4 were used extensively in the analyses done by the teams.

There is no evidence in the case of extensive reliance on customer satisfaction surveys of the type outlined in Chapter 5. It appears that the primary customers from the perspective of hospital management were the employers and the physicians. Management perceived that the physicians would not really want to become heavily involved in the TQM process, and the primary employer expressed an interest in dealing with clinical matters directly through the IPA and its HMO rather than through the CQI process at Holston Valley. We leave it to the reader to judge whether the hospital should have accepted that division of duties among the health care players in Kingsport.

Top management support at the level of the CEO was very strong. Mr. Bishop had made a very strong personal commitment to CQI. It is hard to tell whether this was perceived by the staff as full top management support. The role of the CEO as the head of the corporate holding company focused on financial matters would have made him relatively remote from operating personnel. Mr. Bishop took every possible occasion to "walk the talk" and emphasize the importance of this effort to his staff, including the celebrations at the weekly staff meetings and the use of outside individuals to reinforce the prominence of their efforts.

Implementation

Many of the planning approaches discussed in various chapters were not evident in the case. The effort seemed to be conceived and implemented pretty much according to Mr. Bishop's conception of the TQM process. There did not seem to be any attempt to involve the hospital board or the medical staff in the planning process, nor evidence of a strong quality council or quality steering committee setting priorities for projects or setting an agenda for the expansion of the effort into more multidisciplinary areas.

The hospital staffed the implementation of CQI fully. Four full-time facilitators were trained and assigned to developing and supporting the teams. The basic training was started in teams at the community college and was experiential. Each team brought an issue from its work environment to start with. As time went on, some efforts were multidisciplinary, but were intended not to be clinical.

The implementation was limited to the administrative side of the hospital, and involvement in clinical activities was studiously avoided. This was motivated by fear that negative physician response to TQM would lead them to send more patients over to Indian Path Hospital. This is not an unrealistic concern, but it kept the hospital from reaping the clinical benefits so important to any TQM initiative. The approach to TQM at Holston Valley was well done technically. We leave it up to the reader to assess whether this effort was a success or a failure strategically.

Regardless of whether the reader agrees with the strategic thrust of this hospital's efforts, there is much to be learned about the details of reinforcing CQI at all levels of the organization. The Friday morning meeting without chairs was used quite skillfully to reinforce management's commitment to the effort. The use of the statistical tools was frequent and intense. The management understood process variation and how to begin to bring it under control and invested heavily in inculcating its administrative staff with those concepts, insights, and values. In many ways, therefore, this case makes an interesting example when studied in parallel with the West Florida Regional Medical Center case that follows it.

CASE 4

West Florida Regional Medical Center

Curtis P. McLaughlin

West Florida Regional Medical Center (WFRMC) is an HCA-owned (Hospital Corporation of America) and operated, for-profit hospital complex on the north side of Pensacola, Florida. Licensed for 547 beds, it operated approximately 325 beds in December 1991 plus the 89-bed psychiatric pavilion and the 58-bed Rehabilitation Institute of West Florida. The 11-story office building of the Medical Center Clinic, P.A. was attached to the hospital facility, and a new cancer center was under construction.

The 130 physicians practicing at the Medical Center Clinic and its satellite clinics admitted mostly to WFRMC, whereas most of the other physicians in this city of 150,000 practiced at both Sacred Heart and Baptist hospitals downtown. Competition for patients was intense, and in 1992 as many as 90 to 95 percent of patients in the hospital would be admitted subject to discounted prices, mostly Medicare for the elderly, CHAMPUS for military dependents, and Blue Cross/Blue Shield of Florida for the employed and their dependents.

The CQI [continuous quality improvement] effort had had some real successes over the last four years, especially in the areas where package prices for services were required. All of the management team had been trained in quality improvement techniques according to HCA's Deming-based approach, and some 25 task forces were operating. The experiment with departmental self-assessments, using the Baldrige Award criteria and an instrument developed by HCA headquarters, had spurred department heads to become further involved and begin to apply quality improvement techniques within their own work units. Yet John Kausch, the Center's CEO, and his senior leadership sensed some loss of interest among some managers, whereas others who had not bought into the idea at first were now enthusiasts.

THE HCA CQI PROCESS

John Kausch had been in the first group of HCA CEOs trained in CQI techniques in 1987 by Paul Batalden, M.D., corporate vice president for medical care. John had become a member of the steering committee for HCA's overall quality effort. The HCA approach was dependent on the active and continued participation of top local management and on the Plan-Do-Check-Act (PDCA) cycle of Deming. Figure 4.1 shows that process as presented to company employees. Dr. Batalden told the case writer that he does not work with a hospital administrator until he is convinced that that individual is fully committed to the concept and is ready to lead the process at his or her own institution—a responsibility that includes being the one to teach the Quality 101 course on site to his or her own managers. John Kausch also took members of his management team to visit other quality exemplars, such as Florida Power and Light and local plants of Westinghouse and Monsanto.

In 1991 John Kausch became actively involved in the Total Quality Council of the Pensacola Area Chamber of Commerce (PATQC), when a group of Pensacola area leaders in business, government, military, education, and health care began meeting informally to share ideas in productivity and quality improvement. From this informal group emerged the PATQC under the sponsorship of the Chamber of Commerce. The vision of PATQC was "helping the Pensacola area develop into a total quality community by promoting productivity and quality in all area organizations, public and private, and by promoting economic development through aiding existing business and attracting new business development." The primary employer in Pensacola, the U.S. Navy, was using the total quality management (TQM) approach extensively, was quite satisfied with the results, and supported the Chamber of Commerce program. In fact, the first 1992 one-day seminar presented by Mr. George F. Butts, consultant and retired Chrysler vice president for quality and productivity, was to be held at the Naval Air Station's Mustin Beach Officers' Club. Celanese Corporation (a Monsanto division), the largest nongovernmental employer in the area, also supported PATQC.

The CQI staffing at WFRMC was quite small, in keeping with HCA practice. The only program employee was Ms. Bette Gulsby, M.Ed.,

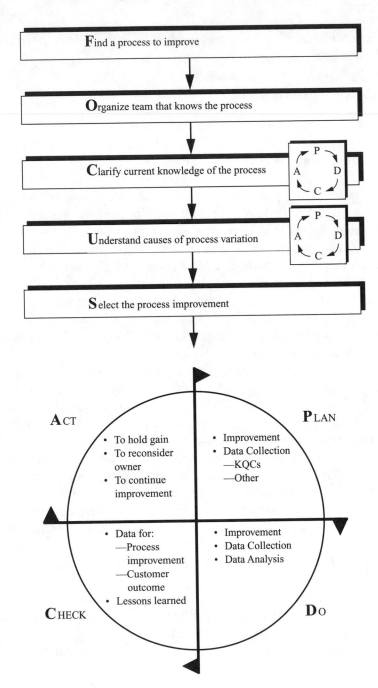

Figure 4.1 HCA's FOCUS-PDCA® Cycle

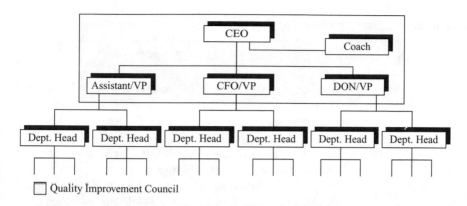

Figure 4.2 Organization Chart with Quality Improvement Council

director of quality improvement resources, who served as staff and "coach" to Mr. Kausch and as a member of the quality improvement council. Figures 4.2 and 4.3 show the organization of the council and the staffing for Quality Improvement Program (QIP) support. The "mentor" was provided by headquarters staff, and in the case of WFRMC was Dr. Batalden himself. The planning process had been careful and detailed. Exhibit 4.1 shows excerpts from the planning processes used in the early years of the program.

WFRMC has been one of several HCA hospitals to work with a self-assessment tool for department heads. Exhibit 4.2 shows the cover letter

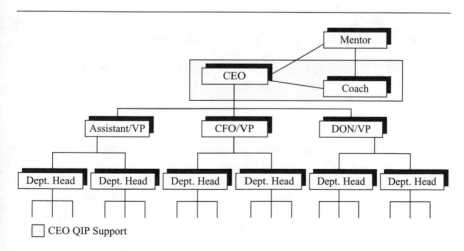

Figure 4.3 Organization Chart with CEO QIP Support

Exhibit 4.1 Planning Chronology for CQI

Initiation Plan—3 to 6 months, starting May 25, 1988

May 25:	Develop initial working definition of quality for WFRMC.
May 25:	Define the purpose of the Quality Improvement Council and set schedule for 2–4 PM every Tuesday and Thursday.
May 25:	Integrate Health Quality Trends (HQT) into continuous improvement cycle and hold initial review.
June 2:	Start several multifunctional teams with their core from those completing the Leadership Workshop with topics selected by the Quality Improvement Council using surveys, experience, and group techniques.
June 2:	Department Heads complete "CEO assessment" to identify customers and expectations, determine training needs, and identify department opportunities. To be discussed with assistant administrators on June 15.
June 16:	Present to QIC the Task Force report on elements and recommendations on organizational elements to guide and monitor QIP.
June 20:	Division meetings to gain consensus on Department plans and set priorities. QIC reviews and consolidates on June 21. Final assignments to Department Heads on June 22.
June 27:	Draft initial Statement of Purpose for WFRMC and present to QIC.
June 29–July 1:	Conduct first Facilitator's Training Workshop for 16.
July 1:	Task Force reports on additional QIP education and training requirements for: Team training and team members' handbook Head nurses Employee orientation (new and current) Integration of community resources (colleges and industry) Use of HCA network resources for Medical Staff, Board of Trustees
July 19:	Task Force report on communications program to support awareness, education, and feedback from employees, vendors, medical staff, local business, colleges and universities, and HCA.

---

continues

Exhibit 4.1 continued

August 1:	Complete the organization of the Quality Improvement Council.

Quality Improvement Implementation Plan to June 30, 1989

Fall:	Pilot and evaluate "Patient Comment Card System."
Oct. 21:	QIC input to draft policies/guidelines regarding: forming teams, quality responsibility, and guidelines for multi-functional teams. Brainstorm at Oct. 27 meeting, have revisions for Nov. 10 meeting, and distribute to employees by November 15.
Oct. 27:	Review proposals for communicating QIP to employees to heighten awareness and understanding, communicate on HCA and WFRMC commitments; key definitions, policies, guidelines; HQT; QIP; teams and improvements to date; responsibility and opportunities for individual employees; initiate ASAP.
Nov. 15:	Prepare statements on "On further consideration of HCA's Quality Guidelines;" discuss with department heads, hospital staff, employee orientation; use to identify barriers to QI and opportunities for QI. Develop specific action plan and discuss with QIC.
Dec. 1:	Identify and evaluate community sources for QI assistance—statistical and operational—including colleges, companies, and the Navy. Make recommendations.
Early Dec.:	Conduct Quality 102 course for remaining Dept. Heads. Conduct Quality 101 course for head nurses and several new Dept. Heads.
Jan. 1, 1989:	Develop and implement a suggestion program consistent with our HCA Quality Guidelines, providing quick and easy way to become involved in making suggestions/identifying situations needing improvement, providing quick feedback and recognition; and interfacing with identifying opportunities for QIP.

QIP Implementation Plan, July 1989–June 1990

Aug. 1:	Survey Department Heads to identify priorities for additional education and training.

continues

Exhibit 4.1 continued

Sept. 14–15:	Conduct a management workshop to sharpen and practice QI methods. To include practice methods; to increase management/staff confidence, comfort; to develop a model for departmental implementation; to develop process assessment/QIP implementation tool; to start Quality Team Review.
September:	Develop a standardized team orientation program to cover QI tools and group process rules.
Fall:	Expand use of HQTs and integrate into Health Quality Improvement Process (HQIP)—improve communication of results and integration of quality improvement action plans. Psychiatric Pavilion to evaluate and implement HQT recommendations from "Patient Comment Card System"—evaluate and pilot.
October:	Incorporate QIP implementation into existing management/communication structure. Establish division "steering committee functions" to guide and facilitate departmental implementation. Identify QI project for each Department Head/Assistant Administrator. Establish regular Quality Reviews into Department Manager meetings.
December:	Evaluate effectiveness of existing policies, guidelines, and practices for sanctioning, supporting, and guiding QI teams. Include Opportunity Form/Cross Functional Team Sanctioning; Team leader and Facilitator responsibilities; Team progress monitoring/guiding; Standardized team presentation format (storyboard). Demonstrate measurable improvement through Baxter QI team.
Monthly:	Monitor and improve the suggestion program.
January:	Pilot the Clinical Process Improvement methodology.
All Year:	In all communications, written and verbal, maintain constant message regarding WFRMC commitment to HQIP; report successes of teams and suggestions; and continue to educate about principles and practices of HQIP strategy.
January:	Successfully demonstrate measurable improvement from focused QIP in one department (Medical Records).

continues

Exhibit 4.1 continued

Spring:	Expand use of HQTs and integrate into HQIP.
	Pilot HQT in Rehab Center.
	Evaluate and implement Physicians' HQT.
	Pilot Ambulatory Care HQT.
Summer:	Expand use of HQTs and integrate into HQIP.
	Human Resources—Pilot HQT.
	Payers—Pilot HQT.

sent to all department heads. Exhibit 4.3 shows the Scoring Matrix for Self-Assessment. Exhibit 4.4 shows the Scoring Guidelines, and Exhibit 4.5 displays the five assessment categories used.

Four Examples of Teams

IV Documentation

The nursing department originated the IV Documentation Team in September 1990 after receiving documentation from the pharmacy department that over a 58-day period there had been $16,800 in lost charges related to the administration of intravenous (IV) solutions. Pharmacy attributed the loss to the nursing staff's record keeping. This was the first time that the nursing department was aware of a problem or that the pharmacy department had been tracking this variable. There were other lost charges, not yet quantified, due to recording errors in the oral administration of pharmaceuticals as well.

The team formed to look at this problem found that there were some 15 possible reasons why the errors occurred, but that the primary one was that documentation of the administration of the IV solution was not entered into the medication administration record (MAR). The MAR was kept at the patient bedside, and each time that a medication was administered the nurse was to enter documentation into this record.

The team had to come to understand some terms as they went along. The way that pharmacy kept its books, anything that was sent to the floors but not billed within 48 to 72 hours was considered a "lost charge." If an inquiry was sent to the floor about the material and what happened and a correction was made, the entry was classified as "revenue recovered."

Exhibit 4.2 Departmental Quality Improvement Assessment

In an effort to continue to monitor and implement elements of improvement and innovation within our organization, it will become more and more necessary to find methods which will describe our level of QI implementation.

The assessment or review of a quality initiative is only as good as the thought processes which have been triggered during the actual assessment. Last year (1990) the Quality Improvement Council prepared for and participated in a quality review. This exercise was extremely beneficial to the overall understanding of what was being done and the results that have been accomplished utilizing various quality techniques and tools.

The Departmental Implementation of QI has been somewhat varied throughout the organization and although the variation is certainly within the range of acceptability, it is the intent of the QIC to better understand each department's implementation road map and furthermore to provide advice/coaching on the next steps for each department.

Attached please find a scoring matrix for self-assessment. This matrix is followed by five category ratings (to be completed by each department head). The use of this type of tool reinforces the self-evaluation which is consistent with continuous improvement and meeting the vision of West Florida Regional Medical Center.

Please read and review the attachment describing the scoring instructions and then score your department category standings, relative to the approach, deployment, and effects. This information will be forwarded to Bette Gulsby by April 19, 1991, and following a preliminary assessment by the QIC, an appointment will be scheduled for your departmental review.

The review will be conducted by John Kausch and Bette Gulsby, along with your administrative director. Please take the time to review the attachments and begin your self-assessment scoring. You will be notified of the date and time of your review.

This information will be utilized for preparing for the next Department Head retreat, scheduled for May 29 and 30, 1991 at the Perdido Beach Hilton.

Thus the core issue was not so much one of lost revenue as one of unnecessary rework in pharmacy and on the nursing floors.

The team developed Pareto charts showing the reasons for the documentation errors. The most common ones were procedural—for example, patient moved to the operating room, or patient already discharged. Following the HCA model, these procedural problems were dealt with one

Exhibit 4.3 A Scoring Matrix for Self-Assessment

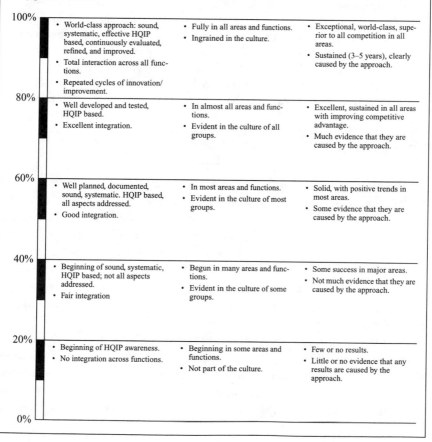

TO BE USED IN EVALUATING EXAMINATION CRITERIA

APPROACH	DEPLOYMENT (Implementation)	EFFECTS (Results)
• HQIP design includes all eight dimensions[*] • Integration across dimensions of HQIP and areas of operation	• Breadth of implementation (areas or functions) • Depth of implementation (awareness, knowledge, understanding, and applications)	• Quality of measurable results

[*]The eight dimensions of HQIP are: leadership constancy, employee mindedness, customer mindedness, process focussed, statistical thinking, PDCA driven, innovativeness, and regulatory proactiveness.

	APPROACH	DEPLOYMENT	EFFECTS
100% 80%	• World-class approach: sound, systematic, effective HQIP based, continuously evaluated, refined, and improved. • Total interaction across all functions. • Repeated cycles of innovation/improvement.	• Fully in all areas and functions. • Ingrained in the culture.	• Exceptional, world-class, superior to all competition in all areas. • Sustained (3–5 years), clearly caused by the approach.
80% 60%	• Well developed and tested, HQIP based. • Excellent integration.	• In almost all areas and functions. • Evident in the culture of all groups.	• Excellent, sustained in all areas with improving competitive advantage. • Much evidence that they are caused by the approach.
60% 40%	• Well planned, documented, sound, systematic. HQIP based, all aspects addressed. • Good integration.	• In most areas and functions. • Evident in the culture of most groups.	• Solid, with positive trends in most areas. • Some evidence that they are caused by the approach.
40% 20%	• Beginning of sound, systematic, HQIP based; not all aspects addressed. • Fair integration	• Begun in many areas and functions. • Evident in the culture of some groups.	• Some success in major areas. • Not much evidence that they are caused by the approach.
20% 0%	• Beginning of HQIP awareness. • No integration across functions.	• Beginning in some areas and functions. • Not part of the culture.	• Few or no results. • Little or no evidence that any results are caused by the approach.

Exhibit 4.4 Departmental Quality Improvement Assessment Scoring Guidelines

In order to determine your department's score in each of the five categories, please review the Scoring Matrix for self-assessment. The operational definitions for Approach, Deployment, and Effects are listed in the small boxes on the top of the scoring matrix. Each criteria is divided into percent of progress/implementation (i.e., 0%–100%). For example, you may determine that your departmental score on category 3.0 (QI Practice) is:

APPROACH	DEPLOYMENT	EFFECTS
20%	*20%*	*20%*

This means that your departmental approach has fair integration of QIP practice, your departmental deployment is evident in the culture of some of your groups, and your departmental effects are not actually evidence that they are caused by the approach.

Please remember that this is a self-assessment and only you know your departmental progress. This assessment is not a tool to generate documentation. However, if you would like to bring any particular document(s) to your review, please do so. This is only meant to provide a forum for you to showcase your progress and receive recognition and feedback on such.

Remember, review each of the self-assessment criteria of approach, deployment, and effects and become familiar with the levels or percentages described. You have three scores for each Departmental QI Assessment Category (categories 1.0–5.0).

at a time to get the accounting for unused materials right. The next step in the usual procedures was to get a run chart developed to show what was happening over time to the lost charges on IVs. Here the team determined that the best quality indicator would be the ratio of lost charges to total charges issued. At this point pharmacy management realized that it lacked the denominator figure and that its lack of computerization led to the lack of that information. Therefore the task force was inactive for three months while pharmacy implemented a computer system that could provide the denominator.

Ms. Debbie Koenig, assistant director of nursing who was responsible for the team, said that the next step would be to look at situations where the MAR was not at the patient bedside but perhaps up at the nursing station so that a nurse could not make the entry at the appropriate time. This was an especially bothersome rework problem because of nurses working various

Exhibit 4.5 Departmental QI Assessment Categories

1.0 DEPARTMENTAL QI FRAMEWORK DEVELOPMENT

The QI Framework Development category examines how the departmental quality values have been developed, how they are applied to projects in a consistent manner, and how adoption of the values throughout the department is assessed and reinforced.
Examples of areas to address:

- Department Mission
- Departmental Quality Definition
- Departmental Employee Performance Feedback Review
- Departmental QI Plan
- QI Methods

APPROACH	DEPLOYMENT	EFFECTS
———%	———%	———%

2.0 CUSTOMER KNOWLEDGE DEVELOPMENT

The Customer Knowledge Deployment category examines how the departmental leadership has involved and utilized various facets of customer-mindedness to guide the quality effort.
Examples of areas to address:

- HQT Family of Measures (patient, employee, etc.)
- Departmental Customer Identification
- Identification of Customer Needs and Expectations
- Customer Feedback/Data Review

APPROACH	DEPLOYMENT	EFFECTS
———%	———%	———%

3.0 QUALITY IMPROVEMENT PRACTICE

The Quality Improvement Practice category examines the effectiveness of the department's efforts to develop and realize the full potential of the work force, including management, and the methods to maintain an environment conducive to full participation, quality leadership, and personal and organizational growth.
Examples of areas to address:

- Process Improvement Practice
- Meeting Skills
- QI Storyboards
- QI in Daily Work Life (individual use of QI tools, i.e., flow chart, run chart, Pareto chart)
- Practice Quality Management Guidelines
- Departmental Data Review
- Plans To Incorporate QI in Daily Clinical Operations
- Identification of Key Physician Leaders

APPROACH	DEPLOYMENT	EFFECTS
———%	———%	———%

continues

Exhibit 4.5 continued

4.0 QUALITY AWARENESS BUILDING

The Quality Awareness Building category examines how the department decides what quality education and training is needed by employees and how it utilizes the knowledge and skills acquired. It also examines what has been done to communicate QI to the department and how QI is addressed in departmental staff meetings.

Examples of areas to address:

- JIT Training
- Employee Orientation
- Creating Employee Awareness
- Communication of QI Results

APPROACH	DEPLOYMENT	EFFECTS
——%	——%	——%

5.0 QA/QI LINKAGE

The QA/QI Linkage category examines how the department has connected QA data and information to the QI process improvement strategy. Also examined is the utilization of QI data-gathering and decision-making tools to document and analyze data. (How the department relates the ongoing QA activities to QI process improvement activities.)

Examples of areas to address:

- QA Process Identification
- FOCUS-PDCA Process Improvement
- Regulatory/Accreditation Connection (Joint Commission)

APPROACH	DEPLOYMENT	EFFECTS
——%	——%	——%

---

shifts and because occasionally an agency nurse had been on duty and was not available to consult when pharmacy asked why documentation was not present for an IV dose of medication.

Universal Charting

There was evidence that a number of ancillary services results, "loose reports," were not getting into the patients' medical records in a timely fashion. This was irritating to physicians and could result in delays in the patient's discharge, which under DRGs [diagnosis-related groups] meant higher costs without higher reimbursement. One employee filed a suggestion that a single system be developed to avoid people running over other people on the floor doing the "charting." A CQI team was developed and led by Ms. Debbie Wroten, medical records director. The 12-member team included supervisors and directors from the laboratory, the pulmonary lab, the EKG lab, medical records, radiology, and nursing. They developed the following "Opportunity Statement":

> At present six departments are utilizing nine full-time equivalents 92 hours per week for charting separate ancillary reports. Rework is created in the form of repulling of inhouse patient records creating an ever-increasing demand of chart accessibility. All parties affected by this process are frustrated because the current process increases the opportunity for lost documentation, chart unavailability, increased traffic on units creating congestion, prolonged charting times, and provides for untimely availability of clinical reports for patient care. Therefore an opportunity exists to improve the current charting practice for all departments involved to allow for the efficiency, timeliness and accuracy of charting loose reports.

The team met, assessed, and flowcharted the current charting processes of the five departments involved. Key variables were defined as follows:

- Charting timeliness—number of charting times per day, consistency of charting, and reports not charted per charting round
- Report availability—indicated by the number of telephone calls per department asking for reports not yet charted
- Chart availability—chart is accessible at the nurses' station without interruption
- Resource utilization—man-hours and number of hours per day of charting

Each department was asked to use a common "charting log" track for several weeks of the number of records charted, who did the charting, when it was done, the preparation time, the number of reports charted, the number of reports not charted (missed), and the personnel hours consumed in charting. The results are shown in Table 4.1.

Table 4.1 Charting Log

Department	Mean Records Per Day	Range	Mean Hours Per Day	Range	Comments
Medical Records	77.3	20–140	1.6	0.6–2.5	Daily
Pulmonary Lab	50.3	37–55	1.0	0.7–1.5	MWF
Clinical Lab	244.7	163–305	3.2	1.9–5.4	Daily
EKG Lab	40.2	35–48	0.8	0.1–1.0	Weekdays
Microbiology	106.9	3–197	1.4	0.1–2.2	Daily
Radiology	87.1	6–163	1.5	0.1–2.9	Daily

These data gave the team considerable insight into the nature of the problem. Not every department was picking up the materials every day. Two people could cover the whole hospital in three-quarters of an hour each or one person in 1.5 hours. The clinical chemistry laboratory, medical records, and radiology were making two trips per day, whereas other departments were only able to chart every other day and failed to chart over the weekends.

The processes used by all the groups were similar. The printed or typed reports had to be sorted by floors, given room numbers if missing, taken to the floors, and inserted into patient charts. If the chart was not available, they had to be held until the next round. A further problem identified was that when the clerical person assigned to these rounds was not available, a technical person, who was paid considerably more and was often in short supply, had to be sent to do the job.

A smaller team of supervisors who actually knew and owned the charting efforts in the larger departments (medical records, radiology, and clinical chemistry) was set up to design and assess the pilot experiment. The overall team meetings were used only to brief the department heads to gain their feedback and support. A pilot experiment was run in which these three departments took turns doing the runs for each other. The results were favorable. The pilot increased timeliness and chart availability by charting four times per day on weekdays and three times per day on weekends. Report availability was improved, and there were fewer phone calls. Nursing staff, physicians, and participating departments specifically asked for the process to be continued. The hours of labor dropped from 92 weekly to less than 45, using less highly paid labor.

Therefore the team decided that the issues were important enough that they should consider setting up a separate Universal Charting Team to meet the needs of the entire hospital.

However, an unanticipated hospital census decline made impractical the possibility of requesting additional staffing, etc. Consequently the group reevaluated the possibility of continuing the arrangement developed for the pilot using the charting hours of the smaller departments on a volume basis. It was discovered that this had the effect of freeing the professional staff of the smaller departments from charting activities and a very minimal allocation of hours floated to the larger departments. It also increased the availability of charters in the larger departments for other activities.

The payroll department was then asked to develop a system for allocating the hours that floated from one department to another. That proved cumbersome, so the group decided to allocate charting hours on the basis of each department's volume. "In the event that one or more departments experiences a significant increase/decrease in charting needs, the group will reconvene and the hourly allocation will be adjusted."

The resulting schedule has the lab making rounds at 6:00 AM and 9:00 AM and radiology at 4:00 PM and 9:30 PM Monday through Friday, and medical records at 6:00 AM, 1:00 PM, and 8:00 PM on Saturday and Sunday. Continuing statistics are kept on the process, which is shown in Exhibit 4.6. The system continues to work effectively.

Labor, Delivery, Recovery, Postpartum (LDRP) Nursing

Competition for young families needing maternity services had become quite intense in Pensacola. WFRMC obstetrical (OB) services offered very traditional services in 1989 in three separate units—labor and delivery, nursery, and postpartum—and operated considerably below capacity.

A consultant was hired to evaluate the potential growth of obstetrical services, the value of current services offered by WFRMC, customers' desires, competitors' services, and opportunities for improvement. Focus group interviews with young couples (past and potential customers) indicated that they wanted safe medical care in a warm, homelike setting with the least possible number of rules. Most mothers were in their thirties, planning small families with the possibility of only one child. Fathers wanted to be "actively involved" in the birth process. The message came back, "We want to be actively involved in this experience and we want to make the decisions." The consultant challenged the staff to develop their

Exhibit 4.6 Universal Charting Team FOCUS-PDCA Outline

F   **Opportunity Statement:**

At present, six departments are utilizing 9 full-time equivalents 92 hours a week for charting separate ancillary reports. Rework is created in the form of repulling of inhouse patient records creating an ever-increasing demand of chart accessibility. All parties affected by this process are frustrated because the current process increases the opportunity for lost documentation, chart unavailability, increased traffic on units creating congestion, prolonged charting times, and provides for untimely availability of clinical reports for patient care.

Therefore an opportunity exists to improve the current charting practice for all departments involved to allow for the efficiency, timeliness, and accuracy of charting loose reports.

O   Team members include:
Debbie Wroten, Medical Records Director—Leader
Bernie Grappe, Marketing Director—Facilitator
Joan Simmons, Laboratory Director
Mary Gunter, Laboratory Patient Services Coordinator
Al Clarke, Pulmonary Services Director
Carol Riley, Pulmonary Services Assistant Director
Marlene Rodrigues, EKG Supervisor
Patti Travis, EKG
Debra Wright, Medical Records Transcription Supervisor
Mike West, Radiology Director
Lori Mikesell, Radiology Transcription Supervisor
Debbie Fernandez, Head Nurse

C   Assessed and flowcharted current charting practices of departments.
Clarified and defined key quality characteristics of the charting process:

Charting Timeliness—number of charting times per day, consistency of charting, and reports not charted per charting round.

Report Availability—indicated by the number of telephone calls per department asking for reports not yet charted.

Chart Availability—chart is accessible at nurses' station for charting without interruption.

Resource Utilization—man hours and number of hours per day of charting.

U   Gathered data on departments charting volumes and time spent on charting.

Department:

Charting Log

Date	Charting Tech vs. Clk.	Prep Time	# Reports Charted	# Reports Not Charted	Charting Time (amt)	Hour of Day	Comment

continues

Exhibit 4.6 continued

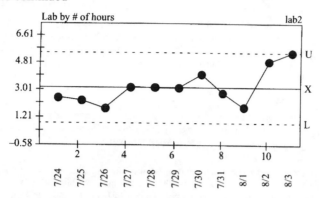

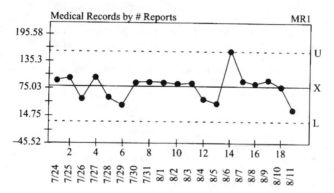

S   Data gained through the pilot indicated that significant gains were available through the effort to justify proceeding with the development of a Universal Charting Team.

P   The team developed a flowchart of the charting process using a universal charting team rather than previous arrangements. In order to pilot the improvement, the group decided to set up a UCT using current charters from the three major charting departments—medical records, laboratory, and radiology. The team also developed written instructions for both the charters and participating departments. A subgroup of the team actually conducted a one-day pilot before beginning extensive education to ensure that the UCT would work as planned and to be sure that the charters from each of the large departments were well versed on possible situations that might occur during the pilot.

D   Piloted proposed Universal Charting Team using current charting personnel from radiology, laboratory, and medical records to chart for all departments.

C   Pilot results were positive and indicated that the UCT concept offered significant advantages over the previous charting arrangements. Results were:

continues

Exhibit 4.6 continued

> Timeliness/Chart Availability—Pilot reduced daily charting to four scheduled charting times daily for all departments. Smaller departments did not chart daily prior to pilot. The charting team also reduced the number of occasions that charters from different departments were on the nursing unit needing the same chart.
>
> Report Availability—Telephone calls were reduced and nursing staff, physicians, and participating departments specifically asked for UCT following the pilot.
>
> Resource Utilization—Number of man hours spent charting and preparing to chart was reduced from 92 hours weekly to less than 45 hours. The improvement also allowed the use of less expensive staff for charting.

 The group reached consensus that the easiest configuration for the UCT would be to set up a separate UCT that would serve the needs of the entire hospital. This was to be proposed to administration by the team as the conclusion of their efforts. However, an unanticipated hospital census decline made impractical the possibility of requesting additional staffing, etc. Consequently, the group reevaluated the possibility of continuing the arrangement developed for the pilot using the charting hours to the smaller departments on a volume basis. It was discovered that this had the effect of freeing the professional staff in the smaller departments from charting responsibilities while a very minimal allocation of hours floated to the larger departments, and it increased the availability of charters in the larger departments for other activities. The payroll department was then involved in order to develop the proper mechanism and procedure for floating hours.

This modification of the previous pilot was piloted for a month with continued good results. Streamlining of the hours floating process may be necessary to place less burden on the payroll department.

Since no major changes were required following the pilot, the group has elected to adopt the piloted UCT format. Allocation of charting hours is based on a monthly review of charting volumes for each department. In the event that one or more departments experiences a significant increase/decrease in charting needs, the group will reconvene and the hourly allocation will be adjusted.

LESSONS LEARNED

Because of the size and the makeup of the team, which included a number of department heads, it was found helpful to set up a smaller team of three supervisors who actually knew and owned the charting efforts in the major departments. This group designed and assessed the initial pilot and actually piloted the pilot before bringing departmental charters into the process. As a result, overall team meetings were used primarily to brief department heads and gain their feedback and consensus.

---

own vision for the department based on the focus group responses, customer feedback, and trends nationally.

It became clear that there was a demand for a system in which a family-centered birth experience could occur. The system needed to revolve around the customers; not the customers following a rigid traditional routine. Customers wanted all aspects of the normal delivery to happen in the same room. The new service would allow the mother, father, and baby to remain together throughout the hospital stay, now as short as 24 hours. Friends and families would be allowed and encouraged to visit and participate as much as the new parents desired. The main goals were to be responsive to the customer's needs and to provide safe, quality medical care.

The hospital administration and the six obstetricians practicing there were eager to see obstetrical services grow. They were open to trying and supporting the new concept. The pediatricians accepted the changes, but without great enthusiasm. The anesthesiologists were opposed to the change. The OB supervisor and two of the three nursing head nurses were also opposed to any change. They wanted to continue operations in the traditional manner. When the hospital decided to adopt the new LDRP concept, it was clear that patients and families liked it but that the nursing staff, especially management, did not. The OB nursing supervisor retired, one head nurse resigned, one was terminated, and the third opted to move from her management position to a staff nurse role. Ms. Cynthia Ayres, RN, administrative director, responsible for the psychiatric and cardiovascular services, was assigned to implement the LDRP transition until nursing management could be replaced.

One of the issues involved in the transition was clarification of the charge structure. Previously each unit charged separately for services and supplies. Now that the care was provided in a single central area, the old charge structure was unnecessarily complex. Duplication of charges was occurring, and some charges were being missed because no one was assuming responsibility.

Ms. Ayres decided to use the CQI process to develop a new charge process and to evaluate the costs and resource consumption of the service. Ms. Ayres had not been a strong supporter of the CQI process when it was first introduced into the organization. She had felt that the process was too slow and rigid, and that data collection was difficult and cumbersome. Several teams were organized and assigned to look at specific areas of the LDRP process.

To reach a simplified charge process, as well as a competitive price, all aspects of the process had to be analyzed. Meetings were held with the nursing and medical staff. Management of OB patient and physician preferences in terms of supplies and practices was analyzed. A number of consensus conferences were held to discuss observed variations. For example, each of the six obstetricians specified a different analgesic for pain control. All of these drugs appeared effective for pain control, but their cost per dose ranged from $10 to $75. The physicians agreed that the $10 product was acceptable since the outcome was the same.

Another standard practice was sending placentas to the pathology laboratory for analysis after every normal delivery. This involved labor time, lab charges, and a pathologist's fee for review. The total procedure cost $196. When questioned about the practice, the current medical staff did not feel it was necessary medically or the current practice nationally, but felt that they were just following the rules. Upon investigation, the team found that an incident involving a placenta had occurred 15 years ago that had led the service chief (since retired) to order all placentas sent to the lab. The obstetricians developed criteria for when it was medically necessary for the lab review of a placenta. This new rule decreased the number of reviews by 95 percent, resulting in cost savings to the hospital and to patients.

The team reviewed all OB charges for a one-year period. They found that in 80 percent of the normal deliveries 14 items were consistently used. The other items were due to variations in physician preferences. The teams and the physicians met and agreed which items were the basic requirements for a normal delivery. These items became the basic charges for package pricing.

The team met weekly for at least one hour for over a year. Some meetings went as long as five hours. Initially, there was a great deal of resistance and defensiveness. Everyone wanted to focus on issues that did not affect him or herself. The physicians objected that they were being forced to practice "cookbook medicine" and that the real problem was "the hospital's big markup." Hospital staff continued to provide data on actual hospital charges, resource consumption, and practice patterns. The hospital personnel continued to emphasize repeatedly that the physicians were responsible for determining care. The hospital's concern was to be consistent and decrease variation.

Another CQI team, the Documentation Team, was responsible for reviewing forms utilized previously by the three separate units. The total number of forms used had been 30. The nursing staff was documenting vital signs an average of five times each time care was provided. Through review of policies, standards, documentation, and care standards, the number of forms was reduced to 20. Nurses were now required to enter each care item only one time. The amount of time spent by nurses on documentation was reduced 50 percent, as was the cost of forms. Data entry errors were also reduced.

The excess costs that were removed were not all physician-related. Many had to do with administrative and nursing policies. Many were due to old, comfortable, traditional ways of doing things. When asked why a practice was followed, the typical response was, "I don't know; that's just the way we've always done it." The OB staff is comfortable with the use of CQI. They recognize that although it requires time and effort, it does produce measurable results. The OB staff is continuing to review its practices and operations to identify opportunities to streamline services and decrease variation.

Pharmacy and Therapeutics Team

In late 1987, a CQI team was formed jointly between the hospital's pharmacy and therapeutics (P&T) committee and the pharmacy leadership. Their first topic of concern was the rapidly rising costs of inpatient drugs, especially antibiotics, which were then costing the hospital about $1.3 million per year. They decided to study the process by which antibiotics were selected and began by asking physicians how they selected antibiotics for treatment. Most of the time they ordered a culture of the organism causing the infection from the microbiology lab. A microbiology lab report would come back identifying the organism and the antibiotics to which it was sensitive and those to which it was resistant. Some physicians reported that they would look down the list until they came to an antibiotic to which the organism was sensitive and order that. That list was in alphabetical order. A study of antibiotic utilization showed a high correlation between use and alphabetical position, confirming the anecdotal reports. Therefore the team recommended to the P&T committee that the form be changed to list the antibiotics in order of increasing cost per average daily dose. The doses used would be based on current local prescribing patterns rather than recommended dosages. The P&T committee, which included attending physicians, approved the change and reported it in their annual report to the medical staff. Figure 4.4 shows what happened to the utilization of "expensive" antibiotics (more than $10 per dose) from 1988 to 1991. These costs were not adjusted at all for inflation in drug prices during this period. The estimated annual saving was $200,000.

Given this success, the team went on in 1989 to deal with the problem of the length of treatment with antibiotics. Inpatients did not get a prescription for 10 days' supply. Their IM and IV antibiotics were continued until the physician stopped the order. If a physician went away for the weekend

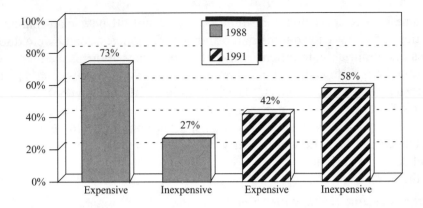

Figure 4.4 Antibiotic Utilization Ratio, Expensive: Inexpensive Doses Dispensed (expensive ≥ $10.00 per dose)

---

and the patient improved, colleagues were very reluctant to alter the medication until he or she returned. The team wrestled with how to encourage the appropriate ending of the course of treatment without hassling the physicians or risking undue legal liability problems. They settled on a sticker that went into the chart at the end of three days that said that the treatment had gone on for three days at that point and that an ending date should be specified if possible. The hospital newsletter and the P&T committee annual report noted that the physician could avoid this notice by specifying a termination date at the time of prescribing. This program seemed to be effective. Antibiotic costs again dropped, and there were no apparent quality problems introduced as measured by length of stay or by adverse events associated with the new system.

In 1990 the team began an aggressive Drug Usage Evaluation (DUE) Program, hiring an assistant director of pharmacy clinical services to administer it. The position had to be rigorously cost justified. DUE involved a review of cases to determine whether the selection and scheduling of powerful drugs matched the clinical picture presented. For example, if the physician prescribed one of three types of antibiotics known to represent a risk of kidney damage in three to five percent of cases, the DUE administrator ordered lab tests to study serum creatinine levels and warn the physician if they rose, indicating kidney involvement. There was a sharp decline in the adverse effects due to the use of these drugs. This program was expanded further to incorporate looking at other critical lab values and relating them to pharmacy activities beyond antibiotics: for example, use of IV solutions and potassium levels. By 1991 the unadjusted antibiotic costs for roughly the same number of admissions had dropped to less than $900,000.

Looking Ahead

One of the things that had concerned John Kausch during 1991 was the fact that implementation had varied from department to department. Although he had written in his annual CQI report that the variation had certainly been within the range of acceptability, he was still concerned about how much variation in implementation was appropriate. If maintaining enthusiasm was a concern, forcing people to conform too tightly might become a demotivator for some staff. This issue and the four mentioned at the beginning of this case study should all be addressed in the coming year.

CASE ANALYSIS

This is a hospital with a large group of physicians closely tied to it, both economically and geographically. It is also operating in an area of intense competition and tight cost controls. The fact that 90 to 95 percent of the hospital's compensation is case-based (DRGs) and not procedure-based has a profound impact on management motivation. Intense support for the CQI process provided by Dr. Batalden and his staff at corporate headquarters also affects motivation.

Introduction

The HCA approach to CQI is a Deming-based approach. The PDCA cycle is at the heart of the approach. So is the quality council, which involves all the top managers in the institution. The process is implemented one hospital at a time, whenever headquarters decides that the CEO is ready to lead the process. The process has been in place several years, and there is no question as to top management commitment on site.

The case shows some major successes in terms of savings and impacts on revenues of the type discussed in Chapter 2. The savings on antibiotics developed by the nursing-pharmacy team are substantial, over $200,000 annually, and the effort is still continuing. Similarly, the utilization of the labor and delivery facilities is up, and the same types of admissions increases were achieved by a team working in the psychiatric pavilion (not reported in the case). Therefore the results are evident to the management and to the employees. They are also evident to the general public since the annual data reported by the Florida Cost Containment Commission, which are based on discharge summary data, show that WFRMC has become the low-priced supplier of obstetric services in the community since these changes were made.

Basics

The hospital uses standard HCA customer satisfaction surveys like those shown in Chapter 5, but these were not particularly relevant to the issues in the case. To revitalize its obstetrical business, the hospital turned to a market research firm to conduct focus groups and surveys of potential patients in the target population. Then it used a combination of management and CQI processes to develop a new approach to service delivery.

The teams used most of the seven tools of TQM as illustrated in the exhibits. They also used other tools such as market research and a sophisticated form of regression analysis to determine the relationship between alphabetical ordering of antibiotic drugs and their utilization. It was also apparent that many of the tools of epidemiology would be applicable in the continuing efforts to avoid the negative side effects of antibiotic utilization.

This case illustrates the classic planning approach outlined in Chapter 1. A detailed plan was developed, reviewed, and implemented annually, as shown in Exhibit 4.1. It was overseen by the quality council. The reader can use the information in those exhibits to gauge how much effort it takes to follow the planning guidelines established in the TQM literature. It is no small investment.

Implementation

Management decision making did not slow down because CQI teams were working on these important processes. For example, in the redesign of obstetrical processes, management studies and those of the teams went forward in parallel. The analyses done by the CQI team enlightened the decisions of management, and the information provided by management enlightened the work done by the team. The same was true of governance processes and the CQI team studying nursing and pharmacy. The P&T committee and the CQI team worked in concert to gather data on antibiotics prescribing practices, to change laboratory reporting procedures, and to win clinician acceptance of those procedures. Other cases in this book also serve to indicate that CQI teams do not work in splendid isolation, but interact regularly with the ongoing management and governance practices of the health care organization.

In this case, it is important to note that the process changes were implemented successfully even at the expense of some clinicians. The anesthesiologists did not like the new labor and delivery setup for normal deliveries. It split their work between the high-tech delivery rooms for non-normal deliveries and the homelike rooms on the floors for normal deliveries. Yet they went along with it because it was clearly in the best interests of their customers, that is, the patients, the obstetricians, and the hospital administration. It is likely that if the process of choosing the new approach had been more participatory, they would have continued to oppose the change—probably indefinitely.

Mr. Kausch emphasizes the fact that the CQI program has had to go through a number of the transitions outlined in Chapter 7. After the first surge of enthusiasm over empowerment, and after work had taken place on the aspects of CQI that bothered people, the quality council had to go to work. It had to plan in detail for the next year, considering the cost and potential value of each effort. This case emphasizes the need for management to focus teams on opportunities, rather than just on problems.

CASE 5

Rex Healthcare and Service Line Teams

Curtis P. McLaughlin and Linda C. Jordan

Rex Healthcare is a private, nonprofit organization founded in 1894 by Raleigh, North Carolina, tanner, John Rex. It provides a wide range of services to the Research Triangle area. The main Rex campus is a 62-acre site in west Raleigh convenient to I-40 and I-440. This campus includes the 394-bed Rex Hospital, 140-bed Rex Convalescent Center, and the Rex Cancer Center. Patients utilizing the Rex Heart Center also have access to the Rex Wellness Centers in Raleigh and Cary. Rex Home Services serves patients in seven counties through approximately 100,000 home health visits a year. Exhibit 5.1 shows the various centers and campuses of Rex Healthcare.

ReXMeD is a physician-hospital organization (PHO) formed in late 1995. By April 1998, ReXMeD had credentialed 45 primary care physicians and over 200 specialty physicians, all of whom were stockholders in this for-profit limited liability company together with the hospital. The Rex primary care network included over 50 board-certified primary care physicians, physician assistants, and nurse practitioners in 12 practices in Raleigh, Cary, Garner, and Wake Forest. Over 800 total physicians are members of the Rex medical staff.

Rex has a long history of innovation, having pioneered in North Carolina in a number of radiological techniques, hospital management training, the comprehensive cancer center, and employee childcare. The introduc-

Exhibit 5.1 Special Centers and Services of Rex Healthcare

In Raleigh:
- Rex Hospital
- Rex Cancer Center
- Rex Convalescent Center
- Rex Same Day Surgery Center
- Rex Wellness Center
- Rex Family Birth Center
- Rex Emergency Department Fast Track Services
- Rex Heart Center
- Rex Breast Care Center
- Rex Primary Care (multiple sites)
- ReXMeD (PHO)
- Healthnet Information and Resource Center
- Rex Senior Health Center (downtown)
- Rex Business Health Services (occupational medicine)
- RexAware (employee assistance program)
- Rex Emergency Response Team
- Rex Urgent Care Centers

In Cary and Apex
- Rex Healthcare of Cary (primary care)
- Rex Wellness Center
- Rex Urgent Care Center
- Rex Convalescent Care Center (107 beds)

In Garner
- Rex Healthcare of Garner/Garner Family Physicians

In Wake Forest
- Rex Healthcare of Wake Forest (primary care)

Regionally
- Rex HomeHealth Services

tion of clinical care service lines in 1996 was a continuation of that history of innovation.

QUALITY AT REX

Rex Hospital has an excellent reputation for quality. A 1995 consumer survey conducted by the Endresen Research Group of Seattle, Washington, identified Rex as the preferred hospital in Wake County. It received National Research Corporation's 1996 and 1997 Quality Leaders awards. This Lincoln, Nebraska-based research organization conducted surveys of 165,000 households in 100 metropolitan areas nationwide with about 2,500 hospitals. Rex was selected as one of the best 119 nationwide based on questions about overall preference, quality of care, best physicians and nurses, best image and reputation, best community health programs, and most personalized care. Rex has consistently earned the Gallup survey's premier rating in several patient categories as well as "Likelihood to Recommend and Likelihood to Choose Again," placing it in the top 20 percent of Gallup hospitals nationwide. In 1997 Rex was honored by *Working Mother Magazine* as one of the "Best 100" workplaces for working women. It has also earned the North Carolina Governor's Award for Excellence for its Workplace Wellness Program.

The hospital's mission/vision statement reads as follows:

> Rex is a patient-centered health care delivery system in working partnership with the medical staff. We are a health care leader, designing innovative and flexible solutions that achieve superior patient outcomes and customer satisfaction. Through the integration of clinical, financial, and administrative systems, we are cost-effective and deliver a continuum of care that meets the dynamic health needs of our community. We are committed to creating a culture that continually improves services, sustains a high-quality team-oriented work environment, and provides for all of our community health care for life.

COMPETITION IN THE RESEARCH TRIANGLE

The Research Triangle area has a population of approximately 1.2 million, about half of whom live in Wake County. It is generally considered to be over-doctored with the University of North Carolina and Duke University medical schools in adjacent Orange and Durham Counties. Wake County and the easterly counties of Johnson, Franklin, and Harnett have a combined population of three-quarters of a million. The market population is growing rapidly, is youthful, and has very low unemployment. There are three substantial hospitals in Wake County—Wake Medical Center, historically the county hospital; Raleigh Community Hospital, formerly Columbia-owned, but purchased in 1998 by Duke Medical Center; and Rex. Wake Medical had a slightly higher share of market than Rex did, but Rex is dominant in ambulatory surgery, women and children's services, and oncology. Rex's payer mix is good with the highest percentage of commercial and managed care patients. The Wake County market in 1997 was:

HMO	43%
Commercial/Other	33%
Medicare	8%
Medicaid	5%
Uninsured	10%

Physician practices were consolidating with MedPartners and FPA Medical Management having practices in the county, with WakeMed having started a medical services organization (MSO) and Rex a physician-hospital organization (PHO), while both Duke and Carolina were developing independent practice associations (IPAs) in the area. In 1997 Wake County hospital discharges per 1,000 dipped below 100 and hospital days per 1,000 below 500.

HISTORY OF QUALITY AND PERFORMANCE IMPROVEMENT EFFORTS AT REX

Exhibit 5.2 provides a chronological list of quality events at Rex. Early efforts to implement clinical pathways were not as successful as hoped, because the software was used for documentation rather than for variance identification, but are again being encouraged and the overall infrastructure to support this effort is being restructured.

Structure for Governance and Implementation

The leaders at Rex established a joint conference committee (JCC) to oversee performance improvement activities. It includes representatives from the board of trustees, medical staff executive committee, and Rex Healthcare executive staff. Its purpose is to direct the selection of organizational measures for important processes, prioritize and reprioritize these

Exhibit 5.2 Chronological Events at Rex Healthcare

Date	Event
1894	Rex Hospital founded in Raleigh, NC
Before 1995	Installs Trendstar cost reporting system
1995	Rex named preferred hospital in Wake County by Endreson Research Group survey
	Case Management and Performance Improvement/Risk Management Departments created (October)
	ReXMeD PHO formed (November)
1996	Case Management Services implemented (January)
	Master Performance Improvement Plan developed (February)
	Service line teams implemented (March)
	Performance Improvement Committee replaces Hospital Quality Assurance Committee (August)
	Mediqual Atlas data collection starts
	Starts using Gallup survey of customer satisfaction
	Starts using Health Management Council Clinical Benchmark cost data
	HCIA hospital discharge benchmarking data set introduced
	Named as one of "Best 100" workplaces for working women by *Working Mother Magazine*
1997	Arthur Andersen report suggests organizational structure for performance improvement with matrix of functional teams and service line teams
	Received National Research Corp.'s Quality Leader Award
	Earned State of North Carolina Governor's Award for Excellence for its Workplace Wellness Program
	MedPartners acquires Cardinal and Piedmont IPA bringing its Raleigh membership to about 500 physicians
1998	Duke University Medical Center announces purchase of Raleigh Community Hospital from Columbia/HCA

measurement activities, and establish performance objectives for them. It receives regular reports from the performance improvement committee (PIC) concerning process improvements and outcomes. This organizational relationship is outlined in Figure 5.1.

The performance improvement committee is an interdisciplinary medical review committee reporting to both the medical staff executive com-

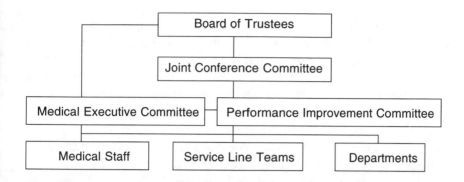

Figure 5.1 Perofrmance Improvement Reporting Structure

mittee and the JCC. Its functions are to oversee organizational compliance with the performance improvement plan adopted by the leadership; identify and recommend priorities and priority changes to the JCC; receive and review regular reports from all of the service line teams, committees, and departments; identify opportunities to improve performance; and recommend and establish "action teams" where indicated. Priorities are based on their potential to enhance patient care, achieve corporate goals, improve the financial strength of the organization, and/or improve quality of work life for employees and physicians.

Introduction of Service Lines

Service lines grouped inpatients according to similar DRGs [diagnosis-related groups] so that the care team can better meet the patients needs. Ten service lines were developed. They are:

1. Oncology
2. Neuroscience
3. Orthopedics
4. Cardiovascular
5. Medicine
6. General Surgery
7. Women and Children
8. Pulmonary/Nephrology
9. Emergency Services
10. Primary Care Division

The objective of the service line team is to promote accountability for the care of their population across the continuum of care. Representation on the teams is multidisciplinary and is determined by the particular needs of the population served. Each team has a physician team leader and a nursing team coordinator. The service line team members assess data on an ongoing basis to identify opportunities for improvement and promote achievable patient outcomes and satisfaction. Each team's charge also includes cost-effective utilization of resources, identification of the need for clinical pathways, and minimization of risks where feasible. It compares internal performance over time, compares Rex's performance with similar facilities, and compares performance to other sources such as practice guidelines as appropriate. It initiates intensive assessments by establishing action teams when variations in performance occur or when opportunities to improve are identified.

The objective of an action team is to provide intensive assessment, analysis, and recommendations for improvement. The expected outputs are recommendations, an implementation plan, and a measurement plan. Rex has adopted the FOCUS-PDCA methodology of process improvement. It is included in the leadership development core training program offered to all employees. Education includes the use of performance improvement tools, analysis of data, and leading and facilitating teams. New employee orientation includes an introductory session on this process improvement methodology.

1995–1996 Reorganization

The reorganization into service line teams highlighted the need to change the way that the staff services that support quality improvement are organized. Rex Hospital had traditional and separate departments of utilization review/quality assurance, social work, and continuous service improvement (also responsible for pathway development). Pathway implementation had not been as successful as hoped except for orthopedics. To prepare for an environment of more risk-based reimbursement and to counter reduced margins, these departments were intensified, reengineered, and integrated to have greater impact on clinical and financial outcomes without adversely affecting existing high quality levels.

In October 1995, two new departments were created: case management and performance improvement/risk management. Case management combined utilization review/quality assurance and social work and added a pre-entry case management function. Within three months the new case management model with concern for clinical, financial, and quality improvement was implemented in the inpatient setting. RN case managers and medical social workers were assigned to each of the eight inpatient core specialties and became core members of the service line teams. By 1998 the case management program included the following:

- Pre-entry coordination
- Screening and referral
- Assessment
- Problem identification
- Care planning
- Utilization management
- DRG analysis
- Variance management
- Discharge planning
- Psychosocial intervention
- Crisis management

At the same time the performance improvement/risk management (PI/RM) department was established to support the organization's quality assurance, quality improvement, outcomes management, risk management, and clinical pathway development. It coordinates, analyzes, and reports improvement data. Wherever possible, measurement activities are incorporated into processes and performed and reviewed concurrently by caregivers. The PI/RM department coordinates systems for the collection of specific data (Atlas, RiskKey) and works directly with other departments to acquire other data (Trendstar, Gallup, National Nosocomial Infection Survey). These data are compiled and initial analysis is performed. Comparison is made to historical experience, reference databases, accreditation guidelines, and practice guidelines. These data and analyses are then presented to service line teams, departments, and committees on a routine basis. Exhibit 5.3 lists the measures regularly collected or acquired. Quality control issues are reported to the performance improvement committee on a "report-by-exception" basis. Regular performance improvement service line reports are issued as well. An example is shown in Exhibit 5.4.

Exhibit 5.3 Reporting Systems Used for Performance Improvement

Atlas
Variance Reports
Clinical Path Variance Reports
Infection Control Surveillance
Comments
Improvement Initiatives
Joint Commission Indicator Monitors
Gallup Satisfaction Results
Department Specific Monitoring Reports
MMI Clinical Indicators
HCIA Comparative Hospital Discharge Summary Data
Trendstar Internal Cost Reports
Sentinel Events
Quality Control in the Organization (= or > 30 cases up to 5% sample quarterly)
• preoperative and postoperative diagnosis discrepancies
• adverse drug reactions
• confirmed transfusion reactions
• adverse anesthesia events
• appropriateness of admissions and hospital stays
• patient satisfaction
• staff views regarding performance and improvement operations
• autopsy results
• restraints
• risk management activities
• quality control activities for clinical labs, diagnostic radiology, dietetic, nuclear medicine, radiation oncology, medication administration equipment, pharmacy equipment used to prepare medications
Additional Measures Identified and Prioritized by Joint Conference Committee:
• patient care functions
• organization functions
• high-risk, high-volume, high-cost, problem-prone procedures/processes

The key coordination mechanism for performance improvement has continued to be the PIC. It has fulfilled a wide variety of roles and its agenda has become extensive and complex. For example, the calendar for the September 1998 meeting called for third-quarter Gallup results, the

Exhibit 5.4 Example of Service Line Report

PERFORMANCE IMPROVEMENT SERVICE LINE REPORT WOMEN AND CHILDREN DATE _____					
Global Indicators	**Benchmark**	Q1	Q2	Q3	Q4
1. C/S	** 20%				
2. APGAR <4 @ 5"	** 18				
3. Meconium aspiration	** 13				
4. NB w/ cerebral hemorrhage	** 1				
5. Pts ≥ 24 wks. gestation who do not receive base-line monitoring	** 5				
6. Use of Pit w/o fetal monitoring	** 11				
7. C/S for fetal ind not started w/in 30"	** 8				
8. Neonates delivered in a Level I or II facility @< 34 wks. & tr. to NICU	** 29				
9. Neonates deliv. ≥34 wks. & tr to NICU	** 130				
10.Maternal deaths	** 0				
11.Neonatal deaths ≥34 wks. < 34 wks. & </= 500 gms.	** 10				
12.Neonatal temp ≤35 C in first 4 hours of life	** 5				
13.Pneumothorax after neonatal resuscitation using ppv	** 1				
14.Neonates w/intubation prior to use of ppv	** 42				
** Based on MMI					
Gallup Survey Results					
Service Line Overall					
Rex Overall		3.59	3.56	3.55	N.A.
Resource Management					
Cost per Case					
Cost Index					

quarterly infection control report, review of quarterly HCIA data, and quarterly informational presentations from the cardiovascular, medical, and surgical service line teams and from the Rex Convalescent Center team. In addition, it included a quarterly report on risk management issues, medical staff review of clinical pathway team recommendations, and review of other procedural changes. Also it would consider additional items that might come up such as sentinel event reports, adverse drug reaction reports, and accreditation concerns. At other meetings, the PIC may also review plans and performance of the performance improvement/ risk management department and reports required by the hospital's liability insurance carrier, analyze safety issues, pathway utilization and variance reports, review proposals for new action teams, approve forms for reporting, and review Atlas Mediqual, Trendstar, and other benchmarking systems. Table 5.1 shows the schedule of reviews planned for each of the monthly PIC meetings during the fourth quarter of 1998.

Table 5.1 Quarterly Schedule for PIC Presentations

October 1998	November 1998	December 1998
Safety	Procedure Review	Gallup Customer Satisfaction Survey
Pharmacy & Therapeutics Committee	Pulmonary Service Line Team	Infection Control
Risk Management	Orthopedics Service Line Team	Cardiovascular Service Line Team
Oncology Service Line Team	Women and Children's Service Line Team	Medicine Service Line Team
Neuroscience Service Line Team	Nursing Performance Improvement Team	Surgery Service Line Team
Rex Home Services		
Emergency Department Service Line Team		
Blood Utilization Committee		
Cancer Committee	.	

Future Plans

By mid-1998 the assessment of the services showed that service line team leadership was in place with adequate staff support and was functioning with clear targets. The next step was to begin to involve the service line teams (SLTs) in the 1999 budget process to allow service line savings to track back to the bottom line. In 1999 the hospital would try to develop an affordable team reward system that could be implemented in 2000. This would have to be coordinated with the development of job description changes reflecting the new organizational structure and support through a new communication plan to explain the changes to all the Rex community. Beyond that the leadership saw the need to increase medical staff involvement in SLTs and action teams, to move the program beyond acute care, and balance the focus on outcomes, satisfaction, and cost-effectiveness. They also saw needs to develop mechanisms and/or incentives for following protocols, to streamline the approval process of SLT actions, and to streamline and clarify data sources and processes for decision making.

CASE ANALYSIS

This case shows the organizational complexities introduced by the need for outcomes measurement as well as process enhancement. This hospital is much further down that route than most, but it still has a number of issues to deal with in the future, such as the roles of the administration, of the performance improvement committee, and of the medical staff in this transition period and in the long run.

Introduction

Chapter 2 refers to the need to adapt to new standards such as Oryx and to remain competitive. The competitive environment of Rex Healthcare is clearly outlined here and it calls for the organization to be able to show that it is more cost-effective than the competing academic medical centers. The performance improvement process encompasses the efforts of the CQI [continuous quality improvement] teams and the service line teams and also the efforts of this organization to set up benchmarking and internal data gathering systems to support that effort. It also shows the amount of planning and coordination that will be necessary when the outcome measures are available to motivate behavioral changes.

Basics

This organization is committed to the outcomes approach to quality (Chapter 3) even while it maintains the required QA [quality assurance] functions. A number of approaches are used from Chapter 4 at both the macro and micro levels. Training in CQI techniques is available broadly throughout the organization. Teams are set up to implement the approach, although it is not clear how the concept of the quality council is really functioning. Many of the issues of maintaining physician participation in teams (Chapters 6 and 7) are available. The Gallup organization is used and followed here in order to follow up on customer satisfaction (Chapter 5). This organization is in the midst of implementing the complete system.

Implementation

We see that this is not an easy or rapid transition to implement. Issues of physician participation (Chapters 7 and 8) loom large. Issues of having the right information systems in place are also evident (Chapter 9). You will find that there is much to think about here in both of those sets of issues. One sees the cost of having such an organization and wonders about the cognitive complexity of the issues addressed by the performance improvement committee. Note that people are now talking about simplifying things, but unfortunately the issues and the institution and its medical community are extremely complex. One must move with both urgency and deliberation through the various implementation steps that are necessary. Chapters 12, 13, 16, and 17 on clinical innovation bring home the issues that are ahead, if clinical behavior in this community is to change, since this is not an organization employing most of the physicians practicing there. Because this is a teaching hospital, there are also a number of issues of professional education that are to be addressed in this process, but these were beyond the scope of this case.

Application

This is a community hospital making the transition from hospital to health system in a complex, highly fluid medical marketplace. All of the players will need to think how to address the issues of academic training noted in Chapter 16 and then think about the possibilities raised by Chapter 17. Because Rex Healthcare does maintain and operate primary care centers, the experiences discussed in Chapter 12 will also be relevant to the organization, although there may have to be a separate effort there, since those clinics are dispersed from the hospital. This is a very rich application and one which points the way that many organizations will have to follow in the future, each with its own process enhancement process.

CASE 6

Dr. Johnson,
Network Medical Director

William Q. Judge and Curtis P. McLaughlin

Charles A. Johnson, DO, MBA, reviewed his six months of experience as a network medical director for the Southeast region of Vigilant—Xtra Mile HealthCare located in Atlanta, Georgia. He was one of two physicians responsible for developing and managing the professional medical network of providers and hospitals serving this market which included the states of Alabama, Georgia, and Mississippi. His duties involved recruiting providers, negotiating contracts, promoting the company's disease management approaches, credentialing physicians, maintaining NCQA [National Committee on Quality Assurance] accreditation, reviewing cost and quality data as well as provider report cards, arranging education efforts for outliers, and controlling the unit cost side of the firm's medical loss ratio in that market.

Dr. Johnson had a full plate of responsibilities that were new to him and his organization. Furthermore, he had limited staff to delegate duties to and there were overlapping responsibilities with two other medical directors in his office that needed to be coordinated carefully. Despite these challenges, he felt fortunate to have a supportive and powerful boss and he was convinced that Vigilant—Xtra Mile HealthCare was the wave of the future. His immediate challenge was fundamentally a matter of time

Source: This case was prepared by Professor William Q. Judge, College of Business Administration, University of Tennessee, Knoxville, and Professor Curtis P. McLaughlin, Kenan-Flagler Business School, University of North Carolina, Chapel Hill, for use at both universities as a basis for class discussion rather than to illustrate the effective or ineffective handling of an administrative matter. Copyright © 1998 by the Kenan-Flagler Business School of the University of North Carolina, Chapel Hill, NC 27599-3490. All rights reserved. Not to be reproduced without permission.

management. Although Dr. Johnson was highly organized, he felt he was constantly "putting out unexpected fires" and these urgent projects tended to push out longer-term strategic issues. For example, in the last month, his schedule had been consumed by several unexpected activities including (1) supervising a database cleanup, (2) addressing open enrollment administrative glitches in January, (3) being available for audits of the Medicare program by HCFA [Health Care Financing Administration] and the state of Georgia, (4) preparing for a mock NCQA audit, and (5) dealing with supervisory and human relations issues within his unit. These issues tended to get in the way of refining his network of providers and overseeing quality, but they had to be addressed. Dr. Johnson hoped that with time things would settle down.

BACKGROUND

When Charles Johnson graduated in 1970 from Baldwin-Wallace College in Berea, Ohio with a BS in zoology and philosophy, he went to work as a pharmaceutical salesman in Ohio and western Pennsylvania. He was successful there, but he wanted direct patient contact, so he decided to pursue a medical degree. In 1973, he entered the Midwestern University-Chicago College of Osteopathic Medicine. Graduating in 1977, he interned at HCA [Hospital Corporation of America] Northlake Hospital in Tucker, Georgia. In 1979, he founded the East Cobb Family Practice in Marietta, Georgia and joined the staff of the Archway Hospital. He became board certified by the American Board of Osteopathic Family Practitioners and a fellow of the American Academy of Family Practice in 1986 and a diplomat of the American Board of Medical Management in 1997.

In the late 1980s, Dr. Johnson and his partner differed markedly over the importance of managed care. His partner did not want to participate, while he was convinced it was the wave of the future. When he witnessed the loss of 20 percent of his patients after Lockheed Marietta moved all of its employees to managed care, he was convinced that he needed to change his practice. He had been participating in management workshops provided by the American College of Physician Executives (ACPE) and decided to enter Emory University's weekend executive MBA program. He found this to be a valuable learning experience, particularly his thesis project, which involved a study of methods of valuation for small medical practices. When he graduated in June 1991, he installed a total quality management effort in his family practice and asked his partner to leave within 90 days. After his partner left, Dr. Johnson increased the volume of the practice 83 percent within 12 months while accepting managed care patients and adding a new partner, two physician assistants, and a nurse practitioner.

Dr. Johnson tried to start a group practice without walls in conjunction with other providers, but it "failed within six months due to lack of capital and physician management skills and involvement." Then in late 1994 he received four offers to sell his practice. One of the offers came from an organization that was connected to the hospital where he practiced. Ultimately, he decided to harvest his practice to this organization and become involved in the management of the resulting organization. Thus, he became one of the founding members and chief of family medicine for Dominion Northwest Physician's Group, a group with 180 physicians and 60 locations with affiliations with 13 hospitals in the greater Atlanta region. There he spent half time in management and half time in patient care delivery.

The job with Dominion Northwest was a useful transition for him. He negotiated contracts for the physicians and was involved in developing methods for equitably dividing capitated payment among the specialists and primary care physicians. He was on the contracting committee of the Dominion PHO [physician-hospital organization] and the Physician's Group, and on the strategic planning and the informatics committees as well as the physicians' advisory board. He learned more about working in large organizations with hours spent in committee meetings and dealing with larger bureaucracies. With time, however, he became convinced that this organization did not have sufficient physician involvement in decision making to satisfy him in the long run, but he kept on learning about medical management and leadership.

Then one day an executive recruiter called him about the job at Vigilant—Xtra Mile HealthCare [Vigilant—XMHC]. Dr. Johnson felt he had nothing to lose in looking at it, especially since it was in Atlanta. He concluded that it was the type of job that would allow him to make a difference at a higher level. Vigilant—XMHC was looking for a physician with management skills, with a good reputation and credentials, and well connected to the local network. Dr. Johnson had been very active in the Georgia Academy of Family Practice, was on the board of directors of Blue Ridge Area Health Education Center (AHEC) and of a couple of managed care plans in addition to his involvement with administrative duties within Dominion.

In 1994 Governor Zell Miller had appointed Dr. Johnson to the nine-member Georgia Joint Board of General Practice which oversees the allocation of $50,000,000 in state residency and training funds. Dr. Johnson worked with the other members to formulate state policy on funding of graduate medical education and to redesign all state funding mechanisms for medical education. He was currently secretary/treasurer of the board. He has also served as a preceptor for Emory University and the West Virginia College of Osteopathic Medicine and on the 6th District (Newt Gingrich's [former] district) Medicare Advisory Board Task Force on Alternative Plans for Medicare. In short, his connections and experience were ideal for the job.

The job carried with it a salary comparable to a good primary care practitioner income with major upside potential in the long run. There were very good benefits and he was part of the regional management team. Fortunately, Dominion Northwest allowed Dr. Johnson to opt out of the remaining two years of his employment contract and he joined Vigilant—XMHC in August 1997.

His counterpart, Chris Donovan, M.D., was a native of the West Indies who had previous experience as a medical director with Domina in Charlotte, North Carolina. He was also new to the organization as he joined Vigilant—Xtra Mile HealthCare about the same time as Charley Johnson did. Drs. Johnson and Donovan had a good working relationship. Their responsibilities were basically the same, except for different parts of the market.

Corporate Background

Vigilant and Xtra Mile HealthCare merged in April 1996, bringing together two quite different firms. Vigilant was a traditional full-line insurance company founded in 1899 with 48 highly decentralized HMO operations and a rather conservative business outlook. It was headquartered in Boston. In contrast, Xtra Mile HealthCare was founded in Wheeling, West Virginia in 1978. It was a highly centralized and entrepreneurial company developed and managed by physicians. For example, Vigilant had 50 different claims processing centers, while XMHC had only one. In addition to structural differences, their growth strategies were also quite different. Vigilant had been buying primary care practices, while Xtra Mile HealthCare did not buy any practices.

The resulting merger was a giant company with revenues in excess of $17 billion, more than half of which was in health care products. It divided the nation into six regions, which are depicted in Figure 6.1. In 1998, Vigilant—Xtra Mile HealthCare provided health care services to 23 million Americans in 50 states through networks involving 300,000 physicians and 3,000 hospitals. Roughly one insured American in 12 was covered for health care by the resulting organization.

The merged company developed a number of strategies aimed at capitalizing on its extensive asset base and unique array of competencies. First and foremost, it would offer a full line of health care insurance products (e.g., indemnity, PPO [preferred provider organization], POS [point-of-service] plan, HMO, senior HMO) on a national basis to offer "one-stop shopping" to nationally based organizations. The firm would not purchase medical practices or facilities, but would maintain an open panel of physicians and nonexclusive contracts with hospitals and ancillary providers. Its basic HMO contracting model called for primary care physicians (PCPs) to serve as gatekeepers on quality-based capitation, with specialists paid on a discounted fee-for-service or capitated basis and hospitals paid at a negotiated rate by the case or per diem.

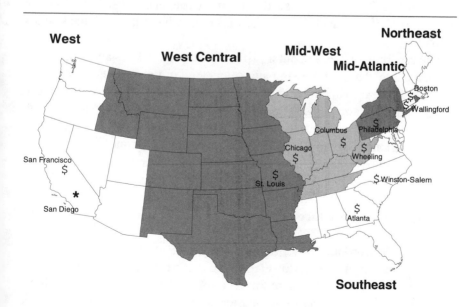

Figure 6.1 Six Regions of Vigilant—Xtra Mile HealthCare

By 1997, Vigilant—XMHC had an approved HMO in 23 states and the District of Columbia covering 73 percent of the population and had applications pending in the rest. Each physician recruited to the network was expected to service all Vigilant—XMHC health care products under one contract. This consistent national presence and full range of health care products allowed the company to approach large national employers on a highly competitive basis. The fact that they could also supply disability insurance, group life, retirement plans, 401k's, dental insurance, and variety of other products to the same benefits managers nationwide was considered a strong competitive advantage. The company is a leading provider of Medicare managed care services and could also service the company's retirees.

The two companies had been highly profitable in 1995 and 1996. However, profit margins narrowed and medical loss ratios rose sharply in 1997. The stock had dropped sharply from 1996 levels. The economies in operations and from scale that had been expected took much longer to achieve. Dr. Johnson talked about the loss of human capital during the reorganization that cost it dearly. According to Dr. Johnson: "In our efforts to reengineer the organization, a lot of administrative help was eliminated. In so doing, we let go of a lot of Ms. Smiths. You know, Ms. Smith was the one in the local office who knew that Dr. Jones never checked box 30 on the HCFA 1500 form, but checked it for him rather than sending it back to his office."

The resulting delays and other glitches with new offices and employees slowed down claims processing and overstated initial earnings, with costs catching up later. However, the new organization was now getting more integrated and claims processing was functioning better in 1998. The new Vigilant—Xtra Mile HealthCare organization was partially decentralized into six regions. The Southeast region consisted of four markets stretching from Mississippi to Florida to Maryland.

Organizational Structure

The overall corporate headquarters was located with Vigilant in Boston, while the health care operations were headquartered at XMHC in Wheeling. The six regional offices reported to the Wheeling corporate offices. There were three medical director hierarchies in the company. Network medical directors, of whom Dr. Johnson was one, reported to the general manager for each market who reported in turn to the regional manager. Patient management medical directors were involved with utilization management, pre-authorizations, length-of-stay reviews, case management development, retrospective reviews, and disease management enrollment. Patient managers came under the regional medical director who reported directly to the core team at Wheeling. Finally, there was also a regional quality medical director who reported to quality management in Boston. A detailed comparison of these three types of medical directors is listed in Exhibit 6.1.

Dr. Johnson supervised a team of eight individuals: two provider relations managers who in turn led five professional service coordinators, and an administrative assistant shared with Dr. Donovan. The professional service coordinators were the ones out on the firing line with the providers. There were numerous dotted line relationships among the various medical directors. In fact, when he was hired, Dr. Johnson had only dotted line relationships and no direct reports, so he recommended a reorganization in which he took on budgetary and supervisory responsibility for a portion of the provider services staff. He also made a determined effort to be seen as a contributor to the management team of the market and the region. For example, he hosted a weekend strategic planning session for the regional management team at his summer home at Lake Lanier.

This meant considerable added workload due to supervision, performance review, objective setting, and process improvement. He typically worked from 7:00 AM to 6:00 PM two days a week, and 9:00 AM to 6:00 PM the other three and then usually had a couple of dinner meetings each week. Weekend activities such as a strategic planning retreat or a mock NCQA site visit exercise might tie up one weekend a month. Typically, he responded to about 60 internal e-mail messages a day and a large number of telephone calls. A two-month review of his calendar showed that he spent on average four hours a day in meetings about 60 percent in the office and 40 percent outside. When he took the job, he was told to expect to be traveling four days a week. However, this market's business was very heavily concentrated in Georgia and in Atlanta in particular.

Management of Quality

In 1990, XM Data Driven, Inc. (XMDD) was established as a XMHC quality measurement subsidiary. With over 280 employees, it had access to a data warehouse of claims information from hospitalization, outpatient

Exhibit 6.1 Excerpts from the Job Descriptions of Medical Directors at Vigilant—Xtra Mile HealthCare

Job Characteristics	Patient Management Director & Quality Management Director	Network Medical Director
Fundamental Role	Develop and manage a health services organization focused on reducing medical cost and improving clinical outcomes, member satisfaction, and provider satisfaction	Develop and manage a health services organization focused on reducing medical cost and improving clinical outcomes, member satisfaction, and provider satisfaction
Central Activities	Implement utilization and quality management programs through timely policy interpretation and local application	Provide strategic and operational direction for the delivery of performance-based medical management
	Manage budget	Manage budget and risk drivers
	Provide marketing support through sales presentations, site visits, and support for requests for proposals	Analyze and report business performance data to customers and colleagues
	Render medical necessity determinations	Handle Vigilant funds as if they were his/her own
	Chair committees in accordance with market and contractual needs	Participate in internal and external health industry development efforts
	Participate in national, regional, local work groups as required	Participate in management of local profit and loss
	Serve as liaison between field organization, home office, and governmental agencies	Serve as liaison with regulatory and accrediting agencies and other business units within the company
	Develop local medical review and coverage policies	Develop and maintain strong provider relationships
Leadership	Maintain a customer-driven passion for excellence and commitment to action and change	Maintain a customer-driven passion for excellence and commitment to action and change
Direction Setting	Make timely and high-quality decisions as well as implement them	Make timely and high-quality decisions as well as implement them
Selection	Hire, develop, and reward staff to effectively support the company's strategy	Hire, develop, and reward staff to effectively support the company's strategy
Communication	Excellent verbal and written skills as well as negotiation and conflict resolution skills	Excellent verbal and written skills as well as negotiation and conflict resolution skills
Business Knowledge	In-depth knowledge of managed care, financial, business processes, and strategies and objectives	In-depth knowledge of managed care, financial, business processes, and strategies and objectives
	Job-specific technical knowledge	Job-specific technical knowledge
Other Requirements	Board certification is highly desired; state license must be active & unencumbered	Board certification is optional
	Demonstrated commitment to professional development (e.g., CME, conferences)	Demonstrated commitment to professional development (e.g., seminars)

visits, pharmacy claims and laboratory reports of 15 million enrollees. It was a pioneering and innovative unit with Xtra Mile HealthCare, developing clinical algorithms, identifying and risk-stratifying seriously ill members for disease management interventions, providing risk-adjusted performance reporting systems, maintaining a disease registry for members with any of more than 65 chronic illnesses, and working with participating academic medical centers to conduct applied research. A fuller description of XMDD is provided in Exhibit 6.2. An example of the type of report cards that they provide to management and to providers is shown in Exhibit 6.3.

Exhibit 6.2 XMDD (XM Data Driven, Inc.) Description

The XMDD's health services research program is the dedicated research and development unit of Vigilant—Xtra Mile HealthCare.™ Physicians, Ph.D.-level researchers, methodologists, nurses, statisticians, programmers, medical coders, and other experienced professionals make up this unit. Staff conduct applied research and develop methodologies that measure and improve the quality and efficiency of health care services for Vigilant—Xtra Mile HealthCare's membership. One of the main goals of the Health Services Research Program is to evaluate the outcomes and cost-effectiveness of managed care programs.

The XMDD Health Services Research Program has access to an abundance of health-related data on more than 14 million insured members throughout the United States, and routinely analyzes both primary and secondary data for hundreds of practical applications. Research conducted by this unit is designed to benefit four primary customers which include: (1) individual members, (2) providers, (3) plan sponsors, and (4) the Vigilant—Xtra Mile HealthCare system.

When working with external organizations on collaborative research, XMDD staff provide methodological, data acquisition, and technical support, and assist with the grant application process as well.

Examples of XMDD Health Services Research

- Health Profiling—Using a number of different data sets, clinical logic has been created to identify individuals with any of 65 chronic diseases. Each individual's disease-specific health status can be categorized and used in a number of applications. For instance, an individual's health profile is used as a predictor in risk-stratification models to determine who should be entered into disease management programs. Health status is also used as a risk adjuster in physician performance compensation models. Furthermore, these profiles are used to calculate employer group disease-specific prevalence rates, which help employers determine the best benefits package to purchase from Vigilant—Xtra Mile HealthCare.
- Risk-Stratification Modeling—XMDD has created empirically driven risk-stratification models designed to identify individuals who are at high risk for certain types of disease-specific acute exacerbations. These multivariate predictive models use previous utilization patterns to assign chronically ill individuals into one of five risk strata. After extensive cross-validation, these models are used to determine appropriate disease

continues

Exhibit 6.2 continued

> management resources that are consistent with the health needs of each category of individuals.
> - Clinical Outcomes Studies and Program Evaluation—Both pilot and long-standing managed care programs are evaluated to determine their impact on members' health status. A number of different econometric, epidemiological and statistical quasi-experimental models have been employed to evaluate these programs while controlling for important confounding variables.
> - Severity-Adjusted Performance Measurement—Severity-adjusted performance measurement models have been developed for hospitals, specialists, and primary care providers. These multivariate statistical models are used to provide feedback to providers and institutions about their performance relative to others in their field. Additionally, performance measurement information is used to determine a portion of each provider's reimbursement. By accounting for differences in patient mix by factoring in characteristics such as age, gender, and co-morbidities, the playing field is leveled between providers, and performance results are more valid.
> - Health System Research—A number of research projects are under way to further investigate the health system overall. Cost-effectiveness and practice pattern variation studies, for example, have been undertaken to more fully understand costs and utilization of the country's health system. Additionally, the impact of different insurance arrangements on utilization and health status are being studied. Results from these studies will help Vigilant—Xtra Mile HealthCare better understand how to resource high-quality health services.

Vigilant—Xtra Mile HealthCare believed that ultimately the market would be defined by quality. This was so important to Vigilant—XMHC that the company had established a unique quality-driven compensation system for primary care physicians. The incentives in this system are balanced to attempt to avoid both over- and under-utilization. Each practice receives a capitation payment, which is adjusted for the age and gender of the covered population. This payment is further adjusted by a quality factor that is revised every six months. The example below in Exhibit 6.4 illustrates how the quality factor is determined.

Offices that failed to make a score of at least 2 percent received a 10 percent reduction in capitation payments during the subsequent six months. Those that maintained a score of at least two percent received an increase in their semi-monthly capitation payments equal to the percentage score.

Exhibit 6.3 Sample XMDD Report Card for Asthma

Practice Type: Family Practice   Region: XX   Office Number: XX
Office Address: 1 Street, Anytown, PA 19074   Reporting Period: 10/1/94-9/30/95
Number of our current insureds identified with asthma: 232

PREVALENCE MEASURES	Office	XMHC Average
1. Estimated overall prevalence of asthma	4.5%	4.0%
2. Estimated overall prevalence of asthma age 0-9	9.0%	7.9%
3. Estimated overall prevalence of asthma age 10-19	7.2%	6.8%
4. Estimated overall prevalence of asthma age 20-39	5.7%	4.0%
5. Estimated overall prevalence of asthma age 40+	2.5%	2.8%
ASTHMA TREATMENT PATTERNS		
6. Asthmatics on prescription drugs for asthma	65.8%	66.4%
7. Asthmatics receiving sympathomimetics	58.3%	58.3%
8. Asthmatics receiving theophylline	6.4%	11.0%
9. Asthmatics receiving only theophylline	0.0%	0.7%
10. Asthmatics receiving cromolyn	8.0%	8.7%
11. Asthmatics receiving inhaled steroids	21.4%	18.8%
12. Average annual number of beta agonist prescriptions for asthmatics receiving any beta agonist	4.29	3.72
13. Asthmatics on beta agonists receiving 2 or more prescriptions in one month	18.3%	17.9%
14. Asthmatics receiving one or more course of oral steroids	17.1%	18.3%
ACCESS MEASURES		
15. Asthmatics seeing the PCP at least once	92.5%	86.9%
16. Average number of annual PCP visits per asthmatic	5.74	4.69
17. Asthmatics seeing a pulmonologist	8.8%	7.0%
18. Asthmatics seeing an allergist	14.5%	11.7%
PROCESS MEASURES		
19. Asthmatics with an outpatient chest X-ray	8.4%	8.9%
20. Asthmatics age 8+ receiving pulmonary function tests	8.3%	10.1%
21. Asthmatics receiving allergy testing	3.1%	4.8%
22. Asthmatics receiving allergy immunotherapy	7.5%	8.0%
23. Asthmatics using a home nebulizer	2.2%	2.4%
24. Asthmatics with at least one antibiotic prescription	63.1%	71.3%
25. Asthmatics on theophylline who have at least one theophylline level drawn	10.0%	18.9%
26. Average annual number of theophylline levels in asthmatics on theophylline	0.10	0.29
27. Asthmatics receiving at least one home care visit	3.5%	3.4%
OUTCOME MEASURES		
ASTHMA RELATED CONDITIONS		
28. Emergency room visits specifically for asthma/1,000 asthmatics/year	57	86
29. Total admissions (acute) specifically for asthma/1,000 asthmatics/year	44	40
30. Total inpatient days (acute) specifically for asthma/1,000 asthmatics/year	273	177
ALL CONDITIONS FOR ASTHMATIC MEMBERS		
31. Total emergency room visits for all conditions/1,000 asthmatics/year	154	242
32. Total admissions (acute) for all conditions/1,000 asthmatics per year	128	149
33. Total inpatient days (acute) for all conditions/1,000 asthmatics/year	493	572
SATISFACTION MEASURES*		
34. Overall satisfaction with medical care at the PCP office of asthmatic members	100.0%	95.9%
35. Satisfaction with the ability to make appointments for illnesses	95.4%	92.1%
36. Satisfaction with the response to an emergency call within 30 minutes	98.6%	93.0%

*Percent of respondents with Good, Very Good, or Excellent

Thus the ABC Practice would have received a 14.55 percent increment in its capitation payments.

Each practice also received a six-month quality-factored distribution based on its three utilization components (hospital, specialist, and ER) year-to-date, which was adjusted by the Quality Review and Comprehensive Care components (in the example above 4.25 percent + 8.50 percent = 12.75 percent). If the practice had achieved a combined Quality Review and Utilization component score of at least 4 percent (4.25 + 1.80 percent = 6.05 percent), it was eligible for an office status payment of 5 percent, if it had remained open for XMHC enrollment throughout the period or if it had accepted current patients as XMHC members throughout that period.

Exhibit 6.4 Sample Quality Factor Calculation

Based on the quality of care, comprehensive service, and utilization, the ABC Practice earned the following quality factor which is multiplied by their sex- and age-adjusted base capitation payment for the previous two weeks:

Quality Review Components:

a. Member Surveys (compared to others in HMO, range: -0.75 to +3.0)   2.00%

b. Focused Medical Chart Reviews (2/yr., comparative, -0.75 to +3.0)   0.75%

c. Member Transfer Rates (comparative, -0.75 to +1.5)   0.50%

d. Philosophy of Managed Care (cooperation and participation with XMHC quality programs (subjective, -0.75 to +3.0)   1.00%

   Quality Review Subtotal   **4.25%**

Comprehensive Care Components:

a. Membership Size (members/doctor or practice, e.g.: range = 0, 1% at 100/doctor, 1.5% at 200/doctor, 2% at 300/doctor)   1.00%

b. Schedule Office Hours (range = 0, 0.5% for 50–59, 1.0% for 60–69, and 1.5% for >70 hours/week)   0.50%

c. Available Office Procedures (e.g., flexible sigmoidoscopy =1.0%) max.=3%)   1.00%

d. Program Education (completing XMHC educational courses (e.g., Current Concepts in Cancer = 0.5%,) max. sum = 2%)   0.50%

e. Internal Practice Coverage (1% if coverage is by   - practice for continuity)   1.00%

f. Catastrophic Care (practice has greater than the HMO type average total costs for catastrophic cases (e.g.,>$20,000= 1.5%)   1.50%

g. Patient Management (1% if practice supports and participates in XMHC patient management and directs hospital care of own patients)   1.00%

h. Practice Growth (XMHC membership growth (e.g., >10% = 1.0%)   1.00%

continues

Exhibit 6.4 continued

i.	Computer Links to XMHC (transmits encounter and referral data electronically = 1.0%)	1.00%
	Comprehensive Care Subtotal	**8.50%**
Utilization Components:		
a.	Hospital Utilization at the average bracket (range = -0.8 to +1.8%)	0.80%
b.	Specialist Utilization one bracket greater than average (-0.8 to +1.8%)	0.40%
c.	Emergency Room Utilization one bracket less than average (-0.8 to +1.4%)	0.60%
	Utilization Subtotal	**1.8%**
	TOTAL QUALITY FACTOR =	**14.55%**

The large employers that the company sought out tended to insist on NCQA certification. Therefore, one of Dr. Johnson's main performance objectives was to have the network meet NCQA requirement of meeting its own written quality standards. He spent much time and effort making sure that the network conformed to NCQA requirements such as having a certain percentage of members within 15-minutes travel time of a primary care provider in the network and working with practices to help them achieve NCQA's HEDIS [Health Plan Employer Data and Information Set] standards for their patients. Another standard was that of keeping provider turnover below five percent per year.

The costs of achieving these standards can be substantial. In six months, the region had gone through a NCQA audit exercise, a Georgia exercise for Medicare, and a federal exercise for Medicare. Then there were the operational costs of maintaining standards. For example, NCQA standards required recredentialing each network physician every two years. With over 7,000 physicians in their network in Georgia, that was a substantial workload, the cost of which made Dr. Johnson consider strategies for narrowing the network where possible. HMOs in Georgia were licensed county by county by the state. As geographic coverage was expanded, the number of physicians to be credentialed expanded. He found himself having to trade off greater choice for his patients with the costs of providing the larger provider network in the served areas as well as allocating scarce resources between served areas and new target market areas.

One decision that Dr. Johnson had to make was how much time to spend requesting and reviewing report cards on the physicians in the network. XMDD could generate an almost infinite number of reports like the one in Exhibit 6.3. They could also generate statistical reports identifying outlier individuals and practices. Much of the data on over- or under-utilization were of more concern to the regional medical director responsible for patient management, but that medical loss ratio was part of his performance evaluation also.

Dr. Johnson's Observations about the Job

Dr. Johnson had been in the job only six months when this case was written. So far, he was quite happy with the job and with its potential. He observed that the Dominion Northwest had been a useful transition for him to enable him to see the comparative advantages of various types of health care organizations and to get used to working in a large organization. He was no longer seeing patients, but he was comfortable with that fact. He had already "seen enough patients to fill Fulton County Stadium three times" and no longer found practice much of a challenge. He often compared the practice of medicine to flying an airplane: "When you need a skilled pilot, that individual is important and one's skills are critical during the unique takeoff and landing periods. However, in between takeoffs and landings, most of the system is on autopilot and that gets old over time. The same is true of medicine."

There were always the fires to fight and there were always special projects related to process improvement. For example, the company had just gone through a major database cleanup of its provider records. Many physicians had changed their affiliations due to mergers and acquisitions and thus their tax ID numbers, but had not informed their payers. A wrong provider ID number on a claim could hold up payment and distort the company's data on activities and costs. That had been a major effort for his group.

He observed that most physicians would not be comfortable with the length of time that it took to get things done in a large organization. They, like he, were used to dealing with and reaching closure on a presenting problem every 15 minutes. Recruiting a substantial group practice into the network might take as much as a year with a meeting every month to establish a trusting relationship and to work out the details of the contract.

Medical directors also had to be comfortable working as part of a management team, to influence others where possible, but take orders when necessary. They would have to know when to keep quiet and when to speak up. For example, in the disease management arena, the core management at Wheeling would often decide which disease management programs were "network impactable" and he would have to make them work. He noted that he still had more to learn about the politics of large organizations and about the insurance industry in general, about group selection, underwriting, claims management, contracting, and marketing. He certainly felt that he had a better idea of what groups such as independent practice associations [IPAs] could or could not do effectively. Having seen the information system investment that Vigilant—Xtra Mile HealthCare had to support membership enrollment, claims processing, disease management, and utilization review, he saw no way that much smaller, physician-led organizations could compete. On the other hand, he felt that insurance organizations knew relatively little about managing practices or running hospitals and were better off not trying to integrate them.

Dr. Johnson was aware of the high turnover rate among medical directors in the industry. In his own words: "The health care environment is in turmoil and one needs a mentor, someone looking out for them, if one is to survive. One has to be careful to avoid the lose-lose situations that many medical directors had gotten into." By way of example, he cited medical directors of Medicaid managed care organizations when the Georgia State legislature decreed a 20 percent cut in funding, or those whose jobs were eliminated during mergers. He knew a local medical director working for MedPartners who was let go when the merger with Phycor was announced. Now that that merger did not go through, they were recruiting a replacement.

He noted that most physicians are not at all prepared for the practices of large organizations. He had heard them speak quite heatedly about the experience of a terminated medical director at another HMO who was given 20 minutes under observation to clean out her desk, escorted to the door with security person on each side, and asked to hand over her keys at the door. After a few months in a data-driven organization, he fully understood why. Why give anyone a chance to download proprietary information onto a computer disk or destroy a data set? However, no practicing physician would ever expect to be mortified that way.

Dr. Johnson also felt that most physicians would have difficulty with having to clear so many decisions with the legal department or with public relations. Yet, while there were policies and procedures governing most everything, he did not feel that they would constrain his team from setting aggressive goals, developing plans to compete in the markets that they chose, and implementing them quickly and efficiently. However, most physicians would have trouble at first being resource-constrained in what could be accomplished. When he was in practice, if he felt the practice would benefit from a piece of equipment, he bought it. It meant a loss in the profits distributed at the end of the month, but there was still enough. But when he wanted an additional employee to serve as a practice management coordinator, a highly skilled professional services consultant to go into network practices and help them solve billing or cost problems, he had to work hard to justify that position and show how it would contribute to meeting financial targets.

The Future

Dr. Johnson saw the provider community consolidating, which would give them more power in the negotiations with the payer networks. He felt that the payers would have to learn how to do a better job of partnering with the providers so that in sharing the risks they would both succeed. Thus far, providers had had a very poor track record in profiting by taking on risk and he felt that one of his jobs in the future would be in helping them succeed.

He also saw many opportunities for expanding the network. There were many areas of Georgia, Mississippi, and Alabama that did not have rationalized provider networks. He recognized a need to tell the managed care story more effectively given the current hostility in the profession and in the media which was being echoed politically in Georgia and Washington, D.C. He also saw the need to become more effective in negotiating good contracts, closely observing quality and utilization, and moving population to the good providers. There were many opportunities, many issues, and many unknowns to be faced.

CASE ANALYSIS

This case is about the role of medical directors in the quality efforts of large HMO companies and insurers. In this case, the primary focus is on gatekeeper contracts rather than PPO contracts. Dr. Johnson is just one of three types of medical directors in the firm, each reporting to a different level of the organization. The reader can use case data to review the apparent criteria used by the company in recruiting its market medical directors individually and as a team. There is also considerable information about the company's databases and their methods of motivating participating primary care physicians.

Introduction

This case is good when paired with Case 5 to provide a look at two sides of the outcomes measurement issues, since one is about a provider and the other about a purchaser of services. While the ORYX system is very important to the hospital, so is NCQA accreditation to the HMO. Dr. Johnson notes that he still has a ways to go in figuring out how to use the report cards that could be provided to him at the provider level, but the potential is clearly there. Much of the analysis and decision making about clinical quality in the aggregate, however, are handled by other units of the corporation at other locations, so that Dr. Johnson's ability to impact best practices is limited to his geographic area and the protocols adopted at the higher level.

Basics

Dr. Johnson talks about a team (Chapter 6) but it is not clear whether it is or is not his role to build one in the quality area. There is a great deal of firefighting going on here, but he does not seem to have a process orientation to what he is planning. There are many possibilities for involving local physicians on problem-oriented teams, if he so chooses. However, it does not seem to be the focus of the current corporate culture as he sees it. The information in Chapter 3 on outcome approaches could be very useful to Dr. Johnson and was not apparently covered in his graduate studies. The basics of CQI analysis in Chapter 4 could be applied to many of the processes in Dr. Johnson's work unit and to the clinical issues that he uncovers in his market area. First, however, he has to define what his area of responsibility will be in the quality arena and go to work on this.

Implementation

Dr. Johnson will have to move away from his individualistic style of management, if he is going to implement any changes. This will require effective managing up, down, and out into the community. This is a highly transitional company, which is in the process of merging two highly different cultures and there is more change likely to come. Maintaining morale and effectiveness during these transitions is his primary requirement as well as keeping the network development moving forward. The advantage that his organization has is in field of organizational learning (Chapter 7) and in the data and information processing areas (Chapter 9), areas where most providers are at a distinct disadvantage. However, one might wonder whether the company is yet fully cognizant of the potentials of either of these. If so, it does not seem to have resulted in disseminating the tools and concepts for action to the market level yet.

Application

This case lines up opposite the concepts presented in Chapter 13, "CQI in Managed Care." However, this is not a system in which the organization directly controls any providers. Everything has to be done indirectly. Therefore, there is an interesting contrast between the methods outlined in Chapter 13 and those implied by the information in the case exhibits. Exhibits 6.2, 6.3, and 6.4 are especially interesting in this regard. However, it is up to the reader to interpret these and to evaluate the quality implications of the two systems.

The Patient Transportation Project at University Hospitals

Sandra K. Evans and Ronald T. Pannesi

Sally Lloyd, vice chair of nursing and assistant director of operations at University Hospitals, had just received the patient transportation statistics for January 1992. She could hardly believe them—7,100 transports. But how good was the system? She called Patient Transportation's new computerized number and within two minutes a transporter was dispatched! "This is quite a change from a year ago when transport response time, defined as the interval between the request for transport and the time a transporter is dispatched, averaged 26–30 minutes and the patient transport project was conceived."

The Patient Transportation Project began when University Hospitals funded a proposal to improve the delivery of inpatient transportation services. The one-year grant funded the purchase of a communications system that primarily consisted of two-way radios and a voice information system. At about this same time and prior to the arrival of the communications equipment, University Hospitals was initiating a pilot quality improvement team to work on the admission-discharge (A/D) process. This pilot program had evolved from University Hospital's participation in the National Demonstration Project on Quality Improvement in Health Care, sponsored by the John A. Hartford Foundation and the Harvard Community Health Plan.

The adage that "timing is everything" certainly proved true here. Patient Transportation was one of the 12 departments/divisions invited to join the A/D continuous quality improvement (CQI) team. The introduction of the new communications technology and the application of quality improvement techniques and methods learned as participants on the A/D CQI team had propelled the operational changes in transport services. In just three months, the average transport response time went from 30 to 15 minutes, and the response times just kept getting better even after the A/D CQI team completed its work.

UNIVERSITY HOSPITALS

University Hospitals is a 665-bed teaching and referral center located at the University of North Carolina at Chapel Hill. As a public academic medical center, its mission is fourfold: (1) providing quality patient care, (2) educating health care professionals, (3) advancing health research, and (4) providing community service.

As a patient care resource, University Hospitals fulfills an important state and regional role by providing comprehensive services and highly specialized treatment for more than 20,000 inpatients and 500,000 outpatient visitors each year. Built in 1952, the Hospitals has continued to grow with the addition of the first Ambulatory Patient Care Facility (APCF) in 1975, two bed towers in 1975 and 1981, and the five-story Anderson wing in 1986. Most of the diagnostic and treatment facilities are concentrated in the original (1952) section of the Hospitals shown in Figure 7.1. The Hospitals' master facility plan projected an expansion of licensed beds to 702 by 1995.

The Hospitals operates its own personnel department subject to the state system of personnel management. Full-time and part-time employees numbered 4,122 in 1991, exclusive of the 510 house staff and the medical staff of 750 attending physicians, almost all of whom were faculty members of the medical school and dental school.

Patient Transportation Service

University Hospitals developed a centralized Patient Transportation Service in 1963 at the request of the Nursing Services. Six transporters were hired to escort stable patients to and from diagnostic and treatment areas throughout the hospital, thus freeing up nursing time. The transport program was managed by the director of Central Supporting Services, a department comprising patient equipment, linen room, and central sterile supply. In 1985, the transportation service became a component of the

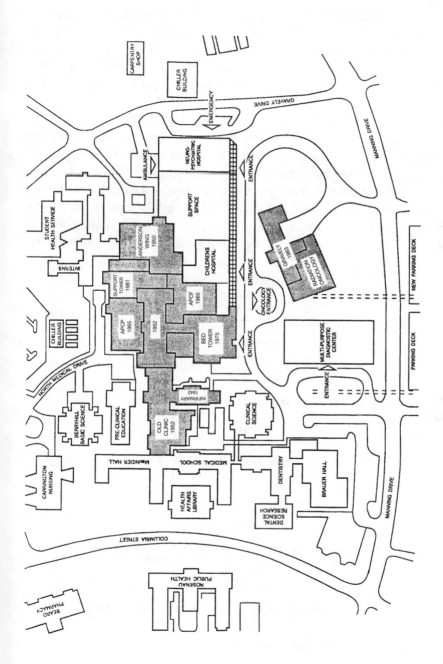

Figure 7.1 Facility Master Plan

Hospitals' overall Materials Management Department. Figure 7.2 shows the organization chart after the 1985 reorganization.

Staff positions were added to the department to keep pace with the Hospitals' growth in services. The patient equipment supervisor provided daily supervision until 1982, when a transporter position was upgraded to a supervisor of daily operations within the service. The position was filled with the promotion of Mr. Ollie Williams, a transporter, to supervisor reporting to the supervisor of patient equipment. Mr. Williams started at the Hospitals in 1978 as a linen room attendant before transferring to a front door attendant position in 1980.

The Patient Transportation Service is housed in a large space on the ground floor in the original section of the Hospitals adjacent to patient equipment and storeroom activities. The space is predominantly used to store wheelchairs, stretchers, portable oxygen tanks, and equipment re-

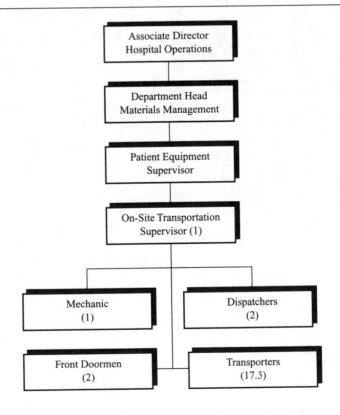

Figure 7.2 Patient Transportation Project at University Hospitals

placement parts. A small space at the back of the room is the staff's congregating point. The room is furnished with old chairs, a dispatcher's desk and phone, staff lockers, and a sink. Leading off this space is the transportation supervisor's small office.

The Transport Staff

At the time the project started, Patient Transportation had 23.5 full-time equivalent [FTE] positions, which included 17.5 full-time and part-time transporters, a supervisor, two transporter/dispatchers, a mechanic, and two front door attendants. Of the 17.5 actual transporters, 5 were assigned Monday through Friday to Radiology according to a prior agreement. Transporters were reassigned from the central pool to cover all absences among the Radiology transporters. Transporters serviced all areas of the Hospitals except the Critical Care and Emergency departments, operating and recovery rooms, and inpatient psychiatric units. Transporter job functions required completion of an eighth-grade education. The work force included both males and females. The pay scale for transporters was among the lowest in the state's health care system. Dispatchers, front door attendants, and the mechanic were classified in higher pay grades.

Mr. Williams, the first and only Transportation Service supervisor, viewed his role as that of a day shift supervisor. He readily acknowledged that the department did not function as well in his absence, but felt there was not a lot he could do about that. He displayed a strict, authoritarian management style, and his 6'4" stature often intimidated the transporters. Mr. Williams was accused of "showing favoritism," and he freely admitted that he liked those he could "rely on to come to work and do the job." Mr. Williams interviewed, hired, scheduled, and evaluated the transporters. He rotated dispatch functions among the "better" transporters on the day shift and had two dispatchers for evenings and weekends. As higher paying positions opened up in his department, Mr. Williams typically promoted transporters.

The department was plagued with significant morale and behavioral problems. Relationships with users of transport services as well as among the transporters were often strained. The transporters, many of whom had never worked in a hospital before, were provided on-the-job training by the most available peer. Nurses, physicians, patients, and their families expressed dissatisfaction with the inconsistent and often long waits (30-

minute average response times, with recorded response times as long as 129 minutes). A number of users had given up on the service and regularly performed their own transports. Complaints about discourteous service, careless transport techniques, or sloppy appearance were not uncommon. Lost transport equipment resulted in replacement costs averaging $20,000 annually.

In 1990, 16 employees from Patient Transportation agreed to participate in a hospital-wide attitude and opinion survey conducted by the Gallup Organization. Results showed that Patient Transportation's average scores for the 10 dimensions measured ranked below those of all other hospital departments. Transporter attitudes toward their work environment, opportunities for professional growth and development, and organizational integration ranked among the lowest in the Hospitals (see Figure 7.3). In spite of these morale and performance problems, 11 of the employees had been with Transportation Services between 6 and 20 years. Each year, approximately one to two employees transferred to higher paying jobs and two or three resigned.

Reassigning Transport Services to the Nursing Department

The Nursing Department had over 1,400 employees in clinical, educational, and administrative positions to provide and support the delivery of patient care services across 37 inpatient units, operating and recovery rooms, and the emergency department. The Nursing Department became administratively responsible for Transportation Services in 1989. The department's chairperson, Brenda Reynolds, and Ms. Lloyd, vice chair of nursing and assistant director of operations, were reluctant to take on this additional responsibility, given the nurses' staffing situation at the time. The national nursing shortage was at its peak locally. Although the nursing shortage presented significant operational challenges, it also created opportunities for improvements that consumed much of nursing management's time. The Nursing Department was actively engaged in a two-year state legislative pilot project to manage licensed nurse positions and compensation separately. The pilot study had considerable potential for alleviating the Hospitals' nursing shortage and in establishing a permanent model for autonomy desired by Hospitals' executive management. Its implementation was receiving top priority among executive and middle-level nurse managers.

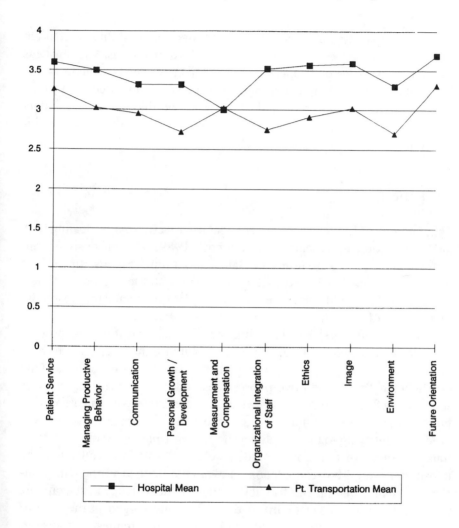

Figure 7.3 Results of Gallup Poll: Comparison Graph of Patient Transportation Department Attitudes vs. Those of Overall Hospital Staff

The transfer of administrative responsibility for Transportation Services, although unwelcome, was not entirely unexpected. Nursing, a major user of Transportation Services, had grown increasingly dissatisfied with the inefficiencies in transporting patients. Nursing management perceived these problems as stemming from employees with low self-esteem and little interest in their work.

Initially, Ms. Reynolds assumed direct line responsibility for Patient Transportation Services in order to evaluate the unit's needs. Mr. Williams continued to manage daily operations, referring personnel problems to Ms. Reynolds. Behavioral problems continued and were addressed one by one. Two employees were terminated in 1989 for performance and conduct reasons; others were moved into various stages of the Hospitals' disciplinary process.

The Project

Reynolds and Lloyd were at first caught in a reactive mode, dealing with the same problems repeatedly throughout 1989. The most significant recurring problems were user complaints about long response times. The two administrators believed that if they could shorten response times, everything else would more or less improve. They contacted the Hospitals' Management Engineering Department for assistance.

Just one morning spent observing the dispatch and transport process convinced Management Engineering and Nursing that there had to be a more efficient way of providing patient transportation services. One dispatcher with access to two phone lines handled all incoming calls. A staff member requesting service—usually a clerk on a patient care unit or in a diagnostic area—phoned in a request at the time a transport was needed, identifying to the dispatcher the patient's name, location, destination, and mode of transport. The dispatcher informed the caller that the transporter would be sent as soon as available, logged in the call, transcribed the information on a trip ticket, gave the ticket to the next available transporter on his or her return to the office, and logged in the time of dispatch. The transporter would then retrieve the requested transport equipment from the adjacent storage area. Equipment was frequently not returned to the storage area during the day, in which case the transporter would have to search throughout the Hospitals for a wheelchair or stretcher. Stretcher patients could require two transporters.

Occasionally, wrong information was communicated from the unit clerks. For example, the unit clerk might request a wheelchair when a stretcher was actually needed, or neglect to identify the need for a portable oxygen tank too. Communication errors often resulted in conflicts between clerks, nurses, and dispatchers as to who was wrong.

Benchmarking

The first action that Nursing management took was to look externally to see how other hospital transportation programs operated. Health Care Advisory Board, a national consulting group based in Washington, D.C., was contracted to conduct a survey of transport communication methods in 400+ bed teaching hospitals. The survey showed that two hospitals had improved services by equipping their transporters with two-way radios.

In pursuing the idea of two-way radios with a vendor, the administrators learned that a local community hospital's transporters were already equipped with two-way radios. A brief observation of patient transport services at the local hospital reinforced their interest. That department completed an average of 7,000 transports per month with 13 full-time equivalent transport positions. The supervisor, who also functioned as dispatcher, reassigned transporters as soon as they called in a completed transport. Space for transport equipment had been identified on each floor of the hospital, eliminating the transporter's need to return to the dispatch area between transports. One could not help noticing the teamwork displayed among the transporters. They readily responded to their peers' calls for assistance with a particular transport or with equipment search. The transporters seemed to enjoy their jobs. One transporter who had worked in another hospital's transportation department commented, "I would not do this job without walkie-talkies. It really cuts down on walking."

The supervisor also praised the system. "Before radios, I had no control over dispatch times. Now, we respond rapidly to all calls. The nurses are our greatest fans. They know we will come within a few minutes of their calls." A nursing manager said, "Before the radios, we never knew when a transporter would show up. Now, a transporter comes soon after we call. Patient transportation is the most efficient and reliable support service we have." Yet the pay was comparable to University Hospitals. The University Hospitals' administrators were sold on the system.

Soon after the site visit, they shared their findings with Mr. Williams. In discussing their observations, they emphasized the benefits to dispatchers, transporters, and users of the system. Mr. Williams, however, was not easily sold. He raised concerns that they had not considered, namely, that his dispatchers would have difficulty managing a combination of phone lines, radios, and activity logs. An automated order-entry system would resolve Mr. Williams' concerns, but this type of hospital-wide system was still in the planning stage and would not be ready for at least another three or four years.

Innovative Project Grant

Every spring, University Hospitals sponsors a competitive Innovative Project Program and awards 10 to 12 one-year grants. Projects are selected for funding based on innovation and potential for operational improvements. Nursing and Management Engineering planned to submit a proposal to fund the purchase of two-way radios; however, they needed to address Mr. Williams' concerns.

A management engineer, Ms. Karen McCall, pursued the potential of automation with various telephone companies and after a few inquiries learned of a computerized voice information system to answer all incoming calls 24 hours a day. The system's literature appeared simple enough. Users responded by touch-tone telephone to computer-activated questions concerning the transport. The system recorded and downloaded all incoming calls, transmitted messages via hard copy or computerized voice and maintained a database of activities. The UNC administrators thought that the voice information system offered definite advantages: (1) minimizing miscommunications between caller and dispatcher, (2) eliminating caller frustrations associated with delays in answering, and (3) affording the dispatcher more time to schedule transporter assignments by location and availability of equipment. Mr. Williams still wasn't convinced that the new communications system would offer any advantages. He expressed concern that transporters might lose radios, but he seemed willing to give the new system a try.

In 1990, Nursing and Management Engineering submitted a proposal to fund the purchase of two-way radios and a voice information system. The goal was to achieve measurable improvements in employee productivity. Based on the review of the transports in a one-month period, response times (defined as the interval from the time of the request to the time of the dispatch) averaged 30 minutes with a range of 26 to 33. The monthly volume of transports ranged between 4,600 and 5,300. Any time saved at the front end of a transport would increase the department's capacity for additional activity, but it was difficult to estimate how much capacity would increase, given the variability in each transport. A project to increase capacity without hiring more staff was both attractive and timely since University Hospitals forecasted increased patient volumes in 1991. The proposal was funded.

Project Implementation

Equipment delivery was anticipated in November-December 1990. In the interim, planning focused on the implementation process. It was becoming increasingly apparent that successful implementation would require on-site management support to assist Mr. Williams. Ms. Virginia Anderson, the critical care transport R.N., was the first choice. Although she had no formal management training or experience, she did have excellent people skills, teaching abilities, and first-hand knowledge of transport responsibilities and problems. She agreed to this promotion with a redefinition of responsibilities to include 40 percent time spent on management of Patient Transportation Services. Mr. Williams appeared receptive to Ms. Anderson's appointment. In preparation for her role change, Ms. Anderson attended basic management classes offered by the Hospitals' Human Resource Development Center and a national meeting for managers of Patient Transportation Services. In January, Ms. Anderson and Mr. Williams spent a morning at the local community hospital observing the dispatcher and transporters in action.

In February 1991, the transportation staff began using the two-way radios, with the expectation that the dispatcher would schedule transporter assignments by location and availability of equipment. Transporters could now be dispatched without returning to the office. Information was put in the Hospitals' employee newsletter announcing the system's implementation. A series of unanticipated problems (equipment delivery, programming, approval of a specific telephone number, and printing publicity flyers) delayed implementation of the voice information system until August. A flyer advertising the service and phone number (6-PACE) was sent to all users (see Exhibit 7.1).

Linkage with the CQI Team

As efforts were underway to purchase the communications equipment, the Hospitals' director of operations announced the establishment of a cross-functional team to improve the A/D process on the Medicine inpa-

Exhibit 7.1 Flyer Advertising New Voice Response System for Patient Transportation Service Users

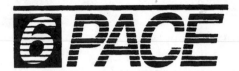

Now there is a fast and efficient way to order patient transportation services!

Call 6-PACE and the Voice Response System will ask you the following questions about the transport:

- patient's full name
- unit location
- transport destination
- time of appointment
- method of transport (i.e., wheelchair, stretcher or discharge cart, oxygen, IV pole)

At the end of the call, the system will play back your responses for you to verify and correct if necessary.

> The new Voice Response System is available for scheduling transport appointments 24 hours a day, 7 days a week.
> The transportation department is open from 7 a.m. to 7 p.m.

For "STAT" transportation requests, call 6-5252.

tient units. Invitations to join the team were extended to 12 departments/ divisions, including Nursing and Patient Transport. The A/D team held its first meeting in October 1990.

Although the CQI process had not been introduced formally in the Hospitals, the A/D team leader, Dr. Anna Organ, served as facilitator and educated the members about the CQI process and provided just-in-time training in quality improvement techniques. The first two months were spent flowcharting and collecting data on the A/D process.

The six subgroups (cross-functional teams) were formed in January 1991 to analyze specific A/D problems and processes on the Medicine service. The subgroups were expected to complete their work by May 1991 and were empowered to implement policy and procedural changes to improve the A/D process. Patient Transportation was designated as one of the six subgroups. The A/D team suggested that the subgroup address the following issues: lack of priority designation for discharge orders, transporter work schedules, communications with unit clerks, and implementation of the two-way radios.

Patient Transport Subgroup Activities

Ms. Lloyd convened the Patient Transportation subgroup. The members represented Patient Transportation, Medicine's clerical and nursing staff, and Admitting, all departments with ownership in the process. All levels of personnel were represented, from patient transporters to nurse managers. The management engineer working on the Innovative Project also joined the team. A supervisor from Radiology joined later. The group met biweekly from January through May 1991. Although the initial charge was to focus improvement efforts on processes for discharge patients on the inpatient Medicine units, the agenda was soon expanded to improving the transport services for all patients because many of the changes could not be restricted to one area of the Hospitals.

Understanding the Process

Findings from an October 1990 study of 50 discharged patients from one 25-bed Medicine inpatient unit were shared with the A/D team in December. Response times ranged from 12 to 22 minutes and arrival times (from time of call to arrival on the unit ranged from 21 to 31 minutes. These transport data showed a surprising improvement over data collected hospital-wide earlier in the year. The findings may have been influenced by the fact that Patient Transportation was aware of the study and may have prioritized discharge transports from the study unit. Additionally, transporters participated in the data collection. An analysis of the transport logs in January 1991 indicated that the average response time had not changed from the original average of 30 minutes measured in early 1990. The subgroup agreed to the following goals with the implementation of the two-way radios.

- For nonscheduled transports: Decrease response time from 30 minutes to 20 minutes on average.
- For scheduled transports: Achieve "on time" patient arrivals, defined as being in a range of 15 minutes before and 5 minutes after scheduled appointments.

The first few subgroup meetings were spent clarifying the process and developing the flowcharts in Figure 7.4, identifying breakdowns in the system, and educating the group on the new communications system's benefits. In the group as it analyzed the process, Medicine nurses and clerks were quick to point out Patient Transportation's problems: busy phone lines, inconsistent response times, and the dispatcher's inability or unwillingness to estimate when a transporter would be available. Mr. Williams and his transporters attributed delays to time spent in search of equipment, time wasted because patients weren't ready when the transporter arrived, and incomplete or inaccurate information about the patient's mode of travel, necessitating repeat trips. Maintaining the group's focus on process was difficult, given the negative feelings that existed between transporters and nursing personnel. It seemed as though the group was going nowhere.

The next meeting's discussion focused on the Radiology transport process. Radiology transport comprised 30 to 40 percent of all patient transports Monday through Friday. The nurses and clerks were unaware that those transporters were based in Radiology and dispatched by the Radiology clerk. With the exception of diagnostic procedures requiring patient fasting or premedication, Radiology had no scheduling system. Trip tickets were prepared by the Radiology clerk and placed in a basket in no particular order. Transporters selected trip tickets randomly, retrieved transport equipment in Radiology, and then went after the patient. Following the x-ray or other procedure, the patient was handed the trip ticket and moved to a back corridor to await a transporter. Transporters were supposed to monitor this corridor closely, but patients frequently complained of long waits. Medicine nurses commented that patients scheduled for discharge were particularly inconvenienced by Radiology's lack of a scheduling system. Physicians on the Medicine service frequently ordered chest films the evening before or the morning of planned discharge. Radiology was usually unable to do the predischarge films until after the more complex prescheduled procedures were completed in the late morning. Patients needing routine films were fitted in as scheduling windows

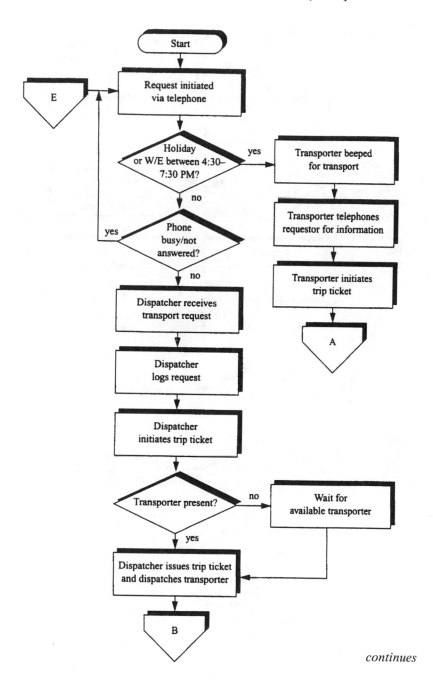

continues

Figure 7.4 Patient Transportation Department, Original Process, 1990

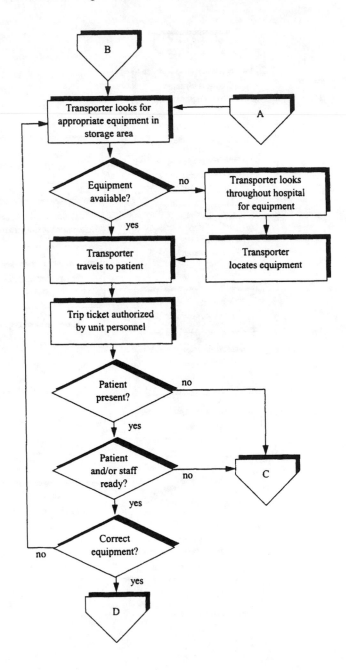

Figure 7.4 continued

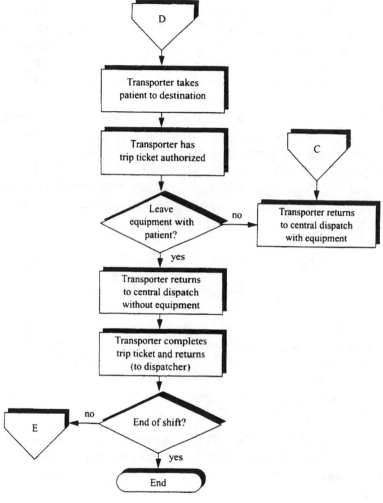

Figure 7.4 continued

opened. A Radiology supervisor was invited to join the subgroup. He participated in the subgroup for the remainder of the meetings.

During this discussion, Medicine nurses and clerks expressed their anger and frustration with transporter attitudes when patients were not immediately ready to leave the unit. A transporter who knew the system well responded that when they took too long getting a patient to X-ray, the Radiology staff got angry. She added, "It looks bad for us transporters." A nurse responded, "Then have X-ray call us before you come, because we don't even know the patient is scheduled to go anywhere! The physicians schedule with X-ray, not with us." Mr. Williams fell back in his chair and asked, "You mean you don't have any idea we are coming?" The nurses and clerks agreed. A head nurse replied, "If we knew patients were scheduled, of course we would try to have them ready." Mr. Williams acknowledged that as long as he had been supervisor, he had thought that the nurses were aware of the scheduled tests and were just being uncooperative with the transporters. The nurses and clerks were just as surprised to learn of the transporter perceptions. Mr. Williams vowed to "set it straight" with his transporters. This realization was the first step in resolving years of friction between nursing staff and transporters. Ms. Lloyd observed, "We really lucked out! From that moment, the tone of the meetings changed. I am convinced that this air-clearing enabled the subgroup to move forward."

Opportunities for Improvement and Testing Remedies

The subgroup tackled a number of process issues over the next few months, but the work did not stop with their final meeting in May 1991. Nursing, Management Engineering, and Patient Transportation continued to pursue opportunities for improving the system and the work group's performance. Along with the development of the voice information system and the two-way radios, the following steps were taken.

To Reduce Response Time. The assignment of a block of transporters to Radiology ended in May 1991 with the concurrence of Radiology. Radiology transporters had various amounts of "downtime" which they spent in Radiology's lounge. Centralization of personnel, together with the two-way radios, held potential for productivity gains while maintaining the same levels of service to Radiology.

Mr. Williams' role as supervisor was revised to include 80 percent time as dispatcher from Monday to Friday. Nursing management recognized the dispatcher role as pivotal to efficient operations and thought it especially important that Mr. Williams model the role. Based on his experiences, he and Ms. Anderson established performance standards for the off-shift dispatchers.

Transport equipment was decentralized to identified sites in the two bed towers and the Anderson wing with the intention of decreasing return trips to the dispatch area. If equipment was unavailable, the ability to stay in communication with peers was expected to facilitate an equipment search.

Work schedules were adjusted in accordance with workload rather than employee preference. Meal breaks were staggered over 2.5 hours instead of 1.5 hours. Limitations were placed on the amount of personal leave that could be taken on any given day.

To Reduce Patient Care Unit Delays. A policy was established limiting the time to five minutes that a transporter waited if a patient was not ready for transport. After five minutes, the transporter radioed the dispatcher. If another transport was waiting, the transporter was reassigned; if not, the transporter waited for the patient. On returning the patient to the unit, the transporter waited five minutes, if necessary, for assistance and then radioed the dispatcher for help. The dispatcher paged the appropriate nurse manager to intervene. Ms. Anderson met with the inpatient nurse managers and clerical supervisors to discuss the rationale for the new policy.

To Reduce Discharge Delays in Radiology. The dispatchers started placing a priority on discharge transports. The only patients that received higher priority were fasting and premedicated patients scheduled for invasive diagnostic procedures.

The patient transportation subgroup worked with Radiology's medical director and staff and physicians on inpatient Medicine units to expedite same-day requests for discharge x-rays. Radiology agreed to do these procedures weekdays between 6:00 PM and 9:00 PM and between 7:00 AM and 7:30 AM if transporters were available. In response, transporter schedules were adjusted slightly to expand coverage from 12 hours to 14 hours on weekdays. Radiology developed and published a scheduling system for these patients. With prenotification, nurses were expected to have patients ready for transport and to notify X-ray and Transportation of any anticipated delays (see Exhibit 7.2).

To Reduce Equipment Replacement Costs. Wheelchairs were typically left in a designated alcove off the main lobby following patient discharges. The front door attendant would access this supply of wheelchairs for arrivals needing assistance. At this end of the shift, the front door attendant returned any excess chairs to the patient transportation storage area. The alcove area could be accessed by any employee or visitor after the front door attendant left in the late afternoon. The process improvement team

Exhibit 7.2 University Hospitals Department of Radiology

PRIORITIZATION FOR DISCHARGE RADIOLOGY ORDERS

Policy:

The department of radiology will prioritize and expedite requests for examinations on the Hospitals' patients scheduled for discharge contingent upon radiologic findings.

Procedure:

1. The physician will write the anticipated discharge order and the radiology/procedure order in the patient's chart the day before discharge.
2. For routine films (non-contrast):
   a. Unit clerk will write "pending discharge" in red ink at the top of the requisition. (Note: If the requisition exam can be performed only in the a.m. of the day of discharge, the unit clerk will write "pending discharge—perform in early AM" in red ink at the top of the requisition.)
   b. Requisition will be sent to radiology before 5:00 PM of the day prior to discharge.
   c. Evening shift radiology clerk will process the requisitions for exam completion between 6:00 and 9:00 PM, unless early AM is indicated.
   d. Evening shift radiology supervisor will ensure the completion of the exam prior to 9:00 PM.
   e. If the exam is not completed during the evening shift, the evening shift radiology supervisor will discuss with the unit's charge nurse and will give the requisition to the night shift radiology supervisor with instructions to perform in the early AM.
   f. If the exam is not completed by the radiology night shift prior to 7:30 AM of the day of discharge, the night shift radiology supervisor will give the requisition to the day shift radiology supervisor with instructions as to when the exam will be performed.
   g. "Discharge pending" requisitions for routine exams that cannot be sent to radiology by 5:00 PM on the day prior to discharge should be tubed to radiology as quickly as possible. Please call the radiology supervisor to ensure receipt of the requisition and to negotiate an expected time for the exam.

felt sure that they could reduce equipment loss by securing this space after hours, so a locked gate was installed.

To Improve Staff Behavior and Morale. Job descriptions and standards of performance were revised. The old standard, which expressed the expectation that there would be 18 transports per employee per eight-hour day, was replaced with a statement not focusing on numbers, but emphasizing continuing improvement and teamwork.

A dress code was established. Transporters, many of whom had been wearing T-shirts and jeans to work, were involved in the selection of the uniforms.

Ms. Anderson developed the Patient Transportation Department's first orientation program and provided classes for all employees on safety (body mechanics, falls prevention, and oxygen transport), infection control, radio communications, and guest relations. The program was piloted on the current transporters. In January 1991, Ms. Anderson initiated monthly staff meetings on day and evening shifts to keep transporters informed of new and changing events and to encourage constructive discussion of problems and possible solutions. One of the staff meetings was devoted to the review and discussion of the Gallup survey results. The staff showed no surprise with the Gallup results and comparative Hospitals data and offered few ideas for improving the situation. Updates on transportation subgroup meetings and monthly activity statistics were provided at each meeting. Year-to-date graphs showing the number of transports, average response times, and longest waits were posted in the dispatch area after each meeting.

Project Results

The radios were an immediate success. By March, the average transport response times had dropped to 15 minutes (based on a random sample of 155 weekday log entries each in January and March 1991), and they just kept getting better (see Figure 7.5). Prioritizing discharges made little difference once the process had been improved. In July, average response times were calculated separately for weekday, weekend (7:00 AM to 3:30 PM) and all evening transports. The response times were five, eight, and seven minutes, respectively. Figure 7.6 shows improvements made in reducing the longest waits until a transporter could be dispatched.

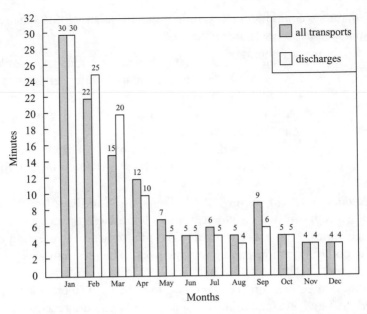

Figure 7.5 Average Transport Response Times, January through December 1991

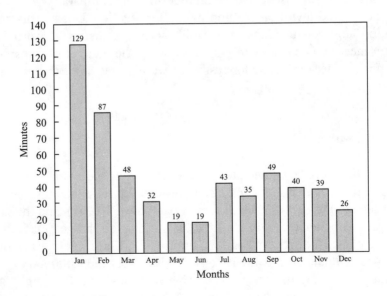

Figure 7.6 Longest Wait Times for Transport Services, January through December 1991

The volume of completed transports increased steadily during the first six months of 1991. After May, as Figure 7.7 shows, transports soared with the centralization of the transporters and with the expansion of bed capacity. Other areas were asking for transport services and although the transporters were reluctant at first, services were extended to the 63-bed inpatient psychiatric unit and the postanesthesia care unit. By the end of 1991, Radiology's Diagnostic Imaging Department suggested transferring their two full-time transporter positions to Patient Transportation. This added another 30 to 35 transports to each weekday shift and represented the first increase in the FTE base.

The voice information system was used predominantly when the transport office was closed. Few diagnostic and treatment departments had scheduling systems in place. For the few with schedules, the system

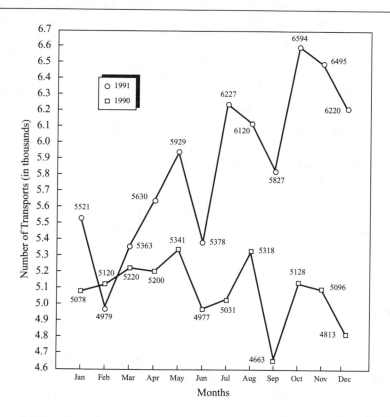

Figure 7.7 Number of Patient Transports, January through December 1990 and 1991

worked well. Approximately 10 to 15 transports were scheduled daily. All discharge films were accomplished the evening before or early on the morning of discharge. Transporters were dispatched 15 to 20 minutes in advance of appointments to ensure "on time" patient arrivals.

Busy telephone lines were no longer a problem for callers. Stabilization of the dispatcher's role and decreased personnel activity in the dispatch area had increased dispatcher efficiency and accuracy.

The idea of decentralizing wheelchairs and stretchers throughout the hospital was a disaster! The hallway alcoves were not large enough to store more than a few wheelchairs at any one time, so equipment was rarely there when a transporter needed it. The equipment was also used by other ancillary staff and visitors. After one month of the new system, the general feeling among transporters was that dispatchers were assigning trips in such a way as to avoid frequent return trips to the dispatch area. The transporters monitored the radios and initiated peer assistance when a dispatched transporter needed equipment.

Contrary to initial concerns, no radios were lost or broken. The Fiscal Year 1993 capital budget request of $20,000 was reduced to $3,700. Transporters were keeping up with the equipment, and the secured storage area in the lobby helped reduce the loss of equipment to the public and other departments. The gate did create unanticipated problems for the Emergency Room (ER), which relied on this area for replenishing their supply of wheelchairs during the night. Without notifying anyone, the ER staff began taking wheelchairs from the dispatch area, sometimes resulting in transport start-up delays the next morning. Tensions between Mr. Williams and the ER aides escalated before management was aware of the problem. Giving the ER staff a key to the gate solved that problem.

Satisfaction Levels

Transporters and dispatchers both liked the radios. Ms. Anderson commented, "At first, it was like a new toy. Transporters talked with each other all the time—even in the presence of patients." Some transporters consistently neglected to radio in completed transports, especially when Mr. Williams was not the dispatcher. Transporter performance improved as individual behaviors were addressed and as the novelty of the radios wore off.

Patient satisfaction with transport services improved, and the number of concerns submitted to patient relations decreased, as shown in Figure 7.8. Nursing staff perceptions of transport services for clinic and inpatient areas were surveyed for the first time in October 1991. (Nurses and clerks on each unit were requested to collaborate by completing one survey form per patient unit). Forty-five of the surveys shown in Exhibit 7.3 were returned, for a response rate of 88 percent. The results are shown in Figures 7.9 and 7.10.

Recognition

The Hospitals senior management council rejected an opportunity to acknowledge the transport team's accomplishments at the end of fiscal year, June 30, 1991. Salary funds were unexpectedly available to award special merit payments. Ms. Reynolds and Ms. Lloyd recommended a

Exhibit 7.3 Patient Transportation Survey Form

Patient Transportation Survey

On a scale of 1 to 5 (with 5 being the highest), please express your degree of satisfaction with the performance of the Patient Transportation Department on the following parameters:

Courtesy of dispatcher when receiving patient information for transport	1	2	3	4	5
Courtesy of transporters to unit staff	1	2	3	4	5
Discretion used by transporters in discussing patient condition with unit staff	1	2	3	4	5
Patient safety precautions followed (ID bracelet checked, side rails secured on stretchers, etc.)	1	2	3	4	5
Trip ticket presented to unit staff for signature upon patient's leaving the floor	1	2	3	4	5
Patient waiting time for transport assistance Average waiting time _____	1	2	3	4	5
Courtesy and respectfulness shown to patients by transporters	1	2	3	4	5
Trip ticket presented to unit staff for signature upon patient's return to floor	1	2	3	4	5
Medical charts returned to unit desk upon patient's return from transport	1	2	3	4	5

Additional comments/suggestions: _____

_____

_____

Patient Care Unit: _____ Department # _____
(10/91)

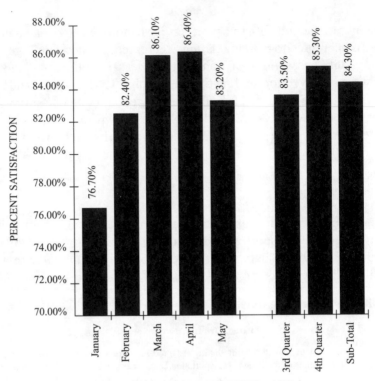

Patient Concerns	1990	1991
January	0	2
February	11	1
March	2	2
April	4	1
May	5	5
June	3	2
July	2	3
August	0	0
September	4	6
October	7	0
November	6	5
December	4	3
Totals	48	30

Figure 7.8 Patient Satisfaction with Transport Time

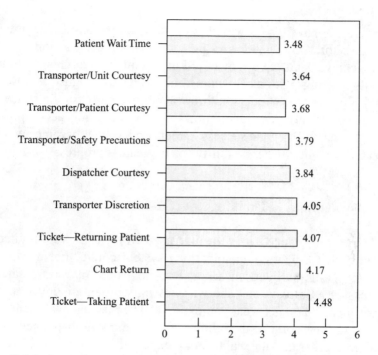

Note: Satisfaction rated on a scale of 1 to 5, with 5 being the highest score.

Figure 7.9 Patient Transportation Satisfaction Survey Results on Various Measures

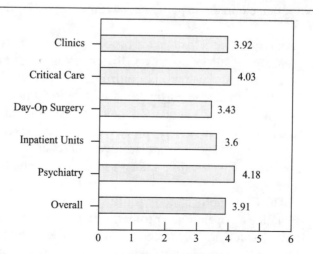

Note: Satisfaction rated on a scale of 1 to 5, with 5 being the highest score.

Figure 7.10 Patient Transportation Satisfaction Survey Results, by Department team award, but the idea was supported by only one other member—the CQI director. Although the transporters did not receive a monetary award, their achievements were showcased in a number of forums, including the CEO's meetings with all Hospitals employees. In August, Ms. Reynolds, Ms. Lloyd, and Ms. Anderson threw a surprise party for the entire staff at the change of shift. The celebration to honor the team's accomplishments since January was a great success. Other service areas became aware of the event, achieving greater visibility for the team's progress.

The Turnaround in Thinking

The original expectations for increased efficiencies were limited to the benefits that a new communications system could offer a work group stereotyped as dull and uncaring. Recently, one transporter said, when discussing a problem that she was having with an employee in another department, "You get what you expect!" The message was clear!

The turning point in the administrators' thinking happened when the CQI progress was made real through experience with the A/D project and particularly the Patient Transportation subgroup. Although Ms. Lloyd had studied CQI theory and its application to manufacturing settings, she was skeptical about its successful translation to complex medical settings. Ms. Lloyd reflected on the experience, saying,

> As an active participant in the process, I worked closely with staff members at all levels to try to understand processes and the problems and frustrations confronting them on a daily basis. Employees became participants in solutions, instead of recipients of mandates. I witnessed their interest and pride as response times and activity levels improved. Their achievements in performance and staff morale are even more surprising in view of the state's FY 1991/92 salary freeze for all employees except nurses.
>
> The CQI approach took more time than I was accustomed to spending on operational problems. It required an unusual level of detail, which initially tested my patience. However, my enthusiasm for the process grew with each small gain. I am convinced that without the timely introduction of CQI the Innovative Project would have been nothing more than an expensive Band-Aid.

One Problem Leads to Another

It had been almost a year since the radios were implemented and the numbers on the charts looked good. Yet the transporters were experiencing more and more delays on the inpatient units. Ms. Anderson's follow-up with nurse managers resulted in only brief periods of improvement. Nurses were annoyed when transporters were reassigned after five-minute delays. Patients awaiting discharge transports and procedural areas awaiting patients often attributed the slow response times to transporters. After a year of steady gains, patient transport was still taking the heat.

Ms. Lloyd and Ms. Anderson studied the current flowchart, Figure 7.11, again. As Ms. Lloyd contemplated the next step, she observed, "There's no end. This whole thing leads to so many other things we need to fix."

CASE ANALYSIS

This case centers on the changes made in the transporter system in a large teaching hospital owned by the state government. Concern with the discharge planning process led to the development of the transportation CQI effort. Clearly, this was an area where there had long been unnecessary friction in the institution. But it was an area that management had seemed reluctant to address, probably because they had little expectation of improvement. As you have read, the effort was quite successful.

One of the impacts of the quality movement started in response to the Japanese quality success has been the realization that one major American quality problem was expectations that were too low, sometimes by an order of magnitude. Here management had expected little from the transporters, and they got it. This case is as much about employee empowerment as it is about quality improvement.

Introduction

CQI provided the impetus and commitment for change. Once into the change process, the teams began to address problem areas that had been left unattended. This hospital, being one of the participants in the National Demonstration Project, has had an ongoing CQI program. The discharge planning project was one of its earliest efforts. However, the decentralized

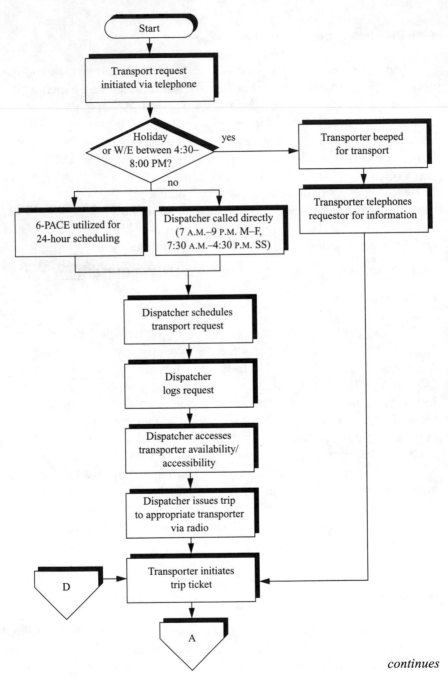

continues

Figure 7.11 University Hospitals' Patient Transportation Department, Current Process, 1991

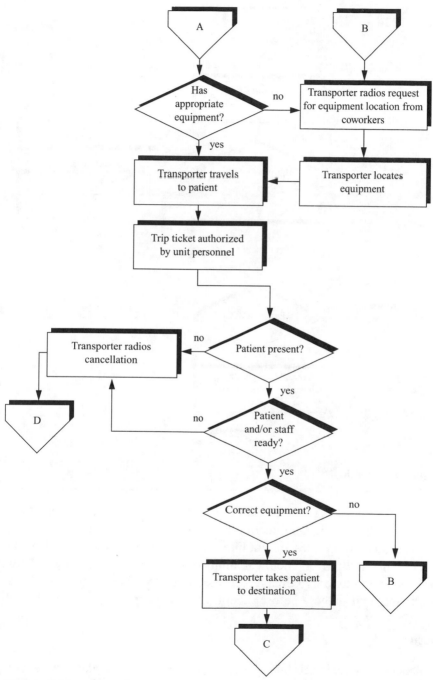

Figure 7.11 continued

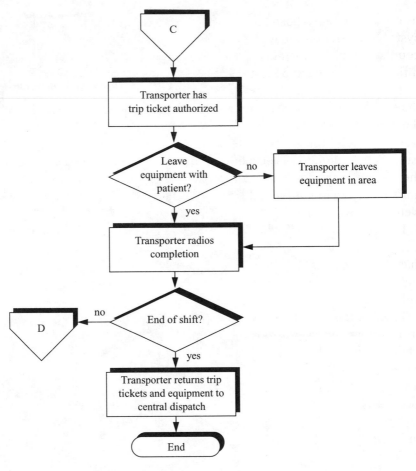

Figure 7.11 continued

nature of decision making in a large teaching hospital staffed by medical school faculty led the administration to start slowly, with a few teams to lead the way. Academics are not likely to adopt something because it has worked in the auto or chemical industries. Given their high need for professional autonomy (Chapter 7), they have to witness successful experiments such as these before accepting the concept.

Basics

This is one case in this book where benchmarking took place. A vendor suggested looking at a communications system used by transporters in a nearby community hospital. Several managers went out to look at this system in operation and were convinced that it was working well there and could work well in their institution. Demonstrations can have a significant influence on pragmatic health care professionals.

This case is a clear illustration of the stages that Chapter 6 describes for the evolution of teams. At first, the representatives of the various groups on the teams blamed the transportation delay problems on each other. This was especially true of the heated discussions about the transportation of patients to Radiology. Then, with further dialogue, people began to realize the sources of their misunderstandings, such as not knowing that the floor units had not been informed of the patient pickups. Realizing that they were poorly informed, the team members began to study the process to try to learn more about what was really happening. That was when the team truly formed. This was followed by some analyses and recommendations that resulted from the team's beginning to set norms for its own behavior and get on with performing the task at hand. The recommendations were followed.

This case also illustrates the fact that teams must continue to follow up on the results of their recommendations. The recommendation to have wheelchairs and carts available on each floor did not work out, and the system had to be revised. Likewise, unanticipated side effects were uncovered, such as issues of access to the same equipment by the emergency room staff at night. The teams must always be alert to the unintended consequences of their system changes. Not every interested party will be on every team, nor can every impact be anticipated. The concepts must be tried out, evaluated, and revised if necessary. Note that there were unintended positive consequences too. The amount spent to replace missing equipment dropped markedly with the changed system as the system came under tighter control.

Implementation

Here again we see that the efforts of management and the work of the teams interact. The organizational change that management made facilitated the changes. It unfroze the transporter system and enabled individuals to switch roles to better fit the new technology. Management provided the capital budget funds to purchase the communications system even before the CQI team came into being. Management had already benchmarked that system. However, the communicators would not have been as effective without the committee's efforts.

The committee delved into the fact that the transporters were split into two groups under separate supervision and analyzed the communications problems between the nursing stations, the transporters, and the ancillary departments. The team analysis provided the occasion for taking Mr. Williams to the community hospital to see how the system could work after he continued to raise objections to the change. Many activities can be made much less threatening when they are presented as a team project effort as opposed to management order. One cannot help wondering whether things might have gone ahead faster if a team had been formed earlier and made that initial benchmarking visit, especially if it had included Mr. Williams.

The planning process cited here is unusual. Basically, those who wish to start teams need to present a proposal to management to have access to resources, including facilitators and capital budget, where necessary. Because this is a large government institution, these approval processes could take quite a bit of time. Furthermore, management was not constrained from addressing the problem while the team process was getting started. Therefore we see that management had already ordered the communicators and moved the transport service under the nursing service before the patient transport team had done its analysis. Therefore one might question what the team accomplished. Mainly, it found solutions to the issues raised by the installation of the communicators and led to the recognition of system improvements that went beyond the province of the transport service. One of these was gaining sufficient trust to merge the two sets of transporters, one in Radiology and one for the rest of the hospital. Such mergers usually improve overall productivity and service responsiveness by 15 percent to 25 percent due to economies of scale in covering each other's calls. The same effects have been seen elsewhere in centralized telephone customer service centers by companies such as Federal Express and American Express.

While not presented in the case, one important role of the team was to publicize the positive results. The transporters, unlike most hospital employees, had a negative image. Their performance improved, but the team served as a vehicle by which that positive effect was talked about around the hospital and by which the attitudinal changes in the transporters were responded to and reinforced. Do not ignore the importance of the CQI team as a means of disseminating, reinforcing, and rewarding positive outcomes.

Applications

This case took place in a teaching hospital, but there is no indication that the effort was associated with any of the teaching objectives of the institution. The reader should refer to Chapter 16 for some ideas about how the academic medical center might well respond to CQI and incorporate CQI into its teaching tasks.

Case 1 focuses on the use of CQI in the laboratory. In this case, the Radiology Department played a major role, but it was not represented in the team effort until later. We suspect that this happens fairly often, that ancillary services are not thought of as having as much impact on processes as they really do. As health care organizations learn more about the complex and interdependent nature of their own processes, we would expect to see the ancillary departments become increasingly involved in CQI efforts.

APPENDIX A

Malcolm Baldrige Award 1999 Health Care Criteria for Performance Excellence

Curtis P. McLaughlin

The year 1999 became the first time that health care organizations were eligible to apply for the Malcolm Baldrige National Quality Award. There was a pilot program in 1995 in which 46 health care organizations and 19 educational institutions participated. Each organization received feedback on its application from the Baldrige National Quality Program. The Health Care Criteria are intended to have the same framework as the Business and Education criteria but with health-care-specific issues and language. The 1999 program is outlined in a Baldrige National Quality Programs document entitled, *1999 Health Care Criteria for Performance Excellence* (Hertz 1999). This publication outlines the program's administration, criteria, core values and concepts, definitions of key terms, application instructions, and scoring guidelines. It urges health care organizations to start early on with the application as a self-evaluation tool.

ITEMS FOR 1999 HEALTH CARE CRITERIA

The items used in the 1998 and 1999 drafts of the criteria are as follows:

Categories and Terms	Point Values
Leadership	
1.1 Leadership System—how leadership is exercised at top and throughout the system	80

Source: Adapted from National Institute of Standards and Technology, U.S. Department of Commerce, Washington, D.C., 1998, http://www.quality.nist.gov.

587

1.2   Public Responsibility and Leadership—how the
      organization contributes to the community and to the health
      of its community   30

Strategic Planning

2.1   Strategy Development Process–how the organization sets
      strategic direction and deploys plans, implements and tracks
      strategic performance   40
2.2   Organizational Strategy–how strategy is being translated into
      plans and projections compared to other similar organizations   40

Focus on Patients, Other Customers, Markets

3.1   Patient/Customer and Health Care Market Knowledge—how
      the organization learns from actual and potential customers
      about needs and opportunities   40
3.2   Patient/Customer Satisfaction and Relationship
      Enhancement—how the organization measures and uses
      customer satisfaction data to support market development   40

Information and Analysis

4.1   Selection and Use of Information and Data—how information
      is developed, secured, and used by the organization   25
4.2   Selection and Use of Comparative Information and Data—
      benchmarking and target setting   15
4.3   Analysis and Review of Organizational Performance—
      collecting and using performance measures to improve and
      innovate throughout the organization   40

Staff Focus

5.1   Work Systems—how all staff contribute to performance
      and learning through work design, compensation and
      recognition   40
5.2   Staff Education, Training and Development—how these
      staff activities support organizational and staff needs and
      potentials   30

5.3   Staff Well-Being and Satisfaction—how to maintain a safe
      and healthy environment and include ergonomics and staff
      satisfaction into improvement priorities   30

Process Management

6.1   Design and Delivery of Health Care—how clinical services
      are designed and improved   70
6.2   Management of Support Processes—how these processes
      including supplier and partnering relationships are managed
      and improved   30

Organizational Performance Results

7.1   Patient/Customer Satisfaction Results—absolute and
      comparative measures of satisfaction by segment   100
7.2   Health Care Results—levels and trends of absolute and
      comparative outcomes, service delivery results, and
      functional status as they relate to 3.1 and 6.1   120
7.3   Financial and Market Results—financial ratios, bond
      ratings, market share, new markets   80
7.4   Staff and Work System Results—staff satisfaction, training
      and development, and participation in improvement efforts   50
7.5   Organization-Specific Results—results of other improvement
      efforts that support the above results   100

TOTAL   1,000

One requirement when applying for the Baldrige National Quality
Award is the submission of a five-page Business Overview that describes
the organization, the services that it provides, key marketplace requirements, supplier and partnering relationships, the strategic context or
strategic activities of the organization, and the competitive environment
being faced. The objective of this information is to state what is "relevant
and important to your organization and its performance" (Hertz 1999, 79).
The brochure explains that the Business Criteria were modified to
address several health care issues, including those listed below.

Mission Specificity

Although health care organizations share common aims, individual organizational missions, roles, and services vary greatly. . . . specific requirements and key drivers of operational performance differ from organization to organization. For this reason, effective use of the Criteria depends upon "personalizing" requirements consistently across all seven categories of the Criteria framework. In particular, the Strategic Planning Category (Category 2) needs to address all key mission requirements, setting the stage for the interpretation of all other requirements. Similarly, results reported in the Organizational Performance Results Category (Category 7) need to reflect results consistent with the organization's mission and strategic objectives.

The Health Care Criteria are most explicit in the area of delivery of health care, since this requirement is common to all organizations, regardless of specific mission. . . .

It is recognized that some, but not all, health care organizations have a significant research and/or teaching commitment as part of their mission. These activities have been noted, as part of process management and operational performance results (Hertz 1999, 102).

Customers

The criteria also had to recognize that some customers such as "physicians, nurse practitioners, midwives, psychologists, and other health professionals" might have multiple roles as staff, suppliers, and customers of the organization (Hertz 1999, 103).

Systems Concept

The Criteria were intended to encourage a systems approach in which measures and indicators were intended to align and link key strategies, processes, and results.

Staff

While the Business Criteria focus on employees, the Health Care Criteria use the word *staff* to include employees. Providers were not employees but still needed to be integrated into the management system and contribute to organizational objectives.

Support Processes

These processes do not involve direct patient care delivery, but support it. These include "information services, facilities management, security, billing, and purchasing" (Hertz 1999, 104).

Primary Focus on Health Care

This primary focus is justified by two main reasons: "(1) improvement of health status is the universal goal of all health care organizations. Thus, sharing health care strategies and methods would have the greatest impact on the nation's health care systems; and (2) those who encouraged the creation of a Baldrige Award category for health care cited improvement in health care quality as their primary or only rationale for such an award" (Hertz 1999, 105).

Nonprofit Health Care Organizations

For-profit health care companies may apply either for the health care award (using health care criteria) or for the service or the small business awards, while nonprofit organizations are limited to the health care category.

Organizations that do not deliver health care directly, but that are considered to be in the health sector, such as dental laboratories, health insurance companies, and social service agencies, can also apply for the health care award.

Item Scoring

Each item is scored either on (1) approach/deployment or on (2) results. Tables A–1 and A–2 show the scoring for each of these. The tables show the criteria for each range. The selection of the range is based on the best fit of the overall item response. Scoring within those limits is left up to examiner discretion based on closeness to the next higher or next lower range.

If you wish to learn more about the Baldrige award application process for the health care sector, contact the Baldrige National Quality Program, National Institute of Standards and Technology, Gaithersburg, Maryland, or the American Society for Quality (ASQ) in Milwaukee, Wisconsin.

Table A–1 Ranges and Criteria for Baldrige Health Care Approach/ Deployment Scores

Score	Approach/Deployment
0%	• No systematic approach evident, anecdotal information
10%–20%	• Beginning of a systematic approach to the basic purposes of the item • Major gaps exist in deployment that would inhibit progress in achieving the basic purposes of the item • Early stages of a transition from reacting to problems to a general improvement orientation
30%–40%	• A sound, systematic approach, responsive to the basic purpose of the item • Approach is deployed, although some areas of work units are in early stages of deployment • Beginning of a systematic approach to evaluation and improvement of basic item processes
50%–60%	• A sound, systematic approach, responsive to the basic purpose of the item • Approach is well-deployed, although deployment may vary in some areas or work units • A fact-based, systematic evaluation and improvement process is in place for basic item processes • Approach is aligned with basic organizational needs identified in the other Criteria Categories
70%–80%	• A sound, systematic approach, responsive to the multiple requirements of the item • Approach is well-deployed with no significant gaps

continues

Table A–1 continued

- A fact-based, systematic evaluation and improvement process and organizational learning/sharing are key management tools; clear evidence of refinement and improved integration as the result of organizational-level analysis and sharing
- Approach is well-integrated with organizational needs identified in the other Criteria Categories

90%–
100%
- A sound, systematic approach, fully responsive to all the requirements of the item
- Approach is fully deployed without significant weaknesses or gaps in any areas or work units
- A very strong, fact-based, systematic evaluation and improvement process and extensive organizational learning/ sharing are key management tools; strong refinement and integration, backed by excellent organizational-level analysis and sharing
- Approach is fully integrated with organizational needs identified in the other Criteria Categories

Table A–2 Ranges and Criteria for Baldrige Award Health Care Results Scores

Score	Approach/Deployment
0%	• No results or poor results in areas reported
10%–20%	• Some improvements *and/or* early good performance levels in a few areas • Results not reported for many to most areas of importance to key organizational requirements
30%–40%	• Improvements *and/or* good performance levels in many areas of importance to key organizational requirements • Early stages of developing trends and obtaining comparative information • Results reported for many to most areas of importance to key organizational requirements.
50%–60%	• Improvement trends *and/or* good performance levels in many areas of importance to key organizational requirements • No pattern of adverse trends and no poor performance levels in area of importance to key organizational requirements

continues

Table A–2 continued

- Some trends *and/or* current performance levels—evaluated against relevant comparisons *and/or* benchmarks—show areas of strength *and/or* good to very good performance levels
- Organizational performance levels address most key patient/customer, market, and process requirements

70%–80%
- Current performance is good to excellent in areas of importance to key organizational requirements
- Most improvement trends *and/or* current performance levels are sustained
- Many to most trends *and/or* current performance levels—evaluated against relevant comparisons *and/or* benchmarks—show areas of leadership and very good relative performance levels
- Organizational performance results address most key patient/customers, market, process, and action plan requirements

90%–100%
- Current performance is excellent in most areas of importance to the key organizational requirements
- Excellent improvement trends *and/or* sustained excellent performance levels in most areas
- Evidence of health care sector and benchmark leadership demonstrated in many areas
- Organizational performance results fully address key patient/customer, market, process, and action plan requirements

BIBLIOGRAPHY

Ackoff, R.L. 1981. *Creating the corporate future.* New York: John Wiley & Sons.

Adams, D.F. et al. 1973. The complications of coronary arteriography. *Circulation* 48, no. 3:609–618.

The Advisory Board Company. 1997. *The great product enterprise: Future state for the American health system.* Washington, DC.

Alemi, F. et al. 1998. Rapid improvement teams. *Joint Commission Journal on Quality Improvement* 24, no. 3:119–129.

American College of Physicians. 1993. *Enhancing the physician's role in patient-centered care.* Philadelphia. Unpublished document. American College of Physicians-American Society of Internal Medicine Online. 1999. *ACP Journal Club* http://www.acponline.org (Last viewed 3 March 1999.)

American Public Health Association. 1992. *Summary of healthy people 2000: National health promotion and disease prevention objectives.* Washington, DC.

American Public Health Association. 1993. *The guide to implementing model standards. Eleven steps toward a healthy community.* Washington, DC.

Ancona, D.G. 1985. Groups in organizations: Extending laboratory models. In *Group processes and intergroup relations.* Vol. 9, *Review of personality and social psychology,* ed. C. Hendrick. Newbury Park, CA: Sage Publications.

Anders, G. 1996. *Health against wealth.* Boston: Houghton Mifflin.

Angell, M., and J.P. Kassirer. 1996. Quality and the medical marketplace: Following elephants. *New England Journal of Medicine* 335, no. 12:883–885.

Argyris, C. 1990. *Overcoming organizational defenses: Facilitating organizational learning.* Needham Heights, MA: Allyn & Bacon.

Argyris, C. 1991. Teaching smart people to learn. *Harvard Business Review* 69 (May-June):99–109.

Argyris, C., and D.A. Schon. 1996. *Organizational learning II: Theory, method and practice.* Reading, MA: Addison-Wesley Publishing Co.

Arndt, M., and B. Bigelow. 1995. The implementation of total quality management in hospitals. *Health Care Management Review* 20, no. 4:3–14.

Arthur Andersen & Co. and the American College of Healthcare Executives. 1991. *The future of medical care: Physician and hospital relationships.* Chicago: American College of Healthcare Executives.

Auerbach S. Report cards found to improve health care. *Washington Post* (6 January 1998).

Baker, E.L. et al. 1994. Health reform and the health of the public: Forging community health partnerships. *Journal of the American Medical Association* 272, no. 16:1276–1282.

Baker, G.R. 1997. Collaborating for improvement: The Institute for Healthcare Improvement's breakthrough series. *New Medicine* 1, no. 1: 5–8.

Baker, G.R. et al. 1998. Collaborating for improvement in health professions education. *Quality Management in Health Care* 6, no. 2:1–11.

Banta, T.W. 1995. Is there hope for TQM in the academy? In *Quality in Higher Education,* ed. B.D. Ruben. New Brunswick, NJ: Transaction Publishers.

Barnsley, J. et al. 1998. Integrating learning into integrated delivery systems. *Health Care Management Review* 23, no. 1:18–28.

Barry M.J. et al. 1995. Patient reactions to a program designed to facilitate patient participation in treatment decisions for benign prostatic hyperplasia. *Medical Care* 33, no. 8:771–782.

Bartlett, L. et al. 1997. *Assessing roles, responsibilities, and activities in a managed care environment: A workbook for local health officials.* Washington, DC: Agency for Health Care Policy and Research, U.S. Department of Health and Human Services.

Batalden, P. 1996a. Vision for change. Presentation at the Interdisciplinary Professional Education Collaborative: Second Milestone Conference, Institute for Healthcare Improvement. Philadelphia. November 1–2.

Batalden, P. 1996b. Collaborative work in health professional education. Paper presented at Interdisciplinary Professional Education Collaborative: Second Milestone Conference, Institute for Healthcare Improvement. Philadelphia. November 1–2.

Batalden, P. 1998. Why focus on health professional development? *Quality Management in Health Care* 6, no. 2:52–61.

Batalden, P.B., and J.J. Mohr. 1997. Building knowledge of health care as a system. *Quality Management in Health Care* 5, no. 3:1–12.

Batalden, P.B., and E.C. Nelson. 1990. Hospital quality: Patient, physician and employee judgments. *International Journal of Health Care Quality Assurance* 3, no. 4:7–17.

Batalden, P.B., and P.K. Stoltz. 1993. Performance improvement in health care organizations. A framework for the continual improvement of health care: Building and applying professional and improvement knowledge to test changes in daily work. *The Joint Commission Journal on Quality Improvement* 19, no. 10:424–452.

Batalden, P.B. et al. 1989. Quality improvement: The role and application of research methods. *The Journal of Health Administration Education* 7, no. 3:577–583.

Batalden, P.B. et al. 1996. Improving health care. Part 4. Concepts for improving any clinical process. *Joint Commission Journal on Quality Improvement* 22, no. 10:651–659.

Batalden, P.B. et al. 1997. Continually improving the health and value of health care for a population of patients: The panel management process. *Quality Management in Health Care* 5, no. 3:41–51.

Bates, D.W. et al. 1998. Effect of computerized physician order entry and a team intervention on prevention of serious medication errors *Journal of the American Medical Association* 280, no. 15:1311–1316.

Beatty, M.J. 1989. Group members' decision rule orientations and consensus. *Human Communications Research* 16:279–296.

Beckhard, R. 1969. *Organization development*. Reading, MA.: Addison-Wesley Publishing Co.

Bellack, J.P. et al. 1996. Collaborating for change in health professions education. *Joint Commission Journal on Quality Improvement* 22:145–236.

Bender, A.D. 1995. The organization of the medical practice and implications for delivering quality care. *Quality Management in Health Care* 3, no. 4:47–53.

Benner, P. et al. 1995. *Expertise in nursing practice: Caring, clinical judgment, and ethics.* New York: Springer Publishing Co.

Berenson, M.J., and D.M. Levine. 1990. *Statistics for business and economics.* Englewood Cliffs, NJ: Prentice-Hall.

Bertalanffy, L.V. 1968. *General system theory: Foundations, development, applications.* New York: George Braziller.

Berwick, D.M. 1989. Continuous improvement as an ideal in healthcare. *New England Journal of Medicine* 320, no. 1:53–56.

Berwick, D.M. 1990. Peer review and quality management: Are they compatible? *Quality Review Bulletin* 16, no. 7:246–251.

Berwick, D.M. 1991. Letter. Peer review and quality management: Are they compatible? *Quality Review Bulletin* 16, no. 12:419–420.

Berwick, D.M. 1993. TQM: Redefining doctoring. *Internist* 34, no. 3:8–10.

Berwick, D.M. 1994. Eleven worthy aims for clinical leadership of health system reform. *Journal of the American Medical Association* 272, no. 10:797–802.

Berwick D.M. 1996. A primer on leading the improvement of systems. *British Medical Journal* 312, no. 7031:619–622.

Berwick, D.M. 1998. Developing and testing changes in delivery of care. *Archives of Internal Medicine* 128, no. 8:651–656.

Berwick, D.M. et al. 1990. *Curing health care: New strategies for quality improvement.* San Francisco: Jossey-Bass, Publishers.

Berwick, D.M. et al. 1992a. Quality management in the NHS: The doctor's role. Part I. *British Medical Journal* 304, no. 6821:235–239.

Berwick, D.M. et al. 1992b. Quality management in the NHS: The doctor's role. Part II. *British Medical Journal* 304, no. 6822:304–308.

Bettcher, D.W. et al. 1998. Essential public health functions: Results of the international Delphi study. *World Health Statistics Quarterly* 51, no. 1:44–54.

Bettenhausen, K.L. 1991. Five years of group research: What we have learned and what needs to be addressed. *Journal of Management* 17, no. 2:345–381.

Bigelow, B., and M. Arndt. 1995. Total quality management: Field of dreams. *Health Care Management Review* 20, no. 4:15–33.

Bishop, P. 1991. Innovation as a team sport: Solutions through partnership. Presentation delivered at *Business Week* Symposium of Health Care CEOs. New York. June 20–21.

Blumberg, M. 1986. Risk-adjusting health care outcomes: A methodological review. *Medical Care Review* 43, no. 2:351–393.

Bluth, E.I. et al. 1982. Improvement in "stat" laboratory turnaround time: A model continuous improvement project. *Archives of Internal Medicine* 152, no. 4:837–840.

Bodenheimer, T. 1996. The HMO backlash: Righteous or reactionary? *New England Journal of Medicine* 335, no. 21:1601–1604.

Borbas, C. et al. 1990. The Minnesota clinical comparison and assessment project. *Quality Review Bulletin* 16, no. 2:87–92.

Boyatzis, R.E. et al. 1995. *Innovation in professional education: Steps on a journey from teaching to learning.* San Francisco: Jossey-Bass, Publishers.

Boynton, A.C. et al. 1993. New competitive strategies: Challenges to organizations and information technology. *IBM Systems Journal* 32, no. 1:40–64.

Brennan, T.A., and D.M. Berwick. 1996. *New rules: Regulation, markets, and the quality of American health care.* San Francisco: Jossey-Bass, Publishers.

Brennan, T.A. et al. 1991. Incidence of adverse events and negligence in hospitalized patients. *New England Journal of Medicine* 324, no. 6:370–376.

Bridges, W. 1994. *Job shift. How to prosper in a workplace without jobs.* Reading, MA: Addison-Wesley Publishing Co.

British Medical Journal. http://www.bmj.com (Last viewed 3 March 1999.)

Brockman, J. 1977. *About Bateson: Essays on Gregory Bateson.* New York: E.P. Dutton.

Brook, R. et al. 1975. A review of the literature on cholecystectomy: Findings, complications, utilization rates, costs, efficacy, and indications. Santa Monica, CA: RAND Corp.

Burns, T., and G.M. Stalker. 1961. The management of innovation. London: Tavistock Publications.

Burrus, W.M. 1993a. How long will CQI take to produce savings? *Quality Matters* 2, no. 3:3–5.

Burrus, W.M. 1993b. Northwest Hospital counting all the way to the bank. *Quality Matters* 2, no. 3:5–7.

Byrne, J. et al. 1993. The virtual corporation. *Business Week* (8 February), no. 3304:98–102.

Caldwell, C. 1998. The role of senior leaders in driving rapid change. *Frontiers of Health Services Management* 15, no. 1:35–39.

Caper, P. 1988. Defining quality in medical care. *Health Affairs* 7, no. 1:49–61.

Carman J.M. et al. 1996. Keys for successful implementation of total quality management in hospitals. *Health Care Management Review* 21, no. 1:48–60.

Carver, P. et al. 1997. A model for collaborative improvement. Presentation at the 9th National Forum on Quality Improvement in Health Care. Orlando, FL. December.

Center Watch. 1997a. Barnett moves monitor training into university setting. *Center Watch Weekly* 1 (15 September), no. 7.

Center Watch. 1997b. Cleveland Clinic and Quintiles sign mutual preferred provider agreement. *Center Watch Weekly* 1 (1 December), no. 18.

Chassin, M.R. 1991. Quality of care: Time to act. *Journal of the American Medical Association* 226, no. 24:3472–3473.

Chassin, M. et al. 1986. Variations in the use of medical and surgical services by the Medicare population. *New England Journal of Medicine* 314, no. 5:285–290.

Chassin M.R. et al. 1996. Benefits and hazards of reporting medical outcomes publicly. *New England Journal of Medicine* 334, no. 6:394–398.

Chassin, M.R. et al. 1998. The urgent need to improve health care quality. *Journal of the American Medical Association* 280, no. 11:1000–1005.

Checkland, P. 1981. *Systems thinking, systems practice.* New York: John Wiley & Sons.

Chessman et al. 1996. Institutionalizing continuous improvement in South Carolina: Taking it "bird by bird." *Joint Commission Journal on Quality Improvement* 22, no. 3:177–187.

Churchman, C.W. 1971. *The design of inquiring systems: Basic concepts of systems and organization.* New York: Basic Books.

Clancy, C.M., and H. Brody. 1995. Managed care: Jekyll or Hyde? *Journal of the American Medical Association* 273, no. 4:338–339.

Clermont, C. et al. 1998. Measuring resource use in the ICU with computerized therapeutic intervention scoring system-based data. *Chest* 113, no. 2:434–442.

The Cochrane Library. Update Software, Ltd. http://www.update-software.com/ccweb/cochrane/cdsr.htm (Last viewed 3 March 1999.)

Coddington, D.C. et al. 1996. *Making integrated health care work.* Englewood, CO: Center for Research in Ambulatory Health Care Administration.

Cotton, P. 1991. Medical schools receive a message: Reform yourselves, then take on health care system. *Journal of the American Medical Association* 266, no. 20:2802–2804.

Counte, M.A., et al. 1992. Total quality management in health care organizations: How are employees affected? *Hospital and Health Services Administration* 37, no. 4:503–518.

Crabtree, B.F. et al. 1998. Primary care practice organization and preventive services delivery: A qualitative analysis. *Journal of Family Practice* 46, no. 5:403–409.

Crosby, P.B. 1979. *Quality is free: The art of making quality certain.* New York: Mentor.

Dalen, J.E. 1996. Managed competition: Who will win? Who will lose? *Archives of Internal Medicine* 156, no. 18:2033–2035.

Damanpour, F. 1991. Organizational innovation: A meta-analysis of effects of determinants and moderators. *Academy of Management Journal* 34:555–590.

Davies, A.R., and J.E. Ware. 1988. Involving consumers in quality of care assessment. *Health Affairs* 7, no. 1:33–48.

Davis, D.A. et al. 1992. Evidence for the effectiveness of CME: A review of 50 randomized controlled trials. *Journal of the American Medical Association* 268, no. 9:1111–1117.

Dean, P., and C.P. McLaughlin. 1998. Personal communication.

Deming, W.E. 1986. *Out of the crisis.* Cambridge, MA: MIT Center for Advanced Engineering Study.

Deming, W.E. 1993. *The new economics for industry, education, government.* Cambridge, MA: MIT Center for Advanced Engineering Study.

DesHarnais, S. et al. 1988. The risk-adjusted mortality index: A new measure of hospital performance. *Medical Care* 26, no. 12:1129–1148.

DesHarnais, S. et al. 1990. Measuring hospital performance: The development and validation of risk-adjusted indexes of mortality, readmissions, and complications. *Medical Care* 28, no. 12:1127–1141.

DesHarnais, S. et al. 1991. Measuring outcomes of hospital care using multiple risk-adjusted indexes. *Health Services Research* 26, no. 4:425–445.

DesHarnais, S.I. et al. 1997. Risk-adjusted quality outcome measures: Indexes for benchmarking rates of mortality, complications and readmissions. *Quality Management in Health Care* 5, no. 2:80–87.

DiBella et al. 1996. Understanding organizational learning capability. *Journal of Management Studies* 33, no. 3:361–379.

Dietrich, A.J. et al. 1992. Cancer: Improving early detection and prevention. A community practice randomised trial. *British Medical Journal* 304, no. 6828:687–691.

Di Masi, J.A. et al. 1991. Cost of innovation in the pharmaceutical industry. *Journal of Health Economics* 10, no. 2:107–142.

Dobyns, L., and C.C. Mason. 1991. *Quality or else: The revolution in world business.* Boston: Houghton Mifflin.

Dolinsky, A.L. 1997. Elderly patients' satisfaction with the outcome of their care complaints. *Health Care Management Review* 22, no. 2:33–40.

Donabedian, A. 1980. The definition of quality and approaches to its assessment. In *Explorations in quality assessment and monitoring.* Vol.1, 95–99. Ann Arbor, MI: Health Administration Press.

Donabedian, A. 1982. *The criteria and standards of quality.* Ann Arbor, MI: Health Administration Press.

Donabedian, A. 1986. Criteria and standards for quality assessment and monitoring. *Quality Review Bulletin* 14, no. 3:99–108.

Donabedian, A. 1990. The seven pillars of quality. *Archives of Pathology and Laboratory Medicine* 114, no. 11:1115–1118.

Donabedian, A. 1993. Models of quality assurance. Leonard S. Rosenfeld Memorial Lecture. School of Public Health, University of North Carolina at Chapel Hill. February 26.

Dotson, M.M., and L. Wallman. 1994. Applying a value-added model to a project management system. Presented at the 30th Annual Meeting of the Drug Information Association. Washington, DC. June.

Dreyfus, H.L., and S.E. Dreyfus. 1996. *The relationship of theory and practice in the acquisition of skill.* New York: Springer Publishing Co.

DrKoop.com. 1999. http://www.drkoop.com (Last viewed 3 March 1999.)

Dumas, R.A. et al. 1987. Making quality control theories workable. *Training and Development Journal* 41, no. 2:30–33.

Duncan, R.B. 1976. The ambidextrous organization: Designing dual structures for innovation. In *The management of organizations*, eds. R.H. Kilmann, L.R. Pondy, and D. Slevin. New York: North-Holland.

Durand, R. et al. 1991. Association between third-year medical students' abilities to organize hypotheses about patients' problems and to order appropriate diagnostic tests. *Academic Medicine* 66, no. 11:702–704.

Dyall, W.W. 1995. Ten organizational practices of public health: A historical perspective. *American Journal of Preventive Medicine* 11(Suppl 2):6–8.

Ebel, K.E. 1991. *Achieving excellence in business: A practical guide to the total quality transformation process.* New York: Marcel Dekker.

Edvinsson, L., and M.S. Malone. 1999. *Intellectual capital: Realizing your company's true value by finding its hidden brainpower.* New York: HarperCollins, Publishers.

Eilbert K. et al. 1996. *Measuring expenditures for core public health functions.* Washington, DC: Public Health Foundation.

Eilbert K.W. et al. 1997. Public health expenditures: Developing estimates for improved policy-making. *Journal of Public Health Management and Practice* 3, no. 3:1–9.

Elliott, R.L. et al. 1996. Quality in residence training: Toward a broader, multidimensional definition. *Academic Medicine* 71, no. 3:243–247.

Ellrodt, A.G. 1993. Introduction of total quality management (TQM) into an internal medicine training program. *Academic Medicine* 68, no. 11: 817–823.

Ellwood, P. 1988. Shattuck Lecture: Outcomes management: A technology of patient experience. *New England Journal of Medicine* 318, no. 23:1549–1556.

Ellwood, P.M., Jr., and G.D. Lundberg. 1996. Managed care: A work in progress. *Journal of the American Medical Association* 276, no. 13:1083–1086.

Ellwood, P.M. et al. 1971. Health maintenance strategy. *Medical Care* 9, no. 3:291–298.

Engelkemeyer, S.W. 1995. Total quality: A mechanism for institutional change and curriculum reform. In *Academic initiatives in total quality for higher education,* ed. H.V. Roberts. Milwaukee, WI: ASQC Quality Press.

Enthoven, A.C. 1988. Theory and practice of managed competition in health care finance. In *Professor F. de Vries lectures in economics.* Vol. 9. Amsterdam: North-Holland.

Evans, C.E. et al. 1986. Does a mailed continuing education program improve physician performance? *Journal of the American Medical Association* 255, no. 4:501–504.

Evans, J.P. 1992. Implication for management education. In *Total quality management. The health care pioneers,* eds. M.M. Melum and M.K. Sinioris. Chicago: American Hospital Publishing.

Feigenbaum, A. 1983. *Total quality control*. 3d ed. New York: McGraw-Hill.

Feinglass, J. et al. 1991. The relationship of residents' autonomy and use of a teaching hospital's resources. *Academic Medicine* 66, no. 9:549–552.

Felkins, P.K. et al. 1993. *Change management: A model for effective organizational performance*. New York: Quality Resources, The Kraus Organization, Ltd.

Ferguson, T. *Self-help central*. Web site: http://www.healthy.net/home/index.html (Last viewed 3 March 1999.)

Ferrini R. 1997. Screening asymptomatic women for ovarian cancer: American College of Preventive Medicine practice policy. *American Journal of Preventive Medicine* 13, no. 6:444–446.

Fetter, R. et al. 1989. *DRG refinement with diagnosis specific comorbidities and complications: A synthesis of current approaches to patient classification*. Final Report to HCFA. New Haven, CT: Health Systems Management Group.

Fielding J.E., and N. Halfon. 1997. Characteristics of community report cards—United States, 1996. *MMWR* 46, no. 28:647–655.

Fischer, L.R. et al. 1997. A process IMPROVEment approach to preventive services: Case studies of CQI demonstration projects in two primary care clinics. *HMO Practice* 11, no. 3:123–129.

Fischer, L.R. et al. 1998. Quality improvement in primary care clinics. *Joint Commission Journal on Quality Improvement* 24, no. 7:361–370.

Fisher, E.S. et al. 1992. The accuracy of Medicare's hospital claims data: Progress has been made but problems remain. *American Journal of Public Health* 82, no. 2:243–248.

Fleming, M.E. et al. 1986. Effect of case mix on provider continuity. *Journal of Family Practice* 23:137–140.

Fletcher, R.H. et al. 1983. Patients' priorities for medical care. *Medical Care* 21, no. 2:234–242.

Flood, A. et al. 1982. Effectiveness in professional organizations: The impact of surgeons and surgical staff organizations on the quality of care in hospitals. *Health Services Research* 17, no. 4:341–366.

Flood A.B., and M.L. Fennell. 1995. Through the lenses of organizational sociology: The role of organizational theory and research in conceptualizing and examining our health care system. *Journal of Health and Social Behavior* (Special no. 154–169).

Flood A.B. et al. 1998. How do HMOs achieve savings? The effectiveness of one organization's strategies. *Health Services Research* 33, no. 1:79–99.

Ford, R.C. et al. 1997. Methods of measuring patient satisfaction.*Health Care Management Review* 22, no. 2:74–89.

Forrester, J.W. 1990. *Principles of systems.* Portland, OR: Productivity Press.

Fortune. 1998. How America stacks up. *Fortune* (21 December), 151–156.

Future HealthCare. 1998. "QI-Tools™." Home page: http://www.futurehealthcare.com.

Galbraith, J. 1973. *Designing complex organizations.* Reading, MA: Addison-Wesley Publishing Co.

Gardner, E.S., Jr., and C.P. McLaughlin. 1980. Forecasting—A cost control tool for health care managers. *Health Care Management Review* 5, no. 3:31–38.

Garg, M.L. et al. 1991. Primary care teaching physicians' losses of productivity and revenue at three ambulatory care centers. *Academic Medicine* 66, no. 6:348–353.

Garvin, D.A. 1990. Afterword: Reflections on the future. In *Curing health care: New strategies for quality improvement,* by D.M. Berwick, A.B. Godfrey, and J. Roessner, 159–165. San Francisco: Jossey-Bass, Publishers.

Gaucher, E. 1994. World class health care. Presentation at the National Conference on Benchmarking. Health Care Forum. San Diego. July14.

Gaucher, E.J., and R.J. Coffey. 1993. *Total quality in healthcare: From theory to practice.* San Francisco: Jossey-Bass, Publishers.

Gelmon, S.B. 1997. *Facilitating academic-community partnerships through educational accreditation: Overcoming a tradition of barriers and obstacles.* Washington, DC: Bureau of Health Professions, Health Resources and Services Administration, U.S. Public Health Service.

Gelmon, S.B., and G.R. Baker, eds. 1994. *A quality improvement resource teaching guide.* Arlington, VA: The Association of University Programs in Health Administration and the Institute for Healthcare Improvement.

Gelmon, S.B., and G.R. Baker. 1995. Incorporating quality improvement in the health administration curriculum. *Journal of Health Administration Education* 13, no. 1:91–107.

Gelmon, S.B. et al. 1995. Performance assessment for health administration education: Applications of the Baldrige criteria. *Journal of Health Administration Education* 13, no. 1:109–127.

Gelmon, S.B. et al. 1997. Formulating the mess: Lessons from building knowledge of health care as a system. *Quality Management in Health Care* 5, no. 3:13–17.

Gerzoff, R.B. 1997. Comparisons: The basis for measuring public health performance. *Journal of Public Health Management and Practice* 3, no. 5:11–21.

Gill, S.L. 1987. Elements of conflict and negotiation. *Clinical Laboratory Management Review* 1:187–192.

Gilutz, H. et al. 1998. The "door to needle blitz" in acute MI: The impact of a CQI project. *Joint Commission Journal on Quality Improvement* 24, no. 6:323–333.

Gitlow, H. et al. 1989. *Tools and methods for the improvement of quality*. Homewood, IL: Irwin.

Glassman, A.M. 1995. Rethinking organization stability as a determinant for innovation adoption and diffusion. *NIDA Research Monograph* 155:132–146.

Goldberg, H.I. 1998. Building healthcare quality: If the future were easy, it would be here by now. *Frontiers of Health Services Management* 15, no. 1:40–42.

Goldberg, H.I. et al. 1998. A randomized controlled trial of CQI teams and academic detailing: Can they alter compliance with guidelines? *Joint Commission Journal on Quality Improvement* 24, no. 3:130–142.

Goldsmith, J.C. et al. 1995. Managed care comes of age. *Healthcare Forum* 38, no. 5:14–24.

Gonnella, J.S. 1981. Patient case mix: Implications for medical education and hospital costs. *Journal of Medical Education* 56, no. 7:610–611.

Gordon, P.R. et al. 1996. A multisite collaborativefor the development of interdisciplinary education in continuous improvement for health professions students. *Academic Medicine* 71, no. 9:973–978.

Gordon, R.L. et al. 1996. Prevention and the reforming U.S. health system: Changing roles and responsibilities for public health. *Annual Review of Public Health* 17:489–509.

Graham, N. 1990. *Quality assurance in hospitals*. Gaithersburg, MD.: Aspen Publishers, Inc.

Grason, H.A., and B. Guyer. 1995. *Public MCH program functions: Essential public health services to promote maternal and child health in*

America. Baltimore, MD: The Johns Hopkins University School of Hygiene and Public Health.

Greene L.W. 1992. PATCH: CDC's planned approach to community health, an application of PRECEED and an inspiration for PROCEED. *Journal of Health Education* 23, no. 3:140–147.

Green, L.W., and M.W. Kreuter. 1991. *Health promotion planning: An educational and environmental approach.* 2d ed. Mountain View, CA: Mayfield Publishing Company.

Greenlick, M.R. 1996. The house that Medicare built: Remodeling for the 21st century. *Health Care Financing Review* 18, no. 2:131–145.

Griffin S.R., and P. Welch. 1995. Performance-based public health in Texas. *Journal of Public Health Management and Practice* 1, no. 3:44–49.

Grove, A.S. 1983. *High output management.* New York: Vintage Books.

Gustafson, D.H. 1997. *Case studies from the quality improvement support system.* iii, 107: no. 97–0022. Rockville, MD: U.S. Department of Health and Human Services, Public Health Service, Agency for Health Care Policy and Research.

Hagen, T. Personal correspondence with author. August 1998.

Halverson, P.K., and G.P. Mays. 1998. Disease management: A public health perspective. In *A health care professional's guide to disease management,* ed. J.B. Couch, 29–51. Gaithersburg, MD: Aspen Publishers, Inc.

Halverson, P.K. et al. 1996. Performing public health functions: The perceived contribution of public health and other community agencies. *Journal of Health and Human Services Administration* 18, no. 3:288–303.

Halverson, P.K. et al. 1997a. Privatizing health services: Alternative models and emerging issues for public health and quality management. *Quality Management in Health Care* 5, no. 2:1–18.

Halverson, P.K. et al. 1997b. Managed care and the public health challenge of TB. *Public Health Reports* 112, no. 1:22–28.

Halverson, P.K. et al., eds. 1998. *Public health and managed care.* Gaithersburg, MD: Aspen Publishers, Inc..

Hand, R. et al. 1991. Hospital variables associated with quality of care for breast cancer patients. *Journal of the American Medical Association* 266:3429–3432.

Handy, C.B. 1989. *The age of unreason.* Boston: Harvard Business School Press.

Harkey, J., and R.A. Vraciu. 1992. Quality of health care and financial performance: Is there a link? *Health Care Management Review* 17, no. 4:55–64.

Harper, A., and B. Harper. 1998. *Skill-building for self-directed team members*. New York: MW Corporation.

Hart, C. 1993. Handout. Northern Telecom-University Quality Forum. Research Triangle Park, NC. June.

Haynes, R.B. 1990. Loose connection between peer-reviewed clinical journals and clinical practice. *Annals of Internal Medicine* 113, no. 9:724–728.

Headrick, L. et al. 1991. Introducing quality improvement thinking to medical students: The Cleveland Asthma Project. *Quality Review Bulletin* 17, no. 8:254–260.

Headrick, L.A. et al. 1992. Teaching medical students about quality and cost of care at Case Western Reserve University. *Academic Medicine* 67, no. 3:157–159.

Headrick, L.A. et al. 1995. Continuous quality improvement and the education of the general physician. *Academic Medicine* 70(1 Suppl): S104–109.

Headrick, L.A. et al. 1996. Working from upstream to improve health care: The IHI interdisciplinary professional education collaborative. *Joint Commission Journal on Quality Improvement* 22, no. 3:149–164.

Headrick, L.A. et al. 1998. Using PDSA to establish academic-community partnerships: The Cleveland experience. *Quality Management in Health Care* 6, no. 2:12–20.

Health Care Advisory Board. 1993. *The components of a hospital's community report card*. Catalog No. 00 I-1 95-372. Washington, DC: Advisory Board Company.

Health Care Financing Administration. *Nursing Home Compare, National Nursing Home Database*. http://www.medicare.gov/nursing/home.asp (Last viewed 3 March 1999.)

Health care report cards. Editorial. *New York Times* (7 July 1995).

The Health Resource, Inc., Conway, AK. http://www.thehealthresource.com (Last viewed 3 March 1999.)

Healthcare Informatics. "Top 100 IS Vendors List." http://www.healthcare-informatics.com/atop.htm (Last viewed 28 August 1998.)

Hebel, J. et al. 1982. Assessment of hospital performance by use of death rates: A recent case history. *Journal of the American Medical Association* 248, no. 23:3131–3135.

Heiniger, S.L. et al. 1997. Improving preventive care services processes in a community clinic. *Medical Journal of Allina* 6:27–34.

Hellinger, F.J. 1998. The effect of managed care on quality: A review of recent evidence. *Archives of Internal Medicine* 158, no. 8:833–841.

Hellman, S. 1991. The intellectual quarantine of American medicine. *Academic Medicine* 66, no. 5:245–248.

Hernandez, G.R., et al. (In Press.) Organization, innovation, change, and learning. In *Health care management, organization design, and behavior*, eds. S. Shortell and A. Kaluzny. Albany, NY: Delmar Publishing Inc.

Hersey, P., and K.H. Blanchard. 1984. *The management of organizational behavior*. 4th ed. Englewood Cliffs, NJ: Prentice Hall.

Hertz, H.S. 1999. *1999 Health care criteria for performance excellence*. Gaithersburg, MD: National Institute for Standards and Technology.

Hertz, H.S. et al. 1994. The Malcolm Baldrige National Quality Award concept: Could it help stimulate or accelerate health care quality improvement? *Quality Management in Health Care* 2, no. 4:63–72.

Hillman, A.L., and N. Goldfarb. 1995. Exemplary quality improvement programs in HMOs. *Joint Commission Journal on Quality Improvement* 21, 457–464.

Hirokawa, F.Y. 1988. Group communications and decision-making performance: A continued test of the functional perspective. *Human Communication Research* 14:487–515.

Hoff T.J., and D.P. McCaffrey. 1996. Adapting, resisting and negotiating. *Work and Occupations* 23, no. 2:165–189.

Hogan, T.M. et al. 1997. Implementing a preventive care services delivery system in a community clinic. *Medical Journal of Allina* 6, no. 2:35–37.

Holzer, J. 1990. The advent of clinical standards for professional liability. *Quality Review Bulletin* 16, no. 2:72–79.

Horn, S.D., and D.S. Hopkins. 1994. *Clinical practice improvement: A new technology for developing cost-effective quality health care*. New York: Faulkner and Gray.

Horn, S.D., and R.A. Horn. 1986. The computerized severity index: A new tool for case-mix management. *Journal of Medical Systems* 10, no. 1:73–78.

Hornbrook, M.C. 1982. Hospital case mix: Its definition, measurement, and use: Part 1. The conceptual framework. *Medical Care Review* 39, no. 1:3–5.

Hsieh, M., and J.D. Kagle. 1991. Understanding patient satisfaction and dissatisfaction with health care. *Health and Social Work* 16, no. 4:281–290.

Hunt, D.L. et al. 1998. Effects of computer-based clinical decision support systems on physician performance and patient outcomes. *Journal of the American Medical Association* 280, no. 15:1339–1346.

Hunt, H.K. 1977. CS/D: Overview and future research directions. In *Conceptualization and measurement of consumer satisfaction and dissatisfaction*, ed. H.K. Hunt. Cambridge, MA: Marketing Science Institute.

Hurley, R. 1997. Approaching the slippery slope: Managed care as the industrial rationalization of medical practice. In *Rationing sanity: The ethics of mental health,* ed. P. Boyle. Washington, DC: Georgetown University Press.

Hynes, D.M. et al. 1992. Evaluating productivity in clinical research programs: The National Cancer Institute's (NCI) community clinical oncology program (CCOP). *Journal of Medical Systems* 16, no. 6:247–267.

Iezzoni, L.I. 1991a. Black box medical information systems: A technology needing assessment. *Journal of the American Medical Association* 265, no. 22:3006–3007.

Iezzoni, L.I. 1991b. Severity standardization and hospital quality assessment. In *Health care: Quality management for the 21st century*, ed. James Couch. Tampa, FL: American College of Physician Executives.

Iezzoni, L.I. 1995. Predicting who dies depends on how severity is measured: Implications for evaluating patient outcomes. *Annals of Internal Medicine* 123, no. 10:763–770.

Imai, M. 1986. *Kaizen: The key to Japan's competitive success.* New York: Random House.

Institute of Medicine. 1999. *Healthy communities: The future of public health.* Washington, DC: National Academy Press.

Institute of Medicine, Committee for the Study of the Future of Public Health. 1988. *The future of public health.* Washington, DC: National Academy Press.

Institute of Medicine, Committee on Using Performance Monitoring to Improve Community Health. 1997. *Improving health in the community: A role for performance monitoring.* Washington, DC: National Academy Press.

Intermountain Health Care, Inc. 1993. *Inpatient perceptions of quality questionnaire.* Salt Lake City, UT.

Ishikawa, K. 1987. *Guide to quality control*, trans. Asian Productivity Organization. White Plains, NY: Kraus International Publications.

Jackson, R.S. et al. 1994. Implementing continuous quality improvement in primary care: Implications for preventive services. *Journal of Ambulatory Care Management* 17, no. 3:8–14.

Jackson, S.E. 1992. Team composition in organizational settings: Issues in managing an increasingly diverse work force. In *Group process and productivity*, ed. S. Worchel et al., 138–180. Thousand Oaks, CA: Sage Publications.

James, B.L. 1989. *Quality management for health care delivery*. Chicago: Hospital Research and Educational Trust of the American Hospital Association.

Johnson, D.E.L. 1990. HCFA's mortality statistics boost teaching hospitals. *Health Care Strategic Management* 8, no. 1:2–3.

Joiner, B.L. 1994. *Fourth generation management. The new business consciousness*. New York: McGraw-Hill.

Joint Commission on Accreditation of Healthcare Organizations. 1992. *Striving toward improvement. Six hospitals in search of quality*. Oakbrook Terrace, IL.

Joint Commission on Accreditation of Healthcare Organizations. 1998. "Performance measurement." http://www.jcaho.org/perfmeas/oryx/dearcol.htm (15 November 1998).

Joint Commission on Accreditation of Healthcare Organizations. 1998. Appendix C in "Performance Measurement" report. 1–15. http://wwwa.jcaho.org/perfmeas/nlhi/appendc.htm (7 December 1998).

Jollis, J.G. et al. 1993. Discordance of databases designed for claims payment versus clinical info systems. Implications for outcomes research. *Annals of Internal Medicine* 119, no. 8:844–850.

Juran, J. 1988. *Juran on planning for quality*. New York: Free Press.

Kaluzny, A.D. 1992. Implementation of prevention and early detection strategies: Selected organizational perspectives. *Proceedings of the second primary care research conference,* 197–202. Washington, DC: Agency for Health Care Policy and Research.

Kaluzny, A.D., and C.P. McLaughlin. 1992. Managing transitions. Assuring the adoption and impact of TQM. *Quality Review Bulletin* 18, no. 11:380–384.

Kaluzny, A.D. et al. 1991. Prevention and early detection activities in primary care: New directions for implementation. *Cancer Detection and Prevention* 15, no. 6: 459–464.

Kaluzny, A.D. et al. 1992. Continuous quality improvement in the clinical setting: Enhancing adoption. *Quality Management in Health Care* 1, no. 1:37–44.

Kaplan, R.S., and D.P. Norton. 1996. *The balanced scorecard, translating strategy into action.* Boston: Harvard Business School Press.

Kasper, J.F. et al. 1992. A methodology for QI in the coronary artery bypass grafting procedure involving comparative process analysis. *Quality Review Bulletin* 18, no. 4:129–133.

Kassirer, J.P. 1995. Managed care and the morality of the marketplace. *New England Journal of Medicine* 333, no. 1:50–52.

Katzenbach, J.R., and D.K. Smith. 1993. *The wisdom of teams: Creating the high-performance organization.* Boston: Harvard Business School Press.

Keener, S. et al. 1997. Providing public health services through an integrated delivery system. *Quality Management in Health Care* 5, no. 2:27–34.

Kelleher, C. 1993. Relationship of physician ratings of severity of illness and difficulty of clinical management to length of stay. *Health Services Research* 27, no. 6:841–855.

W.K. Kellogg Foundation. 1997. *Turning point: Collaborating for a new century in public health.* Battle Creek, MI. http://www.wkkf.org/ProgrammingInterests/Health/TurningPoint/618.htm.

Kelly, J., and F. Hellinger. 1986. Physician and hospital factors associated with mortality of surgical patients. *Medical Care* 24, no. 9:785–800.

Kibbe, D.C. 1998a. Disease management: Who's caring for your patients? *Family Practice Management* 5, no. 9:44–50.

Kibbe, D.C. 1998b. The information reformation: Physicians, patients, and the changing economy of healthcare information. *New Medicine* 2:319–324.

Kibbe, D.C., and K. Johnson. 1998. Do-it-yourself disease management. *Family Practice Management* 5, no. 10:34–47.

Kibbe, D.C. et al. 1993. Continuous quality improvement for continuity of care. *Journal of Family Practice* 36, no. 3: 304–308.

Kilo, C. Personal Communication with author. September 1997.

Kinsinger L.S. et al. 1998. Using an office system intervention to increase breast cancer screening. *Journal of General Internal Medicine* 13:507–514.

Knapp, M., and D. Hotopp. 1995. Applying TQM to community health improvement: Nine works in progress. *Quality Letter for Healthcare Leaders* 7, no. 6:23–29.

Knaus, W. et al. 1986. An evaluation of outcome from intensive care in major medical centers. *Annals of Internal Medicine* 104, no. 3:410–418.

Kochan, T.A., and M. Useem. 1992. *Transforming organizations.* New York: Oxford University Press.

Kongstvedt, P.R. 1997. *Essentials of managed health care,* 2d ed. Gaithersburg, MD: Aspen Publishers, Inc.

Kosecoff, J. et al. 1987. Effects of the National Institutes of Health consensus development program on physician practice. *Journal of the American Medical Association* 258, no. 19:2708–2713.

Kotler, P. 1997. *Marketing management—Analysis, planning, implementation, and control.* 9th ed. Englewood Cliffs, NJ: Prentice-Hall International.

Kotler, P., and G. Armstrong. 1993. Consumer markets and consumer buying behavior. In *Marketing, An introduction.* 3d ed. Englewood Cliffs, NJ: Prentice Hall.

Kotter, J.P. 1996. *Leading change.* Boston: Harvard Business School Press.

Kottke, T.E. et al. 1993. Making "time" for preventive services. *Mayo Clinic Proceedings* 68, no. 8:785–791.

Kottke, T.E. et al. 1997a. Delivery rates for preventive services in 44 Midwestern clinics. *Mayo Clinic Proceedings* 72, no. 6:515–523.

Kottke, T.E. et al. 1997b. Will patient satisfaction set the preventive services implementation agenda? *American Journal of Preventive Medicine* 13, no. 4:309–316.

Kuhn, T.S. 1962. *The structure of scientific revolutions.* Chicago: University of Chicago Press.

LaBarbara, P.A., and D. Mazursky. 1983. A longitudinal assessment of consumer satisfaction/dissatisfaction: The dynamic aspect of the cognitive process. *Journal of Marketing Research* 20:393–404.

Labovitz, G.H., and M. Lowenhaupt. 1993. The internal customer. *Quality Management in Health Care* 2, no. 1:39–45.

Laine, C. et al. 1996. Important elements of outpatient care: A comparison of patients' and physicians' opinions. *Annals of Internal Medicine* 125, no. 8:640–645.

Langley, G.J. et al. 1994. The foundation of improvement. *Quality Progress* 27, no. 6:81–86.

Langley, G.J. et al. 1996. *The improvement guide: A practical approach to enhancing organizational performance.* San Francisco: Jossey-Bass, Publishers.

Lasker, R. 1997. *Medicine and public health: The power of collaboration.* New York: New York Academy of Medicine.

Lawler, E.E., III. 1988. *High-involvement management: Participative strategies for improving organizational performance.* San Francisco: Jossey-Bass, Publishers.

Lawrence, P.R., and J.W. Lorsch. 1967. *Organization and environment.* Boston: Harvard University Press.

Lazovich, D. et al. 1991. Underutilization of breast-conserving surgery and radiation therapy among women with stage I and stage II breast cancer. *Journal of the American Medical Association* 266, no. 24:3433–3438.

Leape, L. 1987. Unnecessary surgery. *Health Services Research* 24, no. 3:351–407.

Leape, L. 1990. Practice guidelines and standards: An overview. *Quality Review Bulletin* 16, no. 2:42–49.

Leape, L.L. et al. 1991. The nature of adverse events in hospitalized patients: Results of the Harvard Medical Practice study II. *New England Journal of Medicine* 324, no. 6:377–384.

Leininger, L.S. et al. 1996. An office system for organizing preventive services. A report by the American Cancer Society Advisory Group on Preventive Health Care Reminder Systems. *Archives of Family Medicine* 5, no. 2:108–115.

Levy, D. 1997. Disease management as patient-centered care. In *The physician's guide to disease management,* ed. J.B. Couch, 265–290. Gaithersburg, MD: Aspen Publishers, Inc.

Lewis, C.E. 1988. Disease prevention and health promotion practices of primary care physicians in the United States. *American Journal of Preventive Medicine* 4 (4 Suppl.):9–16.

Lewis, I., and C. Sheps. 1983. *The sick citadel: The American academic medical center and the public interest.* Cambridge, MA: Oelgeschlager, Gunn and Hain.

Linder, J. 1991. Outcomes measurement: Compliance tool or strategic initiative. *Health Care Management Review* 16, no. 4:21–33.

Linder, J.C. 1992. Outcomes measurement in hospitals: Can the system change the organization? *Hospital and Health Administration* 37, no. 2:143–166.

Linn, S.L. 1975. Factors associated with patient evaluation of health care. *Health and Society* (Fall):531–548.

Localio, A.R. et al. 1995. Comparing hospital mortality in adult patients with pneumonia: A case study of statistical methods in a managed care program. *Annals of Internal Medicine* 122, no. 2:125–131.

Lohr, K.N. et al, eds. 1996. *The nation's physician workforce: Options for balancing supply and requirements.* Washington, DC: National Academy Press.

Lomas, J. et al. 1991. Opinion leaders vs audit and feedback to implement practice guidelines: Delivery after previous Cesarean section. *Journal of the American Medical Association* 265, no. 17:2202–2207.

Longo, D.R. et al. 1997. Consumer reports in health care: Do they make a difference in patient care? *Journal of the American Medical Association* 278, no. 19:1579–1584.

Lowery, D. 1996. Quality infrastructure: The key to implementing a total quality program in a clinical care setting. *Journal of the Society for Health Systems* 5, no. 2:51–64.

Luft, H., and S. Hunt. 1986. Evaluating individual hospital quality through outcome statistics. *Journal of the American Medical Association* 255, no. 20:2780–2784.

Macdonald, M. 1998. Using the balanced scorecard to align strategy and performance in long term care. *Healthcare Management Forum* 11, no. 3:33–38.

Macintyre, K., and C.C. Kleman. 1994. Measuring customer satisfaction. In *Continuous quality improvement in health care,* eds. C.P. McLaughlin and A.D. Kaluzny, 102–126. Gaithersburg, MD: Aspen Publishers, Inc.

Madison, D.L., and T.R. Konrad. 1988. Large medical group-practice organizations and employed physicians: A relationship in transition. *Milbank Quarterly* 66, no. 2:240–282.

Magnan, S. et al. 1997. Primary care, process improvement, and turmoil. *Journal of Ambulatory Care Management* 20, no. 4:32–38.

Magnan, S. et al. 1998. IMPROVE: Bridge over troubled waters. *Joint Commission Journal on Quality Improvement* 24, no. 10:566–578.

Marder, R.J. 1990. Relationship of clinical indicators and practice guidelines. *Quality Review Bulletin* 16, no. 2:60.

Marquardt, M., and T. Carter. 1998. Action learning and research at George Washington University. *Performance Improvement Quarterly* 11, no. 2.

Masters, R.J. 1996. Overcoming the barriers to TQM's success. *Quality Progress* 29:53–55.

Mayer, S.M., and D.A. Collier. 1998. Contrasting the original Malcolm Baldrige National Quality Award and the Health Care Pilot Award. *Quality Management in Health Care* 6, no. 3:12–21.

Mays, G.P. 1998. Case study: Reconfiguring Memphis' public health system for managed care. In *Public health and managed care,* eds. C.K. Halvorsen et al., 243–251. Gaithersburg, MD: Aspen Publishers, Inc.

Mays, G.P. et al. 1998a. Assessing the performance of local public health systems: A survey of state health agency efforts. *Journal of Public Health Management and Practice* 4, no. 4:63–78.

Mays, G.P. et al. 1998b. Collaboration to improve community health: Trends and alternative models. *Joint Commission Journal on Quality Improvement* 24, no. 10:518–540.

Mays, G.P. et al. 1998c. *Developing a model report card of community health: A proposed methodology*. Chapel Hill, NC: School of Public Health, University of North Carolina.

Mays, G.P. et al. 1999a. *The community health report card survey: A cooperative agreement between the Centers for Disease Control and Prevention and the Association of Schools of Public Health*. Chapel Hill, NC: University of North Carolina at Chapel Hill School of Public Health.

Mays, G.P. et al. 1999b. *Local public health practice: Trends and models*. Washington, DC: American Public Health Association.

McAninch, M. 1988. Accrediting agencies and the search for quality in health care. In *Handbook of quality assurance in mental health*, eds. G. Stricker and A. Rodriguez. New York: Plenum.

McCarthy, B.C. et al. 1997. Redesigning primary care processes to improve the offering of mammography. *Journal of General Internal Medicine* 12, no. 6:357–363.

McEachern, J.E., and D.B. Neuhauser. 1989. The continuous improvement of quality at the Hospital Corporation of America. *Health Matrix* 7, no. 3:5–11.

McEachern, J.E. et al. 1995. Medical leadership in an era of managed care and continual improvement. *Health Care Management–State of the Art Reviews* 2, no. 1:19–32.

McGinnis, J.M., and P.R. Lee. 1995. Healthy people 2000 at mid decade. *Journal of the American Medical Association* 273, no. 14:1123–1129.

McGlynn, E.A. 1997. Six challenges for measuring the quality of health care. *Health Affairs* 16, no. 3:7–21.

McIlvain, H. et al. 1998. Using practice genograms to understand and describe practice configurations. *Family Medicine* 30, no. 7:490–496.

McLaughlin, C.P. 1991. Negotiation as a business matter. *Carolina Journal of Pharmacy* 71, no. 10:25–27.

McLaughlin, C.P. 1992. Negotiation and cooperation. *Carolina Journal of Pharmacy* 72, no. 2:26–28.

McLaughlin, C.P. 1995. Balancing collaboration and competition: The Kingsport, Tennessee experience. *The Joint Commission Journal on Quality Improvement* 21, no. 11:646–655.

McLaughlin, C.P. 1996. Why variation reduction is not everything: A new paradigm for service operations. *International Journal of Service Industry Management* 7, no. 3:17–30.

McLaughlin, C.P. 1998. Evaluating the quality control system for managed care in the United States. *Quality Management in Health Care* 7, no. 1:38–46.

McLaughlin, C.P., and S.P. Johnson. 1995. Inherent variability in service operations: Identification, measurement and implications. In *Services management: New directions and perspectives*, eds. C.G. Armistead and G. Teare, 226–229. London: Cassell PLC.

McLaughlin C.P., and A.D. Kaluzny. 1990. Total quality management in health: Making it work. *Health Care Management Review* 15, no. 3:7–14.

McLaughlin, C.P., and A.D. Kaluzny. 1994. *Continuous quality improvement in health care: Theory, implementation, and applications.* Gaithersburg, MD: Aspen Publishers, Inc.

McLaughlin, C.P., and A.D. Kaluzny. 1995. Quality management in health care: Successes and lessons in implementation. *Journal of Continuing Education in the Health Professions* 15, no. 3 (September):165–174.

McLaughlin, C.P., and A.D. Kaluzny. 1997. Total quality management issues in managed care. *Journal of Health Care Finance* 24, no. 1:10–16.

McLaughlin, C.P., and A.D. Kaluzny. 1998. Managed care: The challenge ahead. *OR/MS Today* 25, no. 1:24–27.

McPherson, C., and L.A. Sachs. 1982. Health care team training in US and Canadian medical schools. *Journal of Medical Education* 57, no. 4:282–287.

Melum, M.M. 1990. Total quality management: Steps to success. *Hospitals* 64, no. 23:42–44.

Melum, M.M., and M.K. Sinioris. 1992. *Total quality management—The health care pioneers.* Chicago: American Hospital Publishing.

Mendelson, D.N., and E.M. Salinsky. 1997. Health information systems and the role of state government. *Health Affairs* 16, no. 3:106–119.

Merry, M.D. 1990. Total quality management for physicians: Translating the new paradigm. *Quality Review Bulletin* 16, no. 3:101–105.

Miller, C.A. et al. 1994a. A screening survey to assess local public health performance. *Public Health Report* 109, no. 5:659–664.

Miller, C.A. et al. 1994b. A proposed method for assessing public health functions and practices. *American Journal of Public Health* 84, no. 1:1743–1749.

Miller, L., and L.G. Millstein. 1996. The FDA and the regulatory oversight of the clinical research process in drug development. In *Clinical research in pharmaceutical development,* eds. B. Bleidt and M. Montagne, 79–95. New York: Marcel Dekker.

Miller, R.H., and H.S. Luft. 1994. Managed care plan performance since 1980: A literature analysis. *Journal of the American Medical Association* 271, no. 19:1512–1519.

Miller, R.H., and H.S. Luft. 1997. Does managed care lead to better or worse quality of care? *Health Affairs* 16, no. 5:7–25.

Miranda, D.R. et al. 1996. Simplified therapeutic intervention scoring system: The TISS-28 items-results from a multicenter study. *Critical Care Medicine* 24, no. 1:64–73.

Mitroff, I.I., and L.A. Linstone. 1993. *The unbounded mind. Breaking the chains of traditional thinking.* New York: Oxford University Press.

Mizuno, S. 1988. *Company-wide total quality control.* Tokyo: Nordica International Limited.

Moriarity, J.M. October 1996. A pound of cure. *Minnesota Medicine* 79:8-9, 60.

Morris, A.H. 1992. Protocols, ECOO2R, and the evaluation of new ARDS therapy. *Japanese Journal of Intensive Care Medicine* 16:61–63.

Moses, L., and F. Mosteller. 1968. Institutional differences in postoperative death rates: Commentary on some of the findings of the National Halothane Study. *Journal of the American Medical Association* 203, no. 7:492–494.

Mosser, G. 1996. Clinical process improvement: Engage first, measure later. *Quality Management in Health Care* 4, no. 4:11–20.

Mowen, J.C. 1990. Individual consumer processes III: Postacquisition processes. In *Consumer Behavior.* 2d ed. Indianapolis, IN: Macmillan Publishing USA.

Muckart, D.J. et al. 1997. Validation of an outcome prediction model for critically ill trauma patients without head injury. *Journal of Trauma* 43, no. 6:934–939.

National Association of County and City Health Officials. 1991. *Assessment protocol for excellence in public health* (APEXPH). Washington, DC.

National Asthma Education Program Office of Prevention, Education, and Control, National Heart, Lung and Blood Institute, National Institute of Health. 1992. "Teach Your Patients About Asthma." Publication No. 92-2737. Bethesda, MD. October. http://www.meddean.luc.edu/lumen/MedEd/medicine/Allergy/Asthma/asthtoc.html (Last viewed 3 March 1999.)

National Center for Health Statistics. 1991. Consensus set of health status indicators for the general assessment of community health status—United States. *MMWR* 40, no. 27:449–451.

National Committee on Quality Assurance. 1995. *Report card pilot project.* Washington, DC.

National Committee on Quality Assurance. http://www.ncqa.org (Last viewed 3 March 1999.)

National Committee on Quality Assurance. "State of Managed Care Quality," *Quality Compass* 1998, 1–22. http://www.ncqa.org/QC98/national.htm (7 December 1998).

National Library of Medicine. 1999. NLM online databases and databanks (http://www.nlm.nih.gov/pubs/factsheets/online_databases.html) Bethesda, MD.

Nelson, D.E. et al. 1995. Outcome-based management and public health: The Oregon benchmarks experience. *Journal of Public Health Management and Practice* 1, no. 2:8–17.

Nelson, E.C., and P.B. Batalden. 1993. Patient-based quality measurement systems. *Quality Management in HealthCare* 1, no. 1:18–30.

Nelson, E.C. et al. 1992. The relationship between patient perceptions of quality and hospital financial performance. *Journal of Healthcare Marketing* 12, no. 4:6–14.

Nelson, E.C. et al. 1996a. Improving health care. Part 1: The clinical value compass. *The Joint Commission Journal on Quality Improvement* 22, no. 4:243–258.

Nelson, E.C. et al. 1996b. Improving health care. Part 2: A clinical improvement worksheet and user's manual. *The Joint Commission Journal on Quality Improvement* 22, no. 8:531–548.

Nelson, E.C. et al. 1996c. Improving health care. Part 3: Clinical benchmarking for best patient care. *The Joint Commission Journal on Quality Improvement* 22, no. 9:599–616.

Nelson, E.C. et al. 1996d. Improving health care. Part 4: Concepts for improving any clinical process. *The Joint Commission Journal on Quality Improvement* 22, no. 10:651–659.

Nelson, E.C. et al. 1998. Building a quality future. *Frontiers of Health Services Management* 15, no. 1:3–31.

Nolan, T. 1997. Accelerating the pace of improvement: An interview with Thomas Nolan. *Joint Commission Journal on Quality Improvement* 23, no. 4:217–222.

Norman, L.D., and M. Lutenbacher. 1996. Process of continual improvement in a school of nursing. *Nursing in Health Care: Perspectives on Community* 17, no. 6:292–297.

O'Connor, G. et al. 1996. A regional intervention to improve the hospital mortality associated with coronary artery bypass graft surgery. *Journal of the American Medical Association* 275, no. 11:841–846.

O'Connor, G.T. et al. 1993. Regional organization for outcomes research. *Annals of the New York Academy of Sciences* 703:44–51; discussion, 50–51.

Oshel, R.E. et al. 1997. Use of national practitioner data bank disclosure information for decision making. *Quality Management in Health Care* 5, no. 4:34–42.

Pace, R.C. 1990. Personalized and depersonalized conflict in small group discussions. *Small Group Research* 21, no. 1:79–96.

Pacific Business Group on Health. *California Consumer Healthscope*. http://www.healthscope.org/ (Last viewed 3 March 1999.)

Pappaioanou, M., and C. Evans. 1998. Development of the guide to community preventive services: A U.S. Public Health Service initiative. *Journal of Public Health Management and Practice* 4, no. 2:48–54.

Parenti, C.M. et al. 1994. Reduction of unnecessary intravenous catheter use: Internal medicine house staff participate in a successful quality improvement project. *Archives of Internal Medicine* 154, no. 6:1829–1832.

Parker, D.F. et al. 1995. Incorporating total quality into a college of business. In *Academic initiatives in total quality for higher education,* ed. H.V. Roberts. Milwaukee, WI: ASQC Quality Press.

Pascale, R.T. et al. 1997. Changing the way we change. *Harvard Business Review* 75, no. 6:126–139.

Patel, R., and L. Kinsinger. 1997. Childhood immunizations: American College of Preventive Medicine practice policy. *American Journal of Preventive Medicine* 13, no. 2:74–77.

Paul-Shaheen, P. 1987. Small area analysis: A review of the North American literature. *American Journal of Health Politics, Policy and Law* 12, no. 4:741–809.

Pennsylvania Health Care Cost Containment Council. 1991. *A consumer guide to coronary artery bypass graft surgery: Pennsylvania's declaration of health care information.* Harrisburg.

Perrin, E.B., and J.J. Koshel, eds. 1997. *Assessment of performance measures for public health, substance abuse, and mental health.* Washington, DC: National Academy Press.

Peters, T. 1994. *The Tom Peters seminar: Crazy times call for crazy organizations.* New York: Vintage.

Pew Health Professions Commission. 1995. *Critical challenges: Revitalizing the health professions for the twenty-first century.* San Francisco: UCSF Center for the Health Professions.

Pharmaceutical Research and Manufacturers Association of America. 1998. *Industry profile, 1998.* Washington, DC.

Phys. 1999. CondeNet, Inc., a division of Advance Internet, Inc. http://www.phys.com/a_home/01home/home.htm (Last viewed 3 March 1999.)

Pocock, S.J. 1983. *Clinical trials: A practical approach.* New York: John Wiley & Sons.

Pollack, M. et al. 1987. Accurate prediction of the outcome of pediatric intensive care: A new quantitative method. *New England Journal of Medicine* 316, no. 3:134–139.

Porras, J.I., and S.J. Hoffer. 1986. Common behavior changes in successful organizational development efforts. *Journal of Applied Behavioral Science* 22:477–494.

Pritchard, R.B., and B.W. Karasick. 1973. The effects of organizational climate on managerial job performance and job satisfaction. *Organizational Behavior and Human Performance* 9:126–146.

PubMed Search Service. National Library of Medicine. http://www.ncbi.nlm.nih.gov/PubMed (Last viewed 3 March 1999.)

Quintiles Transnational Corp. 1997. *Annual Report.* Research Triangle Park, NC.

Quintiles Transnational Corp. 1998. Quintiles, Johns Hopkins to collaborate on clinical research. News Release, 7 July. Also, "Welcome to Quintiles Transnational Corporation: Chairman's Corner." 1998. http://

www.quintiles.com/newsroom/articles_1998/article_980727.html (Last viewed 3/3/99.)

Redman, T.C. 1992. *Data quality management and technology.* New York: Bantam Books.

Reed, R., and D. Evans. 1987. The deprofessionalization of medicine: Causes, effects, and responses. *Journal of the American Medical Association* 258, no. 22:3279–3282.

Reeves, C.A., and D.A. Bednar. 1993. What prevents TQM implementation in health care organizations? *Quality Progress* 26:41–44.

Revans, R. 1991. Action learning: Its origins and nature. In *Action learning in practice*, ed. M. Pedler, 3–15. 2d ed. London: Gower Publishing Company.

Revans, R.W. 1964. *Standards for morale: Cause and effect in hospitals.* London: Oxford University Press.

Roberts, H.V. 1995. Grassroots total quality in higher education: Some lessons from Chicago. In *Academic initiatives in total quality for higher education,* ed. H.V. Roberts. Milwaukee, WI: ASQC Quality Press.

Robinson, T.N. 1998. An evidence-based approach to interactive health communication. *Journal of the American Medical Association* 280, no. 14:1264–1269.

Roemer, M.I. et al. 1968. A proposed hospital quality index: Hospital death rates adjusted for case severity. *Health Services Research* 3, no. 2:96–118.

Rogers, E.M. 1995. *Diffusion of Innovations.* New York: Free Press.

Roglieri, J. Personal correspondence with author. June 4, 1998.

Roos, L. et al. 1985. Using computers to identify complications after surgery. *American Journal of Public Health* 75, no. 11:1288–1295.

Roos, L.L. et al. 1991. Comparing clinical information with claims data: Some similarities and differences. *Journal of Clinical Epidemiology* 44, no. 9:881–888.

Rudy, L.J. 1996. The CRO of the future. *Scrip Magazine* (July-August):42–44.

Ruffin, M.T., IV. 1998. Can we change physicians' practices in the delivery of cancer-preventive services? *Archives of Family Medicine* 7, no. 4:317–319.

Sahney, V.K., and G.L. Warden. 1991. The quest for quality and productivity in health services. *Frontiers of Health Services Management* 7, no. 4:2–40.

Sahney, V.K. et al. 1995. *Re-Engineering: Health Care: Building on CQI*. Chicago: Health Administration Press.

Salive, M.E. et al. 1990. Patient outcomes research teams and the agency for health care policy and research. *Health Services Research* 25, no. 5: 697–708.

Sarazen, J.S. 1990. The tools of quality. Part II. Cause and effect diagrams. *Quality Progress* (July):59–62.

Savitz, L.A. 1994. The influence of maternal employment on obstetrical health care seeking behavior. Ann Arbor, MI: UMI Press.

Schmittdiel, J. et al. 1997. Choice of a personal physician and patient satisfaction in a health maintenance organization. *Journal of the American Medical Association* 278, no. 19:1596–1599.

Schwarz, R.M.1989. Understanding and changing the culture of an organization. *Popular Government* 45 (Winter):23–26.

Schweikhart, S.B. et al. 1993. Service recovery in health service organizations. *Hospital and Health Services Administration* 38, no. 1:3–23.

Schweitzer, S.O. 1997. *Pharmaceutical economics and policy*. New York: Oxford University Press.

Scutchfield, F.D. 1997. The presence of total quality management and continuous quality improvement processes in California public health clinics. *Journal of Public Health Management and Practice* 3, no. 3:57–60.

Scutchfield, F.D. et al. 1997. The presence of total quality management and continuous quality improvement processes in California public health clinics. *Journal of Health and Human Services Administration* 18, no. 3:288–303.

Seattle-King County Department of Public Health, Epidemiology, Planning, and Evaluation Unit. 1995. *Vista/PH software for public health assessment: User's guide*. Seattle, WA.

Senge, P.M. 1990. *The fifth discipline: The art and practice of the learning organization*. New York: Doubleday.

Senge, P.M. et al. 1996. *The fifth discipline fieldbook: Strategies and tools for building a learning organization*. New York: Doubleday.

Shea, G.P., and R.A. Guzzo. 1987. Group effectiveness: What really matters? *Sloan Management Review* 28, no. 2:25–31.

Shewhart, W.A. 1986. *Statistical method from the viewpoint of quality control*. Mineola, NY: Dover Publications.

Shortell, S. 1985. The medical staff of the future: Replanting the garden. *Frontiers of Health Services Management* 1, no. 3:3–48.

Shortell, S. 1990. Revisiting the garden: Medicine and management in the 1990s. *Frontiers of Health Services Management* 7, no. 1:3–32.

Shortell, S. et al. 1993. New versus traditional approaches to quality improvement: Implementation processes and perceived impacts. Evanston, IL: Northwestern University. Working Paper.

Shortell, S. et al. 1996. *Remaking health care in America*. San Francisco: Jossey-Bass, Publishers.

Shortell S.M. et al. 1995. Assessing the impact of continuous quality improvement/total quality management: Concept versus implementation. *Health Services Research* 30, no. 2:377–401.

Shortell, S.M. et al. 1998. Assessing the impact of continuous quality improvement on clinical practice: What it will take to accelerate progress. *The Milbank Quarterly* 76, no. 4:593–624.

Shugars, D.A. et al., eds. 1991. *Healthy America: Practitioners for 2005, an agenda for action for U.S. health professional schools*. Durham, NC: The Pew Health Professions Commission.

Silberg, W.M. et al. 1997. Assessing, controlling, and assuring the quality of medical information on the Internet: Caveat lector et viewor— Let the reader and viewer beware. *Journal of the American Medical Association* 277, no. 15:1244–1245.

Silver, G. 1997. Editorial. The road from managed care. *American Journal of Public Health* 87, no. 1:8–9.

Simone, P.M. 1995. Essential components of a tuberculosis prevention and control program: Recommendations of the Advisory Council for the Elimination of Tuberculosis. *MMWR* 44(RR-11):1–16.

Sloan, F. et al. 1986. In-hospital mortality of surgical patients: Is there an empirical basis for standard setting? *Surgery* 99, no. 4:446–454.

Solberg, L. 1993. Improving disease prevention in primary care. Washington, DC: Agency for Health Care Policy and Research. Working Paper.

Solberg, L.I. 1997. Using continuous quality improvement to improve diabetes care in populations: The IDEAL model. *Joint Commission Journal on Quality Improvement* 23, no. 11:581–592.

Solberg, L.I. et al. 1995. Competing HMOs collaborate to improve preventive services. *Joint Commission Journal on Quality Improvement* 21, no. 11:600–610.

Solberg, L.I. et al. 1996. Using CQI to increase preventive services in clinical practice: Going beyond guidelines. *Preventive Medicine* 25, no. 3:259–267.

Solberg, L.I. et al. 1997a. Are physicians less likely to recommend preventive services to low-SES patients? *Preventive Medicine* 26, no. 3:350–357.

Solberg, L.I. et al. 1997b. How important are clinician and nurse attitudes to the delivery of clinical preventive services? *Journal of Family Practice* 44, no. 5:451–461.

Solberg, L.I. et al. 1997c. Clinical preventive services delivery: A study in variation. *Journal of Family Practice* 44, no. 5:451–461.

Solberg, L.I. et al. 1997d. Delivering clinical preventive services is a systems problem. *Annals of Behavioral Medicine* 19, no. 3:271–278.

Solberg, L.I. et al. 1997e. The three faces of performance measurement: Improvement, accountability, and research. *Joint Commission Journal on Quality Improvement* 23, no. 3:135–147.

Solberg, L.I. et al. 1998a. Continuous quality improvement in primary care: What's happening? *Medical Care* 36, no. 5:625–635.

Solberg, L.I. et al. 1998b. Will primary care clinics organize themselves to improve the delivery of preventive services? A randomized controlled trial. *Preventive Medicine* 27, no. 4:623–631.

Solberg, L.I. et al. 1998c. The case of the missing clinical preventive services systems. *Effective Clinical Practice* 1, no. 1:33–38.

Solberg, L.I. et al. 1999. A randomized controlled trial of CQI to create systems to IMPROVE preventive services in primary care. Draft. Minneapolis, MN: Health Partners Research Foundation.

Sollecito, W.A. 1993. Can CROs accelerate the registration process? Presentation at the Conference on Global Product Registration, sponsored by the pharmaceutical division of the Institute for International Research. Washington, DC. December.

Sollecito, W.A., and M.M. Dotson. 1994. Getting the most from a contract research organization. *Proceedings of the Annual Project Management Institute Symposium*. Vancouver, BC. October.

Sollecito, W.A., and M.M. Dotson. 1995. Communications guidelines and networks for drug development teams. *Proceedings of the Annual Project Management Institute Symposium*. New Orleans, LA. October.

Soumerai, S.B., and J. Avorn. 1990. Principles of educational outreach ('academic detailing') to improve clinical decision making. *Journal of the American Medical Association* 263, no. 4:549–556.

Speake, D.L. et al. 1995. Integrating indicators into a public health quality improvement system. *American Journal of Public Health* 85, no. 10:1448–1449.

Starr, P. 1982. *The social transformation of American medicine.* New York: Basic Books.

Starr, P. 1997. Smart technology, stunted policy: Developing health information networks. *Health Affairs* 16, no. 3:91–105.

State of New York, Department of Health. 1998. "Coronary Artery Bypass Surgery in New York State." http://www.health.state.ny.us/nysdoh/consumer/heart/homehear.htm (Last viewed 2 March 1999.)

Steiber, S.R. 1988. How consumers perceive health care quality. *Hospitals* 62, no. 7:84.

Stitt, F.W. et al. 1998. "Severity scoring systems in brain injury." (http://neurosun.medsch.ucla.edu/BMML/Stitt/new.htdocs/severity.html).

Strasser, S., and R.P. Davis. 1991. *Measuring patient satisfaction for improved patient service.* Ann Arbor, MI: Health Administration Press.

Tan, J.K. 1995. *Health management information systems: Theories, methods, and applications.* Gaithersburg, MD: Aspen Publishers, Inc.

Tassignon, J. 1992. *The contract clinical research market.* Brussels: Tassignon and Partners, S.A.

Taylor, R.J., and S.B. Taylor. 1994. *The AUPHA manual of health services management.* Gaithersburg, MD: Aspen Publishers, Inc.

Teboul, J. 1991. *Managing quality dynamics.* Englewood Cliffs, NJ: Prentice-Hall.

Tenner, A.R., and I.J. DeToro. 1992. *Total quality management: Three steps to continuous improvement.* Reading, MA: Addison-Wesley Publishing Co.

Tichy, N. 1997. *The leadership engine.* New York: Harper Business.

Tornatzky, L. et al. with M. Fleischer. 1980. *Innovations and social process: A national experiment in implementing social change.* New York: Pergamon Press.

Tuckman, A. 1992. The yellow brick road: Total quality management and the restructuring of organizational culture. *Organizational Studies* 15:727–751.

Turner, J.C. et al. 1989. Referent informational influence and group polarization. *British Journal of Social Psychology* 28:135–147.

Turnock, B.J. 1997. *Public health: What it is and how it works.* Gaithersburg, MD: Aspen Publishers, Inc.

Turnock, B.J., and A. Handler. 1996. Is public health ready for reform? The case for accrediting local health departments. *Journal of Public Health Management and Practice* 2, no. 3:41–45.

Turnock, B.J. et al. 1994. Local health department effectiveness in addressing the core functions of public health. *Public Health Reports* 109, no. 5:653–658.

Turnock, B.J. et al. 1998. Core function-related local public health practice effectiveness. *Journal of Public Health Management and Practice* 4, no. 5:26–32.

U.S. Agency for Toxic Substances and Disease Registry. 1992. *ATSDR public health assessment guidance manual.* Boca Raton, FL: Lewis Publishers.

U.S. Conference Board. 1996. Total Quality Management Center meeting. Motorola Corporate Headquarters, Schaumberg, IL. July 10.

U.S. Congress, Office of Technology Assessment. 1988. *The quality of medical care: Information for consumers.* OTA-I-I-386. Washington, DC: U.S. Government Printing Office. June.

U.S. Congress, Office of Technology Assessment. 1993. *Pharmaceutical R and D: Costs, risks and rewards.* Washington, DC: U.S. Government Printing Office.

U.S. Department of Health and Human Services. 1990. *Healthy people 2000: National health objectives for the year 2000.* Washington, DC.

U.S. Department of Health and Human Services. 1996. *Health Insurance Portability and Accountability Act of 1996.* (P.L. 104–191). (The full notice of proposed rule making may be viewed and downloaded from the HIPPA Administrative Web site http://aspe.os.dhhs.gov/admnsimp/nprm/regindex.htm.)

U.S. Environmental Protection Agency. 1998. *The changing nature of environmental and public health protection: An annual report on reinvention.* Washington, DC: U.S. Government Printing Office.

U.S. General Accounting Office. 1994. *Report cards are useful but significant issues need to be addressed.* Washington, DC.

U.S. General Accounting Office. 1997. *Performance budgeting: Past initiatives offer insights for GPPA.* Washington, DC.

U.S. Preventive Services Task Force. 1989. *Guide to clinical preventive services: An assessment of the effectiveness of 169 interventions.* Baltimore: Williams & Wilkins.

U.S. Preventive Services Task Force. 1996. *Guide to clinical preventive services: Report of the U.S. Preventive Services Task Force.* Baltimore: Williams & Wilkins.

Van de Ven, A.H. 1974. *Group decision making and effectiveness: An experimental study.* Canton, OH: Comparative Administration Research Institute of the Center for Business and Economic Research, Graduate School of Business Administration, Kent State University.

Van de Ven, A.H., and M.S. Poole. 1995. Explaining development and change in organizations. *Academy of Management Review* 20, no. 3:510–541.

Vaughn, E.H. et al. 1994. An information manager for the assessment protocol for excellence in public health. *Public Health Nursing* 11, no. 6:399–405.

Victor, B., and A.C. Boynton. 1998. *Invented here: Maximizing your organization's internal growth and profitability.* Boston: Harvard Business School Press.

Vinten-Johansen, P., and E. Riska. 1991. New Oslerians and real Flexnerians: The response to threatened professional autonomy. *International Journal of Health Services* 21, no. 1:75–108.

The Virtual Hospital. Electric Differential Multimedia Laboratory. Department of Radiology, College of Medicine, University of Iowa. http://www.vh.org (Last viewed 3 March 1999).

Vladeck, B.C. 1988. Quality assurance through external controls. *Inquiry* 25, no. 1:100–107.

Wagner, D. et al. 1986. The case for adjusting hospital death rates for severity of illness. *Health Affairs* 5, no. 2:148–153.

Walsh, J.P. et al. 1988. Negotiated belief structures and decision performance: An empirical investigation. *Organizational Behavior and Human Decision Processes* 42:194–216.

Walton, M. 1990. *Deming management at work.* New York: G.P. Putnam's Sons.

Wanous, J.P., and M.A. Yautz. 1986. Solution diversity and the quality of group decisions. *Academy of Management Journal* 29:149–159.

Ware, J.E. 1989. The functioning and well being of depressed patients: Results from the medical outcomes study. *Journal of the American Medical Association* 262, no. 7:914–919.

Ware, J.E., and M.K. Snyder. 1975. Dimensions of patient attitudes regarding doctors and medical care services. *Medical Care* 13, no. 8:669–682.

Washington State Department of Health. 1996. *Public health improvement plan: A blueprint for action.* Olympia, WA.

Watson, W.E., and L.K. Michaelsen. 1988. Group interaction behaviors that affect group performance on an intellective task. *Group and Organizational Studies* 13:495–516.

Weick, K.E. 1984. Small wins: Redefining the scale of social problems. *American Psychologist* 39, no. 11:40–49.

Weiner, B.J. et al. 1997. Promoting clinical involvement in hospital quality improvement efforts: The effects of top management, board, and physician leadership. *Health Services Research* 32, no. 4:491–510.

Weingart, S.N. 1996. House officer education and organizational obstacles to quality improvement. *Joint Commission Journal on Quality Improvement* 22, no. 2:640–646.

Weingart, S.N. 1998. A House officer-sponsored quality improvement initiative: Leadership lessons and liabilities. *Joint Commission Journal on Quality Improvement* 24, no. 7:371–378.

Wennberg, J. 1995. Shared decision making and multimedia. In *Health and the new media: Technologies transforming personal and public health*, ed. L.M. Harris, 109–126. Mahwah, NJ: Lawrence Erlbaum Associates Inc., Publishers.

Wennberg, J.E., and A.M. Gittlesohn. 1973. Small area variations in health care delivery. *Science* 182, no. 117:1102–1108.

Wennberg, J.E. et al. 1987. Use of claims data systems to evaluate health care outcomes: Mortality and reoperation following prostatectomy. *Journal of the American Medical Association* 257, no. 7:933–936.

Wennberg, J.E. et al. 1996. *The Dartmouth atlas of health care.* Chicago: American Hospital Association.

Westert, G.P., and R.J. Lagoe. 1995. Evaluation of hospital stays for total hip replacement. *Quality Management in Health Care* 3, no. 3:62–71.

Whittle, J. et al. 1991. Accuracy of Medicare claims data for estimation of cancer incidence and resection rates among elderly Americans. *Med Care* 29, no. 12:1226–1236.

Woodbury, D. et al. 1997. Does considering severity of illness improve interpretation of patient satisfaction data? *Journal for Healthcare Quality* 20, no. 4:33–40.

Young, S.W. et al. 1988. Excellence in leadership through organizational development. *Nursing Administration Quarterly* 12, no. 4:69–77.

Young, W.N. 1984. Incorporating severity of illness and comorbidity in case-mix measurement. *Health Care Financing Review* (Annual Suppl.):23–31.

Zairi, M., and A. Matthew. 1995. An evaluation of TQM in primary care: In search of best practice. *International Journal of Health Care Quality Assurance* 8, no. 6:4–13.

Zifko-Baliga, G.M., and R.F. Krampf. 1997. Managing perceptions of hospital quality. *Marketing Health Services* 17, no. 11:28–35.

Zmud, R.W., and C.P. McLaughlin. 1989. "That's not my job": Managing secondary tasks effectively. *Sloan Management Review* 30, no. 2:29–36.

Zusman, J. 1991. Letter. Peer review and quality management: Are they compatible? *Quality Review Bulletin* 16, no. 12:418–419.

LIST OF SOURCES

CHAPTER 1

Exhibit 1–1 Reprinted from *Out of the Crisis* by W. Edwards Deming by permission of MIT and the W. Edwards Deming Institute. Published by MIT, Center for Advanced Educational Services, Cambridge, MA 02139. Copyright 1986 by The W. Edwards Deming Institute.

Figure 1–1 Adapted with permission from C.P. McLaughlin and A.D. Kaluzny, Managed Care: The Challenge Ahead, *OR/MS Today,* Vol. 25, No. 1, p. 25, © 1998, Lionheart Publishing, Inc.

Figure 1–2 Reprinted by permission of Harvard Business School Press. From *Invented Here: Maximizing Your Organization's Internal Growth and Profitability* by B. Victor and A.C. Boynton. Boston, MA 1998, p. 233. Copyright © 1998 by the President and Fellows of Harvard College; all rights reserved.

Figure 1–4 Adapted with permission from C.P. McLaughlin and A.D. Kaluzny, Managed Care: The Challenge Ahead, *OR/MS Today,* Vol. 25, No. 1, p. 26, © 1998, Lionheart Publishing, Inc.

Figure 1–6 Reprinted from *The New Economics for Industry, Government, Education* by W. Edwards Deming by permission of MIT and the W. Edwards Deming Institute. Published by MIT, Center for Advanced Educational Services, Cambridge, MA 02139. Copyright 1993 by The W. Edwards Deming Institute.

Figure 1–7 Reprinted with permission of the Columbia Healthcare Association, Nashville, Tennessee.

631

CHAPTER 2

Exhibit 2–1 Reprinted with permission from the National Committee of Quality Assurance; "1999 Reporting Set for HEDIS." http://www.ncqa.org.news/h99meas.htm, 11/15/98.

Figure 2–1 Reprinted from J. Harkey and R. Vraciu, Quality of Health Care and Financial Performance: Is There a Link? *Health Care Management Review,* Vol. 17, No. 4, p. 56, © 1992, Aspen Publishers, Inc.

Table 2–1 Reprinted from J. Harkey and R. Vraciu, Quality of Health Care and Financial Performance: Is There a Link? *Health Care Management Review,* Vol. 17, No. 4, p. 59–60, © 1992, Aspen Publishers, Inc.

Table 2–2 © The Oryx Initiative, Planning Schedule. Oakbrook Terrace, IL: Joint Commission on Accreditation of Healthcare Organizations, © 1998, http://www.jcaho.org/perfmeas/oryx/20pct.htm, 11/15/98. Reprinted with permission.

CHAPTER 3

Figure 3–1 Adapted with permission from *Exploration in Quality* Assessment and Monitoring: The Definition of Quality and *Approaches to Its Assessment Volume 1,* by Avedis Donabedian, (Chicago: Health Administration Press, 1980): 95–99.

Figure 3–2 Adapted with permission from S. DesHarnais et al., The Risk-Adjusted Mortality Index: A New Measure of Hospital Performance, *Medical Care,* Vol. 26, No. 12, pp. 1129–1148, © 1988, J.B. Lippincott.

Figure 3–3 Courtesy of Greater New York Hospital Association, 1995, New York, New York.

Table 3–1 Reprinted from C.P. McLaughlin, Evaluating the Quality Control System for Managed Care, *Quality Management in Health Care,* Vol. 7, No. 1, p. 43, © 1998, Aspen Publishers, Inc.

Table 3–2 Adapted with permission from S. DesHarnais et al., The Risk-Adjusted Mortality Index: A New Measure of Hospital Performance, *Medical Care,* Vol. 26, No. 12, pp. 1129–1148, © 1988, J.B. Lippincott.

CHAPTER 4

Figure 4–6 Adapted with permission from Hynes et al., Evaluating Productivity in Clinical Research Programs: The National Cancer Institute's

(NCI) Community Clinical Oncology Program, *Journal of Medical Systems,* Vol. 16, No. 6, p. 252, © 1992, Plenum Publishing Corp.

Figure 4–7 Adapted with permission from Hynes et al., Evaluating Productivity in Clinical Research Programs: The National Cancer Institute's (NCI) Community Clinical Oncology Program, *Journal of Medical Systems,* Vol. 16, No. 6, p. 259, © 1992, Plenum Publishing Corp.

Figure 4–14 Data from S.P. Johnson and F. Alemi et al., Rapid Improvement Teams, *Joint Commission Journal on Quality Improvement,* Vol. 24, No. 3, pp. 119–129, © 1998, Joint Commission on Accreditation of Healthcare Organizations.

Figure 4–15 Data from S.P. Johnson and F. Alemi et al., Rapid Improvement Teams, *Joint Commission Journal on Quality Improvement,* Vol. 24, No. 3, pp. 119–129, © 1998, Joint Commission on Accreditation of Healthcare Organizations.

Table 4–3 © *Joint Commission Journal on Quality Improvement,* Oakbrook Terrace, IL: Joint Commission on Accreditation of Healthcare Organizations, 1998, Vol. 24, No. 3, pp. 119–129. Adapted with permission.

CHAPTER 5

Exhibit 5–1 Adapted with permission from M. Macdonald, Using the Balanced Scorecard to Align Strategy and Performance in Long Term Care, *Healthcare Management Forum,* Vol. 11, No. 3, p. 36, © 1998, Healthcare Management Forum.

Exhibit 5–2 Adapted with permission from D.D. Woodbury et al., Does Considering Severity of Illness Improve Interpretation of Patient Satisfaction Data? *Journal of Healthcare Quality,* Vol. 20, No. 4, pp. 33–40. Copyright © 1993, Intermountain Healthcare Corporation Hospitals, Inc. All rights reserved.

Figure 5–1 MARKETING: AN INTRODUCTION, "Buyer-Decision Process" Figure, 3/E by Kotler/Armstrong, © 1996. Reprinted by permission of Prentice-Hall, Inc., Upper Saddle River, NJ.

Figure 5–2 Data from S.R. Steiber, How Consumers Perceive Health Care Quality, *Hospitals,* Vol. 62, No. 7, p. 84, © 1988, Health Forum-American Hospital Association and SRI Gallup, Princeton, NJ.

Figure 5–3 Data from The Patient-Centered-Care Project, Steps in Office-Based Medical Care, *Enhancing the Physicians' Role in Patient-*

Centered Care, (unpublished document), 1993, and C. Laine et al., Important Elements of Outpatient Care: A Comparison, *Annals of Internal Medicine*, Vol. 125, No. 8, pp.640–645, © 1996, American College of Physicians and the American Society of Internal Medicine and R.H. Fletcher et al., Patients' Priorities for Medical Care, *Medical Care*, Vol. XXI, No. 2, pp. 234–242, © 1983, J.B. Lippincott Co.

Figure 5–4 Copyright © 1991. Hospital Corporation of America Hospital Quality Trends.[SM]

Figure 5–5 A.R. Tenner/I.J. DeToro, TOTAL QUALITY MANAGEMENT, p. 84. © 1992 by the Addison-Wesley Publishing Co., Inc. Reprinted by permission of Addison Wesley Longman.

CHAPTER 7

Figure 7–1 From THE FIFTH DISCIPLINE FIELDBOOK by Peter Senge, Charlotte Roberts, et al. Copyright © 1994 by Peter M. Senge, Art Kleiner, Charlotte Roberts, Richard B. Ross and Bryan J. Smith. Used by permission of Doubleday, a division of Random House, Inc.

CHAPTER 8

Exhibit 8–1 © *JCAHO Journal on Quality Improvement.* Oakbrook Terrace, IL: Joint Commission on Accreditation of Healthcare Organizations, 1998, Vol. 24, No. 7, 361–370. Adapted with permission.

Table 8–1 © *JCAHO Journal on Quality Improvement.* Oakbrook Terrace, IL: Joint Commission on Accreditation of Healthcare Organizations, 1998, Vol. 24, No. 7, 361–370. Adapted with permission.

CHAPTER 9

Table 9–1 Adapted with permission from Healthcare Informatics Top 100 IS Vendors List, *Healthcare Informatics Website,* URL http://www.healthcare-informatics.com/atop.htm, 8/28/98.

CHAPTER 10

Exhibit 10–1 Reprinted from G. Ross Baker et al., Collaborating for Improvement in Health Professions Education, *Quality Management in*

Health Care, Vol. 6, No. 2, p. 6, © 1998, Aspen Publishers, Inc.

Table 10–1 Reprinted from G. Ross Baker et al., Collaborating for Improvement in Health Professions Education, *Quality Management in Health Care,* Vol. 6, No. 2, pp. 9–10, © 1998, Aspen Publishers, Inc.

CHAPTER 11

Exhibit 11–1 Data from P. Benner et al., *Expertise in Nursing Practice: Caring, Clinical Judgment, and Ethics,* © 1995, Springer and H.L. Dreyfus and S.E. Dreyfus, *The Relationship of Theory and Practice in the Acquisition of Skill,* © 1996, Springer.

CHAPTER 12

Table 12–1 L. Kinsinger et al., Using an Office System Intervention to Increase Breast Cancer Screening, *Journal of General Internal Medicine,* Vol. 13, No. 8, pp. 507–514, © 1998. Adapted by permission of Blackwell Science, Inc.

Table 12–2 L. Kinsinger et al., Using an Office System Intervention to Increase Breast Cancer Screening, *Journal of General Internal Medicine,* Vol. 13, No. 8, pp. 507–514, © 1998. Adapted by permission of Blackwell Science, Inc.

CHAPTER 13

Exhibit 13–1 Adapted with permission from L.I. Solberg et al., Delivering Clinical Preventive Services Is a Systems Problem *Annals of Behavioral Medicine,* Vol. 19, No. 3, pp. 271–278, © 1998, Society of Behavioral Medicine.

Exhibit 13–2 Adapted with permission from L.I. Solberg et al., How Important Are Clinician and Nurse Attitudes to the Delivery of Clinical Preventive Services? *Journal of Family Practice,* Vol. 44, No. 5, pp. 451–461, © 1997, Appleton & Lange.

Exhibit 13–3 Adapted with permission from L.I. Solberg et al., Will Primary Care Clinics Organize Themselves to Improve the Delivery of

Preventive Services? A Randomized Controlled Trial, *Preventive Medicine*, Vol. 27, No. 4, pp. 623–631, © 1998, Academic Press, Inc.

Table 13–1 Courtesy of Jeffrey C. Goldsmith, 1995, Charlottesville, Virginia.

CHAPTER 15

Exhibit 15–1 Reprinted from Healthy People 2000: *National Health Objectives for the Year 2000,* 1990, U.S. Department of Health and Human Services.

Exhibit 15–2 Reprinted with permission from *Healthy Communities: The Future of Public Health*. Copyright © 1997 by the National Academy of Science. Courtesy of the National Academy Press, Washington, D.C.

Exhibit 15–3 Adapted from B.J. Turnock et al., Core Function-Related Local Public Health Practice Effectiveness, *Journal of Public Health Management and Practice,* Vol. 4, No. 5, pp. 26–32, © 1998, Aspen Publishers, Inc.

Figure 15–1 Reprinted with permission from *Healthy Communities: The Future of Public Health*. Copyright © 1997 by the National Academy of Science. Courtesy of the National Academy Press, Washington, D.C.

Figure 15–2 Adapted with permission from C.A. Miller et al., A Proposed Method for Assessing the Performance of Local Public Health Functions and Practices, *American Journal of Public Health*, Vol. 84, No. 11, pp. 1743–1749, © 1994, American Public Health Association.

Table 15–1 Reprinted from P.K. Halverson et al., Case Study: Integrated Public Health and Private Health Care Systems in Denver, Colorado, *Managed Care and Public Health*, p. 207, © 1998, Aspen Publishers, Inc.

Table 15–2 Data from G.P. Mays et al., *The Community Health Report Card Survey: A Cooperative Agreement Between the Centers for Disease Control and Prevention and the Association of Schools of Public Health,* 1999, University of North Carolina at Chapel Hill School of Public Health.

CHAPTER 16

Table 16–1 Data from Arthur Andersen & Co. and the American College of Healthcare Executives, *The Future of Medical Care: Physician* *and Hospital Relationships,* © 1991, American College of Healthcare Executives.

CASE 4

Figure 4.1 Reprinted with permission of the Columbia Healthcare Association, Nashville, Tennessee.

APPENDIX A

Table A-1 Adapted from National Institute of Standards and Technology, U.S. Department of Commerce, Washington, D.C., 1998, http:// www.quality.nist.gov.

Table A-2 Adapted from National Institute of Standards and Technology, U.S. Department of Commerce, Washington, D.C., 1998, http:// www.quality.nist.gov.

INDEX

639

Q

ABOUT THE EDITORS

Curtis P. McLaughlin is Professor Emeritus of Health Policy and Administration in the School of Public Health and Professor Emeritus of Business Administration in the Kenan-Flagler Business School as well as Senior Research Fellow of the Cecil G. Sheps Center for Health Services Research at the University of North Carolina. He is also Adjunct Professor in the Physician Executive MBA Program for the College of Business Administration at the University of Tennessee Knoxville.

He has served as a consultant for a number of companies and organizations and various international, federal, and state agencies, including the Ford Foundation, the World Health Organization, and UNFPA. For more than 10 years he was chair of North Carolina's Medicaid Medical Care Advisory Committee.

Dr. McLaughlin is the author of numerous articles and cases, as well as author and co-author of several books, including *The Management of Nonprofit Organizations, Leadership and Management in Academic Medicine* with the late Marjorie Wilson, *Economic Reality and Health Care in Developing Countries* with Joe Kasonde, *Continuous Quality Improvement in Health Care* with Arnold Kaluzny, and most recently *Managed Care and Public Health* with Paul Halverson and Arnold Kaluzny. He has been a member of the editorial boards of *Health Care Management Review*, *International Journal of Service Industry Management*, and *Journal of Service Research*.

Dr. McLaughlin's research has focused on the factors affecting the operational efficiency and strategic success of professional service organizations, including health care providers, research and development facilities, and social service programs. His most recent focus has been on the

657

newer forms of delivery for such services, including surgicenters, merged practices, and disease management companies, as well as administrative and clinical continuous quality improvement efforts.

Dr. McLaughlin received his undergraduate degree in chemistry from Wesleyan University and his MBA and DBA from Harvard. He worked in industry for Union Carbide Corporation and Graphic Controls Corporation and has previously taught at Harvard Business School, Harvard School of Public Health, and London Business School.

Arnold D. Kaluzny is Professor of Health Policy and Administration; Director of the Public Health Leadership Program, School of Public Health; as well as a Senior Research Fellow in the Cecil G. Sheps Center for Health Services Research and a member of the Lineberger Comprehensive Cancer Center at the University of North Carolina at Chapel Hill.

He is a consultant to a number of private research organizations and various international, federal, and state agencies, including Project HOPE, the World Health Organization, the National Cancer Institute, the Joint Commission on the Accreditation of Healthcare Organizations, the Department of Veterans Affairs, and the Agency for Health Care Policy and Research. From 1991 through 1995 he was a member of the Board of Scientific Counselors for the Division of Prevention and Control at the National Cancer Institute and served as Chairman from 1993 to 1995.

Dr. Kaluzny is the author of numerous articles, and co-author of several books, including *Health Care Management* with Steve Shortell, *Evaluation and Decision-making for Health Services* with James Veney, *Partners for the Dance* with Howard Zuckerman and Tom Ricketts, *Continuous Quality in Health Care* with Curt McLaughlin, and most recently *Managing a Health Care Alliance: Improving Community Cancer Care* with Richard Warnecke, and *Managed Care and Public Health* with Paul Halverson and Curtis McLaughlin. He is a member of several editorial boards, including the *Health Care Management Review, Quality Management and Health Care, Journal of the National Cancer Institute*, and is a past chairman of the *Joint Commission Journal on Quality Improvement*.

His research has focused on the organizational factors affecting implementation and change of a variety of health care organizations, with specific emphasis given to cancer treatment, prevention, and control; continuous quality improvement initiatives in both organizational and primary care settings; and, most recently, the study of alliances within health care. In all of these endeavors, Dr. Kaluzny's major focus has been to strengthen the science base of policy and practice.

Dr. Kaluzny received his undergraduate degree from the University of Wisconsin at River Falls, his master's degree in Hospital Administration from the University of Michigan Graduate School of Business, and his doctorate in Medical Care Organization-Social Psychology from the University of Michigan.